SEEING, DOING, AND KNOWING

Seeing, Doing, and Knowing

A Philosophical Theory of Sense Perception

Mohan Matthen

CLARENDON PRESS · OXFORD
2005

OXFORD

UNIVERSITY PRESS

Great Clarendon Street, Oxford OX2 6DP

Oxford University Press is a department of the University of Oxford.
It furthers the University's objective of excellence in research, scholarship,
and education by publishing worldwide in

Oxford New York

Auckland Cape Town Dar es Salaam Hong Kong
Karachi Kuala Lumpur Madrid Melbourne Mexico City
Nairobi New Delhi Shanghai Taipei Toronto

With offices in

Argentina Austria Brazil Chile Czech Republic France Greece
Guatemala Hungary Italy Japan Poland Portugal
Singapore South Korea Switzerland Thailand Turkey Ukraine Vietnam

Oxford is a registered trade mark of Oxford University Press
in the UK and in certain other countries

Published in the United States
by Oxford University Press Inc., New York

British Library Cataloguing in Publication Data

Data available

Library of Congress Cataloging in Publication Data

Matthen, Mohan.
Seeing, doing, and knowing : a philosophical theory of sense perception / Mohan
Matthen.
p. cm.
Includes index.
1. Senses and sensation. 2. Sense (Philosophy) I. Title.

QP431. M295 2005 152.1—dc22 2004026059

ISBN 0–19–926850–9

1 3 5 7 9 10 8 6 4 2

Typeset by Newgen Imaging Systems (P) Ltd., Chennai, India
Printed in Great Britain
on acid-free paper by
Biddles Ltd., King's Lynn, Norfolk

FOR MY DAUGHTERS:
ELAINE, SHEILA, AND PREMALA

With Love, Hope, and Confidence

Acknowledgements

A number of people were kind enough to read and comment on various parts of this book as it took shape. In particular, I should like to thank my Philosophy colleagues at UBC: Melinda Hogan, Dom Lopes, Patrick Rysiew, and Ori Simchen. Colleagues in Psychology and in Linguistics were always ready to offer information and advice: Jim Enns, Brian Gick, Doug Pulleyblank, Joe Stemberger, Richard Tees, Janet Werker, and above all, Vince DiLollo. Ned Block, Richard Heck, and Alison Simmons read parts of the typescript at various stages of its development and made helpful suggestions.

Jonathan Cohen, now at the University of California at San Diego, was special in this regard. Jonathan was 'my' Killam post-doctoral fellow at UBC in 2000–2001, during which we met almost daily to discuss perception. Later, he read a draft of the whole manuscript carefully and offered many valuable suggestions and corrections. I thank the Killam Trust for this opportunity.

In 2003, I read yet another draft of the book with a group of graduate students: Vincent Bergeron, Eric Cyr Desjardins, Martin Godwyn, Selman Halabi, James Kelleher, Harris Kollias, Nola Semszycyn, and Dustin Stokes. This was one of the best discussion groups I have ever been a part of: the criticism, grasp of the whole, and attention to detail were invaluable. My interactions with Vince and Dustin have extended beyond this seminar: they have contributed more than they realize to my thinking about matters of the mind.

At an early stage, I asked Larry Hardin for help. I am always nervous while somebody with as much knowledge and experience as Larry is looking through my work. He was mercifully quick in his response, and offered many corrections and suggestions in the gentlest tone. He also revealed that I was not the only one to ask his opinion of my manuscript: Oxford University Press had done so as well. I am grateful that his comments translated into a favourable report. A second reader for the Press remained anonymous to me for a while, but turned out to be Jim McGilvray. (Who but a Canadian would spell 'colour' with a 'u' *and* print on 8½× 11 paper?) Jim offered many detailed criticisms and suggestions: in many cases, I have brazenly incorporated his suggested wording with no further acknowledgement. Two referees on a later draft also chose not to be anonymous: Jerry Vision and David Hilbert. I thank them for detailed advice on many points, major and minor. My debt to David is particularly large: his writings have influenced my thinking on perception for a long time, and here he not only corrected errors but forced me to adopt a more flexible perspective on sensory content, especially in Parts I and II.

One debt falls into a special category. Catherine Wilson offered opinions, listened, made suggestions, read (often at moment's notice), and corrected. Her help and influence have been continuous in the five years I have worked on this project.

Parts of the manuscript were delivered (at various stages of its evolution) to Green College, the Peter Wall Institute for Advanced Studies, the Department of Philosophy, and the Vision Group in the Department of Psychology, all at the University of British Columbia; the Moral Sciences Club at Cambridge University; the Departments of Philosophy at the Australian National University, Brown, Cambridge, Macquarie, McGill, Queen's, Rutgers, L'Université du Québec à Montréal; the Universities of Adelaide, Alberta, Calgary, Illinois at Urbana-Champaign, Lethbridge, Manitoba, Queensland, Sydney, Victoria, and Wisconsin (Madison); the South African Philosophical Association (Johannesburg, 2000), and the Second Bellingham Summer Philosophy Conference at Western Washington University (2001). Comments received on these occasions were hugely helpful, often in ways that became apparent to me only much later. Late in the preparation of the manuscript, thanks to a Visiting Research Scholarship in July and August 2003, I had the opportunity to exchange ideas with Macquarie University philosophers, especially Tim Bayne, Jordi Fernandes, and John Sutton, and with Max Coltheart and his colleagues at the Macquarie Centre for Cognitive Science. I benefited greatly from this learning opportunity.

I am honoured to acknowledge the financial support of the Social Sciences and Humanities Research Council of Canada.

Paula Wirth prepared the figures for publication.

Contents

Analytic Table Of Contents

1. The Sensory Classification Thesis: Sensory systems are automatic sorting
machines which assign external sensed objects (distal stimuli) to classes.
2. The results of a system's sorting activities are made available to the
perceiver in the form of a conscious sensory state, which can be held in
memory and later recalled.
3. The Sensory Classification Thesis was first articulated by F. A. Hayek,
who strongly emphasized the active nature of sensory processing:
sensory classes are constructed on the basis of commonalities found or
imposed by the system, not passively received.
4. Hayek adopted an extreme nominalism towards sensory classes, but
this neglects evolutionary constraints: not just any classificatory scheme
is useful to an organism.

5. The Sensory Classification Thesis is strongly realistic in one sense: it takes distal stimuli to be the targets of classification. A sensory state attributes a sense feature to such a stimulus.

6. The Sensory Classification Thesis is a simplification. In fact, sensory systems order stimuli in relations of graded similarity. This important complication is suppressed in this book, except in Part II.

7. By contrast with the phenomenalistic tradition, the Sensory Classification Thesis accommodates perceptual error.

1. Sensory experience signals the results of sensory classification: I know that my colour vision has classified something as red because I am in a certain experiential state, namely the state of the thing's looking red to me.

2. Thus, sensory experience follows sensory classification; it is not the basis thereof. Sensory qualities cannot be defined in terms of sensory experience. Evidence for a dissociation between classification and sensation is presented.

3. We are directly aware not of our sensations, but of stimuli. However, the qualitative character of sensation is not exhausted by its representational content; there is more to a sensory state than what it tells us about a stimulus.

4. Appearance follows classification as the record thereof; it follows that differences of classification lead to differences of appearance. Two stimuli that have been assigned to the very same sensory classes will appear the same even though there may be a difference in the quality of our experiences of them.

5. That appearance follows classification shows that dispositionalist theories of sensory qualities have things backwards. These theories do not satisfactorily distinguish between variations in classificatory schemes and variations in the semantic relation between experience and sensory class.

Descartes realized that the retinal image would have to be transformed before it could become material for sensory or mental operations: he discovered what today is called 'transduction'. However, he did not recognize the existence of sensory classification; this is shown by the close correspondence he posits between retinal image and the transduced sensory presentation.

Quine argued that when an animal responds similarly to similar stimuli, it is using an innate 'similarity space', i.e. a scheme of sensory classification. The

Cartesian tradition attributes similarity of response not to any such active process but to the objective similarity of stimuli and the consequent similarity, albeit occasionally degraded, of the sensory processes they evoke. In this tradition, an animal depends for information on fidelity of transmission from receptor to sensation.

This Cartesian account neglects the plethora of similarities available between any two stimuli: relevant similarities have to be selected, not just preserved. The contemporary neurocomputational paradigm in cognitive science sees sensory systems as searching the environment for the occurrence of specific types of events or conditions and discarding all information irrelevant to these.

The results of feature-extraction is recorded in the brain by a series of maps, one for each type of feature. There is a colour map, a shape map, and so on, and in order to see something as having a particular shape as well as a particular colour, the relevant features from the different maps have to be bound together. This act of binding is done by an operation known as 'attention'.

A sensory neuron responds when a particular feature, its 'response condition', is present. Response conditions can be specified in terms of characteristics of the retinal image. They can often be specified in terms of objective characteristics of external things. This opens the door to realism with respect to sensory classification.

Fred Dretske has argued that sensation is analogue while perceptual belief is digital. The central idea he means to convey is that information must be extracted from sensation before the latter can be of any use. Thus, he implies that sensation itself contains no information that is already at the disposal of the organism. This contradicts the Sensory Classification Thesis.

Dretske puts weight on the fact that one cannot visually scrutinize something to determine whether it is *F* without simultaneously receiving other information about it. He concludes that the information about *F* has to be extracted from the visual state. This is a mistake: according to feature integration theory, sensory classifications are first extracted, stored separately, and only then reassembled by 'attention'.

Receptor activity at the 'front end' of a sensory system is always analogue; it is, however, wrong to think that analogue content is always inherited from receptor activity. It may result from numerical data extraction, as well as from how extracted and digitized information is deployed.

Sometimes, what seems to be a single sensation integrates several digitized messages: colour sensation, for instance, contains both information about shades of colour and information about gross colour categories. This makes colour sensation analogue by Dretske's definition, but colour information is processed and extracted information nonetheless. Dretske is wrong to treat analogue form as a sign of unprocessed information.

Some philosophers argue that sensation has no combinatorial structure. In fact, it possesses something parallel to syntactic structure. Other philosophers argue, on the contrary, that sensation *must* be conceptually articulated, but insist that such articulation must be 'spontaneous', and cannot 'well up' from the underlying sub-personal sensory system. It is shown that some degree of spontaneity is indeed found in sub-personally generated sensory concepts.

Richard Heck argues that there are too many sense-features and too many fine distinctions amongst them to pack into a conceptual vocabulary. It is shown that, on the contrary, sensory representation provides us with a means by which to construct such a vocabulary.

The Sensory Classification perspective is congruent with the idea, found in cognitive ethology, that each type of organism seeks out environmental features that are relevant to its peculiar ecological niche. The resultant differences between sensory representations should not be taken as evidence of subjectivism: on the contrary, they argue for Pluralistic Realism.

Part II. Similarity

Part II is an examination of sensory similarity, a more complicated basis for the construction of sense features than the two-valued, in-out classification assumed in Part I.

Sense-features 'generate' their subclasses in an interesting sense noticed by W. E. Johnson: the perceptual grasp of inclusive features such as *red* is based on a grasp of graded similarity relations among the subclasses thereof. This characteristic of sense-features explains some aspects of their abstract structure.

Sensory similarity is quantitatively measured by methods pioneered by the great psychophysicists of the nineteenth century. Similarity measures can be graphically represented in a multidimensional spatial model. These methods give empirical support to Johnson's idea of generability.

Not all the relationships found in a graphical representation of similarity find counterparts in empirical measurements of similarity; some are merely artefacts of how such graphs are drawn. Relationships found in all graphical representations call for explanation: what is the source of the invariance? 'Overall' similarity with respect to several sensory parameters is variable across different graphical representations. This shows that overall similarity is an artefact.

Variation with respect to a single sensory parameter such as colour is invariable in a number of significant ways. Thus, such variation within a single sensory parameter presents a contrast with 'overall' similarity. This calls for explanation.

In the Cartesian paradigm, similarity of sensation is explained by the similarity of receptor state (though the latter can be degraded further downstream). This is a mistake, as empirical studies show. Some suggest that not just receptors but the whole sensory process has to be invoked. It is doubtful that this would *explain* anything. Additional principles are required.

Explanations of similarity are vitiated by vagaries in the logic of similarity, which show that this concept is perspective-dependent. This imposes a constraint on explaining sensory similarity, namely, that it must be accommodated in a manner that relativizes it to the perspective and interests of the organism.

How do sensory systems represent similarity? A suggestion, due to C. R. Gallistel, is that sensory similarity is literally a measure of closeness in a neural map. The system constructs such maps because it needs to resolve imprecision in neural representations and to determine a precise response to the situations represented.

The internal origins of sensory similarity do not preclude realism. Sense-features are physically specifiable. In addition, they serve some purpose in the organism by signalling similarities of functional relevance. These considerations imply that it is possible for an organism to be wrong about similarity, which prefigures a form of realism to be explored further later.

The relationship between a sensation, a sense-feature, and a stimulus is analogous to that between a descriptive word, the attribute it designates, and the individuals that possess this attribute.

Part III. Specialization

Because of perceptual specialization, colour cannot be defined in terms of either the physical properties that human colour vision captures or the sense experiences that it produces in humans.

Some data-processing determinants of colour vision are outlined: opponent processing, metamerism, colour contrast, and colour constancy.

Narrowly anthropocentric theories of colour define particular colour properties (for example, *red*) in terms of the associated colour experiences. These theories produce odd results when applied to species or individuals that possess colour vision systems with different specifications. Defining the general category of colour in these terms undermines comparative studies of colour vision.

David Hilbert and Evan Thompson argue that if colour is not defined in terms of conscious experience, non-representational systems will be included. Their worry is addressed by means of a 'meta-response' schema for sensory representation. This paves the way for a functional definition in terms of how colour vision processes wavelength-sensitive data. One alternative, invoking *resemblance* to human colour experience, inadequately responds to problems posed by perceptual specialization.

Can colour be defined by resemblance to the real properties detected by human colour vision? Successively weaker versions of this idea are explored and found to be incompatible (a) with the ecological variation shown by colour vision systems of different species, and (b) the fact that similarity spaces are generated by sensory systems.

Colour vision has evolved independently in a variety of species. It is widely assumed that this is a case of *convergence*, of the same function appearing in separated phylogenetic paths. It is much more likely to be an instance of Darwin's Principle of Divergence, of a specialized function that enables a species to exploit an environmental resource unavailable to its ancestor. On this account, colour vision has a different function in different occurrences.

It seems that primate colour vision evolved in order to pick out a particular class of vegetation at a distance. It provides the ability to discriminate these fruits in fine detail against a background of green. This tends to explain why colour-blind humans are functionally disabled only with respect to the discrimination of colours in a 'dappled and brindled' background. We use black and white information a lot more than we think.

Intuitively, a person with colour vision experiences a visual image that pixel by pixel is different from that of a colour-blind individual. This intuition is questioned. The visual image of a colour-sighted primate has more in common with that of a colour-blind primate than with that of a colour-sighted insect. The Sensory Classification Thesis makes sense of this; the traditional paradigm does not.

A catalogue of mismatches between experienced colour and the physical counterparts of colour is presented. Does it show that colour is not real?

Different colour vision systems utilize different classificatory schemes. Hardin's catalogue poses a concern about the ontological status of these schemes.
Some argue, on the basis of the idiosyncrasy of colour classification, that colour is an attribute of sensations. This mistakenly shifts the topic of investigation from the ontological status of colour classes to the

identification of which objects bear colour. It has no bearing on the problem posed by Hardin.

Error Theory suggests that colour vision delivers a false message. By comparison with the case of visual illusions, it is shown that this is methodologically dubious.

Colours do not correspond to the quantities that figure in the laws of physics. Some argue that they are therefore unreal. This is a mistake: colours are specifiable in the language of physics.

David Lewis suggests that experienced relations among colours are objective merely in virtue of the fact that they are so experienced. The problem is that organisms of different species experience colours in incompatible ways. How should we accommodate such variation?

It is proposed that a physically specifiable sense-feature is real in the action-relative sense if there is some innate activity that would be disrupted by inconsistent classification. This permits different species to have cross-cutting sensory classifications.

Part IV. Content

The Universalist paradigm casts sensation as a projection of the states of sensory receptors. This implies that, imperfection of transmission aside, sensation is the same across species. Pluralistic Realism claims, by contrast, that sensation is of features and objects in the world beyond the receptors— different features and objects for different species.

Human speech perception is a particularly clear example of a sensory system attuned to features beyond the proximal image, serving a species-specific activity: it is specialized for the detection and differentiation of sounds that in nature emanate only from the human articulatory tract.

Sensory systems do not evolve by adding new items from a preset menu of proximately available sense-features. According to the *Coevolution Thesis* propounded here, they incrementally evolve discriminatory abilities to serve action-modes emerging in parallel. Sensory systems present the world to the perceiver in action-related terms.

Sense perception does not merely serve bodily action. A proper general understanding takes account of the epistemic uses of sense perception. The 'effector organs' that are important for the coevolution of sense perception are units that analyse and store information.

While the primary content or meaning of a sensory state is specified in terms of epistemic action, its secondary content or extension may be specified in physical terms. It is secondary content that is the focus of laboratory psychophysicists and of physicalist theories of sense features.

This chapter examines the role and character of conscious sensory experience.

Sensory classification can lead to action by means of direct manipulation of the effector system. In this case, the output of the sensory system must be causally apt to coerce the effector system.

However, either when a sensory system feeds into many effector systems, or when many sensory systems feed in to a single effector, it is simpler for the sensory systems to be non-coercive. Their output will simply indicate that a particular situation obtains, and the effector system will be left to do what is appropriate.

In the case of non-coercive content, the system will need as many signals as there are response-demanding situations. It is a matter of indifference what signal is linked with which action: in the sense developed by David Lewis, these signals are conventional. The conventionality of sensory signals is overlooked by philosophers who allege an 'explanatory gap' with regard to sensory qualia.

Sensory signals are indications that a certain situation obtains; it is left to effector systems to determine the correct action. Such effector systems are typically epistemic in character. Some philosophers sympathetic to the general approach recommended here fall into error by overlooking epistemic action and assuming that action must involve movement of the limbs.

The present theory is assessed in the context of recent 'teleosemantic' theories of perceptual content.

The senses seem to give us categorical information about distal stimuli with no self-referential element. This chapter attempts to reconstruct this message in a way that respects the Thesis of Primary Sensory Content.

If sensory categories are subjective, how can they be useful for constructing a record of the objective world? If they are objective, how can we possess instinctual knowledge of them? The dilemma has special bite in the case of colour.

A standard philosophical approach to defining colour identifies it with a 'colour look' in standard circumstances. This violates the condition that we should possess instinctive knowledge of colour. A more promising approach is a 'semantic' specification of the meaning of colour experiences, elaborated along the lines of Tarski's semantic theory of truth.

Sensory systems are likened to measuring instruments, which present the user with measurements calibrated in an independently defined scale such as *pounds per square inch*. Sensory systems provide measurements in an 'auto-calibrated' scale: in terms, that is, of something like a reidentifiable pointer position that is not specified by reference to an independently defined scale.

Two things are the same in colour when they should be treated in exactly the same way with respect to the epistemic practices associated with colour. Colour is a superficial property of things; it indicates hidden properties of things, but corresponds to no manipulable characteristic. The superficiality of colour is the key for understanding how colour vision can be useful despite its mismatch with physical colour.

Part V. Reference

Vision presents features as located in environmental things. In this chapter, the structure of this feature-locating scheme is investigated.

There is a difference between the visual presentation of location and that of features like colour and texture. The character of the former can be traced in large part to what Kant called a *formal* element in visual representation.

Austen Clark argues, correctly, that conjunctions of features have to be separated into separate groups according to the subjects to which they are attributed. Clark thinks that these subjects are regions of space: it is argued that they are material objects capable of motion, not mere regions of space.

Vision presents the world in object-feature terms. Other modalities employ different structures.

The differences among sense modalities with regard to their representations of space and their attributions of features argues that a purely a priori or functional treatment will miss philosophically important characteristics of sensation. Empirical science matters to how you understand representation; functionalism is moot.

Bodily action is hierarchically organized; conscious volition specifies goals but is not involved in fine motor control. The visual system that guides fine motor control does not contribute to the conscious descriptive sensory classification that we have been dealing with in Parts I–IV.

Three phases of executing a physical action are identified: information about the descriptive sensory features of the target is required for the first two. Since 'motion-guiding vision' is in charge of the third phase, this must be executable without descriptive information. We show how.

When one looks at a real scene, one generally has a 'feeling of presence' that differentiates real vision from mere visual imaging. This feeling of presence is similar in effect to an assertion operator placed in front of a sentence: in vision it comes from deixis, which serves here as an assertion operator.

When we look at a picture, we see the picture itself and also the thing that is depicted. Our visual experience of the latter can be very similar in descriptive terms to that of seeing the object in real life. However, motion-guiding vision is not engaged by things depicted in the picture.

Prelude: The New Philosophy of Vision

Vision informs us of located features. It tells us of certain qualities—sense-features such as *red, square, moving.* And it tells us *where* these features occur: in which places—red there, movement to the left, and in which objects—that sphere receding, that face flushed. The aim of this book is to examine the nature of these features, and how they and their locations are represented. The examination of visual features will occur in the context of a general treatment of sense-features. The discussion of location will be more specific to vision, for as we shall see different modalities use different systems of feature-location.

I. Perceptual Content and Information

That vision informs us of located features is a central axiom of classic theories of perception by Descartes, Locke, Berkeley, and Hume, and the psychological theories of a host of nineteenth-century scientists including, most prominently, Hermann von Helmholtz and Ewald Hering. This claim received its most elaborate and logically sophisticated treatment in the twentieth-century works of Bertrand Russell, Rudolf Carnap, and Nelson Goodman. However, the attitude taken by these classic thinkers is very different from that presupposed by the framework for visual information proposed in this book. Their attitude is shaped by the philosophical reaction to scepticism. By contrast, the framework that will be presented in this book is motivated by considerations about how animals, including humans, use perception.

What are the features of which vision informs us? What is the nature of the space in which they are seen to be located? The classic theories assumed that sensation is *innocent*, that is, untainted by assumptions about the world. In Descartes and Locke, this assumption came ultimately from reflections on scepticism. From Pyrrho to Sextus Empiricus, the ancient sceptics held that even when I, a normally sighted person, am looking directly at a physical object like a coffee cup in good light, I am able to entertain the thought that the cup is delusional or unreal despite the visual sensations I experience. The cup may not be the colour or shape it looks; indeed, what I am looking at may not even be a cup, but simply a trick of the light, or a hallucination generated by my own derangement. That I can thus be in a sensory state while at the same time entertaining the possibility that it is false shows that ordinary perceptual beliefs are not *logically compelled* by sensation. It follows, so the great philosophers of the seventeenth and eighteenth centuries argued, that sensation does not directly tell us anything about the external world.

Their conclusion is motivated by thinking of the content of sensation in terms of what we now call *information* (Dretske 1981, ch.1). The information carried by something—an event, a signal, the condition of a thing—is what you can deduce from it. Ordinarily, this notion is construed generously. From the mud on a car, you can infer that it has been driven off-road. Thus, the mud carries information about where the car has been. The sceptic points out, however, that it is possible to entertain the possibility that the mud had been put on the car deliberately, perhaps to prepare it for a movie shoot. The sceptic treats inference as logical deduction, and excludes from the information that something carries anything which cannot be logically deduced from it. This is why he holds that sensation does not inform us about the external world.

What then is the content of sensation, if it is not directly the source of commitment to any propositional belief about distal objects? Many of the classic philosophers concluded that it was a mistake to think in such terms. Sensation does not tell us anything at all, they urged: it consists merely of being consciously aware of a subjective *image* from which we extract beliefs about the external world. As David Lewis (1999/1966) has written:

> Those in the traditions of British empiricism and introspectionist psychology hold that the content of visual experience is a sensuously given mosaic of color spots, together with a mass of interpretive judgment injected by the subject. (359)

The thesis is that we segment this colour mosaic into discrete objects and attribute sense-features to these objects on the basis of 'interpretive judgements' that we make by instinct or on the basis of past experience—but, crucially, that we are always directly aware of this image as the background and basis of our added judgements.

What is the source of the sensory image? In a very long tradition stretching from Descartes to the present day, the central philosophical paradigm proposes that sensation corresponds in some way to the physical energy pattern incident upon our outer sensory receptors, that our awareness of visual features, for example, reflects the constantly changing projection of light from the external world focused by the lens of the eye on the retina. As W. V. O. Quine (1960) put it, 'Physical things generally, however remote, become known to us only through the effects which they help to induce at our sensory surfaces' (1)—they are known 'only through impacts at our nerve endings' (2), or 'surface irritations' (26). Quine does not explicitly say, but many philosophers implicitly hold, that sensation is a point by point transformation of these nerve-end impacts into the contents of sensory consciousness, usually called *sensations*, or *qualia*.

Of course, the idea that sensation is merely a transformation of the 'surface irritations' of our sensory receptors is a *paradigm* not a theory, a mental picture or model that influences the way that philosophers think about sensation, rather than an axiom to which they bear explicit allegiance. How could it be anything else? In the tradition we have been speaking about, philosophical theories are meant to abjure empirical assumptions. So these philosophers could not have built the physics of light or sound or the physiology of the sense organs into the foundations of their epistemological theories. It is nevertheless clear when we read the works of even an idealist like Berkeley, that in a physicalist embellishment of the mathematical tradition of Euclidean optics, he thinks of the visual image as if it derived directly from the image of light focused by the lens of the eye on the retina, the 'fund of the eye' as he calls it. Berkeley thinks, in short, that when we open our eyes and look at the world, we come into touch with visual 'ideas' arrayed in the form of a two-dimensional picture.

II. The Outward-Oriented Phenomenology of Sensing

In this book, I shall be arguing that the subjectivist philosophical tradition is fundamentally misguided: sensation is not an image of the retinal (or, more generally, receptoral) image. Indeed, it is nothing like an image.

In the end, the most compelling reason for rejecting the 'image' view is that, as we shall see in Chapter 2, it misconstrues the nature of visual processing in sense-organs and brain. But before we get to that, let's first consider some preliminary reasons for being at least suspicious of this tradition. Consider first the phenomenology of sensing. When we are visually aware of *red*, we are ostensibly aware of a three-dimensional external thing which is red, not of an inner episode of awareness from which we infer the presence of the red thing. The visual features of which sensation informs us *seem* to be located in things outside ourselves. Subjectively, there is clearly more to a visual sensation, then, than a colour mosaic.

Consider the famous Gestalt phenomena of occlusion. A dog behind a picket fence looks like a single occluded object, not like several dog-coloured stripes alternating with picket surfaces. Similarly, as Austen Clark (2000) writes:

Two dimensions do not suffice to describe the gamut of spatial variations in visual experience. Glares, shadows, occluding edges, and reflections pose some obvious problems . . . You see a green pine tree through the window and, overlapping it, a red reflection in the glass. How exactly do we describe this in a two-dimensional visual field? (100)

The eye seems to inform us of a three-dimensional reality—the fence in front, the dog behind; the pine tree distinct from the reflection—not of the planar projection on the retina. But these relations of front and behind are not information carried by the sensation, because having the sensation is compatible with their falsity. Thus, the classic tenet that sensation does not carry information about the external world is at odds with the intuitive truth that it nevertheless conveys, as one might say, a *message* about the external world. This forces us to allow that the sensory message—its subjective significance, as it were—goes beyond the information it carries. Scepticism might lead one to query whether the sensory message is *true*; one might wonder whether it logically compels belief in an external world. Even if the answer in both cases is negative, sensory phenomenology forces us to concede that what we are conscious of is not merely an image.

The perceptual phenomenon misleadingly known as *constancy* furnishes us with another kind of example of the outward orientation of sensation (see Chapter 6, section I, for further discussion). Suppose that you are looking simultaneously at three people, one in bright sunlight, one standing in the shade of a tree, the third standing beside you in the relative darkness of the indoors. These three people send very different signals to your eye; the sharply different illumination conditions in which they stand ensures this. But vision enables you, at least roughly, (a) to determine what illumination each stands in, and (b) to make rough and ready comparisons of their colours. For example, you might be able to tell that the person standing in bright sunlight is darker skinned than the one standing next to you, this despite the fact that the signal he sends to your eye is brighter. Again, despite the greenish tinge of the signal sent by the person standing under a tree, you can tell that she is the same colour as the person standing next to you; you might even be able to tell that she is flushed. In much the same way, you are able to discern the distances, sizes, and shapes of things despite the ambiguity of the signals they send to your eye; you can tell the difference between a loud sound far away and a softer sound close by; you can recognize the voice of a friend in a silent room as well as in a noisy reception room or over the telephone. In all of these cases, what we see and hear is different from the signal received by the eye and ear; we are conscious of something outside of ourselves, and more often than not we are right. Sometimes the message goes beyond the information, and is right nevertheless.

Animals can perform these feats of discrimination too. Suppose for instance that you are able to train a bird or a fish to seek food on yellow-coloured discs. They will not be deterred by lighting conditions different from those that you used during the training: they will recognize yellow even in shadow, in reddish or bluish illumination, discs even at oblique angles, and from far away. Regardless of environmental variations that affect the signal that is received by their eyes, they will forage on yellow discs and ignore other stimuli. Similarly, even new-born babies, who have no prior experience of the world, are able to turn their heads to look at the source of a sound, to reach out in three-dimensional space to grasp a finger, to turn their heads to their mother's breast, and so on. These inarticulate creatures use sensation to function in an objective three-dimensional world.

Sensory awareness does not merely *purport* to be of objects located in three-dimensional space and of stable external visual features: it allows observers, even those without relevant previous experience and without the requisite inferential abilities, to act upon these things and react to these features. Further, it supports induction, reidentification of external objects, and prediction. Our awareness of objects in three-dimensional space similarly affords us the ability to navigate the external world. These facts—the success of induction and of navigation—suggest that visual information must be anchored in *real* observer-independent features located in three-dimensional physical space.

This explains why the phenomenology of sensation is outward-looking. It is so because it gives us, as well as lower animals, the ability to interact with outer objects. A sensation does *not*, then, present itself to us as a 'fancifully fanciless bearer of unvarnished news', to use Quine's rococo phrase (1960, 2); it is not delivered in an idealized protocol language uncommitted to anything concerning the distal environment. On the contrary, it directly provides us with the descriptive sensory concepts and perceptual demonstratives apt for describing three-dimensional objects and their perceiver-independent features.

This is the position taken by many popular treatments of perception in recent years: for example, J. J. Gibson (1950,1979) as a part of his 'ecological approach' to understanding perception, Richard Gregory in influential books like *The Intelligent Eye* (1970), Jerry Fodor in *The Modularity of Mind* (1983), and perhaps most influentially (at least as far as contemporary vision theorists are concerned) the late David Marr in *Vision* (1982). These authors assume that our sensory systems are problem solvers. These systems are not content to pass 'unvarnished news' on to the mind for the operation of innate or learned interpretations. They deliver an interpreted message; this interpreted message constitutes sensory consciousness.

III. Problems to Be Tackled

This is the direction that most recent approaches to the senses take, but there is a problem buried in the conceptual framework that some philosophers take from this turn in psychological theorizing. The problem is that having given up the subjectivity of the classic paradigm, these thinkers resort to describing the content of sensation in terms of properties and locations assumed to exist independently of the perceiver. In so doing, they sometimes go beyond what a perceiver could be expected to know.

As many contemporary philosophers see it, sensory systems are like decoding machines. An encoded signal is the tangled result of two different variables: the code used by the sender, and the message she wishes to send.

How can one extract a message from an encoded message without knowing the code? A code-breaker solves this problem by searching in the encoded text for lexicographic and other invariants—characteristics of all English plain text regardless of meaning. To cite a relatively unsophisticated method, the code-breaker knows that 'e' is the most frequent letter in English, and assumes that the letter that occurs most frequently is likely to decode as 'e'. Such tricks, and inspired guesses, enable her to extract the message from a signal without knowing the code in advance.

In a similar way, sensory signals are the result of several mind-independent physical variables: physical reality, the state of the medium through which a sensory organ receives sensory input, the state of the perceiver herself. In order to guide organisms in their interactions with the external world, sensory systems are faced with disentangling the sources of the signals they receive. In order to solve this problem, sensory systems too use invariants in physical stimuli. For instance, the closer something is, the finer the grain of image it casts. Sensory systems assume that fineness of texture is more or less constant across a scene, and use grain as an indicator of distance. Similarly, the variation of brightness is roughly the same across most brightly lit scenes. Colour vision has evolved to take advantage of this fact: it takes a light signal that results both from illumination and surface reflectance, and using this and other universal characteristics of scenes, it cleverly disentangles these two sources, assigning them separate values. From a signal that is as much a product of the subject's situation as it is of the condition of a distal object, sensory systems extract *representations* of real-world physical variables. The conclusion that some philosophers draw from this account is that we are aware of these physical variables in sensory consciousness. For example, colour vision gives us awareness of both surface reflectance and illumination in the distal scene, though it receives only light that varies in colour and brightness.

This view runs into five interrelated difficulties. I'll review and illustrate these difficulties in the context of the often-propounded thesis that colour vision 'discounts the illuminant' and represents surface reflectances of external bodies.

> The first is that sensory systems only approximately track external features: the constancy of sensory representation is impressive, but it is not absolute. It is possible to make rough and ready comparisons of coloured objects viewed under radically different lighting conditions, but if you want to be sure that your tie matches your shirt, you have to make sure that the lighting conditions in your dressing room are right. To say that colour appearance tracks reflectance is an effective way of saying what is wrong with the traditional subjectivist paradigm. But as a positive statement, it is simply too prone to exceptions to serve as the departure point of a new philosophy of perception.

The second difficulty is that given the approximate character of perceptual constancy, it is hard to determine *what* mind-independent features of the environment are tracked by sensory systems. If colour appearance does not track reflectance precisely, then what exactly is the value of fingering this precise physical quantity as its target? What theoretical advantage does this way of speaking gain us? What is the value of the closely associated claim that colour vision sometimes *mis*represents the world by making a mistake about *this* quantity? Might this imputation of error not be an artefact of focusing on reflectance in the first place?

The third problem is that the structure of our experience of sense-features is in fact quite idiosyncratic. For instance, we see *red* as opposed to and excluding *green*. There is no relationship among reflectances, considered objectively, that corresponds to this relation. How then can we claim that *red* and *green* are objective reflectances?

A fourth challenge for the representationalist framework is that the perceptual capacities of different kinds of animals seem to be different, even within the 'same' sense-modality like vision, or more specifically, colour vision. This is a puzzle if we think that colour is reflectance, and that colour vision decodes reflectance and illumination—for in many organisms, colour vision seems to be decoding something that is of only idiosyncratic significance.

Finally, it is unclear how it can be said that sensory consciousness provides us with a message about things like reflectance. The concept of reflectance is theoretical: one needs to learn some physics before one can use it. But people saw colours long before the requisite physical theory had ever been formulated—Aristotle saw colours, but lacking the wavelength theory of light he know nought about reflectance and illumination spectra. However 'varnished' sensation may turn out to be, it surely has to be more innocent than this. Aristotle surely did not represent the world to himself in terms of the quantities of modern physics. Shouldn't a theory of colour vision be able to offer us a better account of its significance *to the perceiver*?

The upshot of these puzzles is that we need a different and more accommodating way to think about objective sense-features and their locations. We need, in short, a framework within which we can *ask* how exact constancy is in a given case, which means that we should not simply *assume* that constancy or the representation of mind-independent physical variables is the norm. We need a framework, moreover, which is capable of accommodating the idiosyncrasies and specializations of vision as it occurs in various kinds of organisms. Most importantly, we need an account of what exactly we come to know when we see or hear.

IV. The Appeal to Action

This is where the 'doing' in *Seeing, Doing, and Knowing* comes in. The central theme of this book is that perception is for action of two kinds. First, it is for the guidance of the body as it interacts with other material objects. Second, it is for finding out about things in the world, for building up a record of the characteristics of such objects, and forming expectations concerning how they will behave in the future. The main thesis to be advanced builds the content of perception on what it tells us about how objects should be treated with respect to these goals. To put it very briefly, the thesis is that sensory systems are automatic sorting machines that come into direct contact with environmental objects and sort them into classes according to how they should be treated for the purposes of physical manipulation and investigation.

This appeal to action has a great advantage. The problems outlined in the previous section are problems of description. That is, they are questions and doubts about how precisely one should describe the world that is presented to us by the senses. There is also a problem of explanation that needs to be tackled. It is one thing to assert that the phenomenology of sense-perception is outward-looking. It is quite another thing to explain how it can be so: from what in the phenomenology of perception does the idea of externality originate? The fundamental problem here is one that was posed by Kant. In the *Transcendental Deduction* (B), §19, Kant asks how a statement about my own perceptual states such as 'If I support a body, I feel an impression of weight' can possibly be the ground for a statement about the external world such as 'It, the body, is heavy.' We know of features like heaviness and of objects such as bodies through subjective states of ourselves. These states are sometimes expressed in terms of propositions like the following: 'That body feels heavy to me.' And once they are expressed in this way, it might seem obvious that the state *does* offer us awareness ('feels') of a body ('that body') and of one of its properties ('heavy'). But to express the state this way, while not wrong, papers over the explanatory problem. How exactly do we manage to decompose a sensory state into these terms? What in such a state intimates us that it is of something that exists independently of ourselves and the occurrence of a feature that transcends appearance? In other words: how do I detach these ideas from the unitary subjective state I find myself in when something feels heavy?

The connection between perception and action helps us here. It will be argued in Parts IV and V that perception enables us to interact with objects. As we said before, it (a) guides us in our bodily interactions with external objects, and (b) helps us learn about external objects and build over time a record of features that these objects possess. The claim is that these functions are innate in our perceptual abilities, built into them by evolution. Now, when we attempt to act on an object, we are immediately presented with the datum that these objects resist our attempts to act on them: their surfaces resist our probes, effort is required to move them, and so on. Similarly, when we attempt to learn about objects, we find that effort is required: there are gaps in our information that make inference difficult or impossible, mistakes are made, things present inconsistent appearances, and so on. Thus, it is clear to us that the objects we act on are independent of us. In Parts IV and V, the content of sensory states is linked to the bodily and epistemic actions with which these states are innately associated. The idea is that our sensory awareness of object-features amounts to awareness of 'epistemic affordances', or awareness that certain epistemic operations are appropriate. Similarly, awareness of objects amounts to sensing the availability of these objects for attempts at physical interaction. By analysing the subjective content of sensation in this way, we go a long way towards explaining how we come to the idea that sensation informs us of things that exist independently of ourselves.

The aim of this book is to make a start towards a new understanding of located visual features, addressing the problems outlined above. The attempt is to provide new foundations for a representationalist view in which sensations, in and of themselves with no added learning or inference, present us with the materials for propositions concerning the external world that in the traditional view can only be arrived at by higher, more centralized, processing.

Here is a sampling of the problems that will be addressed in what follows:

How can sensation contain the materials from which propositional beliefs are constructed? Is it not merely an image? (Answer: No it is not. See Part I)

In what form is the descriptive content of perception presented to us? What does it mean to say that one perceived object is *similar* in a certain sensory respect to another? (Parts I and II)

Is perceptual content the same across species? (No: Chapter 6.) If not, how are we to understand sense-features in a species-specific way? (Chapter 8)

How exactly are we able to attribute objective content to sensation? What is the evidence needed for this? (Part III)

Is it possible to identify a mind-independent, or organism-independent, realm of which sensation brings us news? (This question in answered by the doctrine of Pluralistic Realism in Chapter 8)

How does sensory consciousness relate to sensory content? That is, what is the relationship between the subjective state that sensory systems put us into and our sensory representations of the external world? (Part IV)

How are the locations of features presented to us? How are we able to act upon and think about external objects on the basis of subjective sensory states? (Part V)

PART ONE

Classification

1

The Sensory Classification Thesis

In the dominant philosophical tradition, conscious *sensation* is a passive record of energy patterns incident on sensory receptors—visible electromagnetic radiation in the case of the eyes, acoustic vibrations in case of the ears, pressure in the case of touch, and so on. This is what expressions like 'raw sensation', 'retinal stimulation', 'proximal stimulus', and so on, allude to. The unprocessed raw material allegedly given us by sensation is usually contrasted with *perceptions* of objects and their properties. In the tradition, we come by the latter when we impose concepts, innate or learned, on the materials furnished us by sensation. Part I of this book argues that this traditional view is rooted in a mistaken conception of the perceptual process. It will be shown that the scientific evidence argues for a very different conception.

I. Sensory Classification

1. Let us begin, eschewing supporting evidence and argumentation for the moment, by outlining some of the basic elements of our theoretical framework.

In Part I we will begin to argue in support of the following position:

The Sensory Classification Thesis
I
a. Sensory systems classify and categorize; they sort and assign distal stimuli (i.e. external sensed objects) to classes.
b. Ideally—i.e. when they are functioning as they should in circumstances to which they are well-adapted—they do so on some consistent basis.
c. The results of this activity have a lasting (not necessarily permanent) effect on the perceiver in the form of conscious memories and changed dispositions with regard to the associative triggering of conscious experiences.

II

A *sense-feature* is a property a stimulus appears to have by virtue of an act of sensory classification. For example, the *colours* are the properties that distal stimuli appear to have when colour vision assigns them to classes in accordance with its own classification scheme. *Red* is the property characteristic of one such class: it is the property a thing appears to have when colour vision assigns it to this class.

Four issues are at stake in the Sensory Classification Thesis:

The Active Role of Sensory Systems. The Sensory Classification Thesis might seem like an uninformative truism: obviously, the redness of things is a feature they share; obviously, *red* is the characteristic property of a class. But the emphasis here is on the *classificatory activity* of the visual system. The analysis does not start, or end, with the *red* that certain visual objects share; it is concerned with the activity of constructing this and other sensory categories. The visual system is classifying these things together—*why*? Why do they belong together? For what purposes are they being classified together?

The Propositional Form of Sensory Awareness. The Sensory Classification Thesis claims, in effect, that sensory awareness can be expressed in terms of a set of singular propositions, messages to the effect that a particular individual is assigned to a certain class, and is identified as exemplifying a certain property. This goes against the traditional distinction between sensation and perception, which implies that the former is more like an *image* from which such propositions may be extracted, but not in itself articulated in such terms, such articulation being attributed to the post-sensory process called *perception*.

The Distal Objects of Sensory Awareness. The Sensory Classification Thesis insists that the targets of sensory classification are distal objects. The theoretical grounding for this proposition is discussed fully in Part V.

Lasting Effects of Sensory Classification. Part IV argues that sensory classification is used for *epistemic* purposes, such as conditioning and learning (including induction, which is a cognitively sophisticated form of these processes), object-comparison, object-identification, and search. Each of these operations requires the perceiver to store the results of sensory classification in a form that permits of conscious recall. Sense-features such as *red* and *round* are storable classifications.

Part I is concerned with the first two of these issues: classificatory activity and propositional form.

2. Classifying stimuli is not all that sensory systems do. They also provide organisms with information that guides the immediate orientation of their

bodies and limbs relative to stimuli—among primates, *vision* is particularly active in this function; in bats and dolphins, *audition* is; *proprioception* (awareness of one's own body and its position) and *haptic* feedback (awareness of how one is affecting environmental objects by touch) are crucial in all.

The sensory processes involved in bodily guidance are, from a perceiver's perspective, crucially different from those that result in sensory consciousness. In the first place, this sort of information—for example, information about where a teacup is, relative to my hand, when I am moving to pick it up—is not of permanent significance. That my hand has to move in such and such a direction to make contact with a cup is information that is useful given my position at the moment. Even if I stay seated at the same table and reach for the cup a few minutes later, subtle differences of position will make it necessary to redetermine the cup's whereabouts for the purposes of picking it up again. This kind of egocentric position is not a lasting characteristic of the cup, and there is no utility in storing it for future use.

A second difference between classificatory sensory systems and those that guide motion is that the former feed into a complex evaluative process. That a thing *looks* a certain way is not the end of the process by which we determine what it is like. Something looks a certain colour. This *may* lead one to believe that it really is this colour. It may also lead one to recall, for purposes of comparison, how it looked on a previous occasion, or to scrutinize it more closely. These investigative procedures may lead to the determination that it is not really the way it looks. Here, a consciously available sensory message contributes to a decision-making process that takes time and has many inputs which have to be weighed against one another. Earlier sensory messages may be recalled to consciousness in order to play their role in such a decision-making process. Consciousness plays the role of a holding area in which recent and earlier messages can be subjected to comparison and analysis.

The sensory guidance of bodily motion is quite different in these respects. The systems involved here act more or less unilaterally. When you reach for something, or walk around an obstacle, the visual information that guides you is not subject to further evaluation. For the most part, you are not even consciously aware of this information. It isn't as if you monitor your hand as it reaches for the cup and consciously guide it on its way there. In fact if a cup that you are in the process of reaching for wobbles or slips, you automatically adjust the trajectory of your hand without necessarily being aware that the cup moved (cf. Goodale, Pélisson, and Prablanc, 1986). Bodily guidance is certainly affected by conscious vision, but not, as it were, moment by moment. The fine control of intentional action is automatic and sub-personal.

So there is a contrast here. As condition Ic of the Sensory Classification Thesis posits, the results of sensory classification are stored for a period of time in a form that permits conscious recall in the short and/or long term. Sensory 'qualia' constitute material for relatively complex processes of evaluation. The body-orienting function of sensory systems, on the other hand, is a one-time only affair which does not employ or demand a lasting record that is accessible to consciousness.

The primary function of sensory classification is, as one might say, 'epistemic'. It is for the construction of a lasting record of information gathered about distal objects and the ways they generally behave. This record is used over time in different ways.

> It may be inserted into, or be used to modify, information 'files' concerning particular individuals.
>
> It may become part of a record of associations among sensory classes themselves, thus assisting conditioning, learning, and 'induction', and creating expectations about unobserved aspects of the environment.
>
> It may alter the subject's dispositions for a short period of time, for example, by 'priming' the subject to expect certain events, or habituating it (damping its reaction) to the presence of certain external conditions.

Parts I to IV of this book are about sensory classification. We will discuss the transient body-orienting function of sensory processes in Part V.

3. The Sensory Classification Thesis (clauses Ia and b) was first articulated (though not under this name) by the University of Chicago economist, Friedrich A. Hayek (1952), in a treatise entitled *The Sensory Order*.[1] Hayek thought of classification as a process that predictably sorts the same (kinds of) objects into the same classes, and then tags or labels these objects so that the user is able to identify them as having been assigned to a particular class. Hayek also insisted, seemingly echoing the McGill University psychologist, D. O. Hebb, and anticipating certain elements of present-day connectionism, that sensation leaves traces in the internal neural network by affecting the strengths of various neural interconnections. (Condition Ic of the Sensory Classification Thesis is stronger: it demands an effect on conscious memory.)

Hayek illustrates the Sensory Classification Thesis by means of the example of a ball-sorting machine:

We may find that the machine will always place the balls with a diameter of 16, 18, 28, 31, 32, and 40 mm. in a receptacle marked *A*, the balls with a diameter of 17, 22, 30, and 35 in a receptacle marked *B*, and so forth. The balls placed by the machine into the same receptacle will then be said to belong to the same class, and the balls placed by it into different receptacles to belong to so many different classes. *The fact that a ball is placed by the machine into a particular receptacle thus forms the sole criterion for assigning it into a particular class.* (1952, 49; emphasis added)

---

[1] I am grateful to Larry Hardin for the reference: in the earlier version of this book that Hardin read, I had formulated the Sensory Classification Thesis without any awareness of Hayek.

In this example, the balls placed in a particular receptacle constitute a class, the diameters the consistent basis for assignment to that class, and the marks—'A', 'B', etc.—the labels that enable the user to identify the class to which a particular ball has been assigned.

Hayek says that the identity of a sensory system's response to stimuli is 'the sole criterion' of co-classification; it is not necessary that there should be some organism-independent natural kind common to co-classified objects.

The phenomena with which we are here concerned are commonly discussed in psychology under the heading of 'discrimination'. The term is somewhat misleading because it suggests a sort of 'recognition' of physical differences between the events which it discriminates, while we are concerned with a process which *creates* the distinctions in question. (ibid., 48)

He quotes Piaget approvingly here (49n): a sensory class is an expression of identity of the subject's response to certain objects. He allows that the word 'grouping', used by George Lewes and Jean Piaget, 'is tolerably free from [these] misleading connotations'. The discriminability of stimuli is no different from their being assigned to different classes: two stimuli are discriminable if they are tagged differently, if, for example, they are assigned to different 'receptacles' in the above example.

4. 'The fact that a ball is placed by the machine into a particular receptacle thus forms the sole criterion for assigning it into a particular class.' One might think that this implies that sensory classification is arbitrary (though consistent). Later in his book, Hayek seems to endorse just this attitude, when he writes:

The characteristic attributes of the sensory qualities, or the classes into which different events are placed in the process of perception, are not attributes which are possessed by these events and which are in some manner 'communicated' to the mind; they are regarded as consisting entirely in the 'differentiating' responses of the organism by which the qualitative classification or order of these events is created. (ibid., 166)

On the face of it, Hayek is an Extreme Nominalist (cf. Woozley 1967, 203)—he believes that there is nothing common to the members of a sensory class other than that they belong to this class, having been assigned to it by the system on some consistent basis.

This is not a correct inference from the Sensory Classification Thesis. To maintain that *red* or *high-pitched* are classifications generated by sensory systems, or that they are based on the sameness of a subject's response to certain objects, is compatible with maintaining that they correspond to perceiver-independent kinds. More generally, it is compatible with the idea that such classifications may be *correct* or *incorrect*, *right* or *wrong*, independently of whether they follow the organism's consistent practice. In real-life situations—putting aside toy examples such as the ball-sorting machine—sensory classification has a function. Acts of classification are useful to the organism that performs them; classificatory dispositions increase the animal's evolutionary fitness by making it better adapted to its environmental niche. Sensory classification is subservient to this general rule.

Now, in certain circumstances, it may well be that a classification is useful only if it corresponds to some externally definable kind. A sensory system that detects the presence of a particular poison would be an example: it would not be doing its job if its classifications did not correspond to the presence of this toxin. More generally, i.e. putting aside correspondence to external kinds, the evolutionary function that a particular classification scheme serves will make it *right* that certain things should fall into a particular class, and *wrong* that others should do so—either generally or on a particular occasion. For we will generally be able to find some activity that is disrupted if the organism consistently adopts a deviant classification scheme, or if it misapplies its species-normal classification scheme on a particular occasion. Since the classification scheme serves this activity, and since the success conditions of the activity are determined by the environmental conditions that the sensory system probes, sensory classification is subject to objective standards of rightness and wrongness. For these reasons, it is appropriate to take from the Sensory Classification Thesis a *constrained* form of nominalism which regards an organism's classification scheme as subject to correction by the external world, given the activities and interests of its species, while at the same time acknowledging that this classification scheme was constructed in evolutionary time, and cannot be understood independently of the organism's history.

We will return to this issue later, in Chapters 8 and 9, where our present cautious stand of Functionally Constrained Nominalism becomes a bolder Pluralistic Realism. The important point to be appreciated here is that even if a classificatory scheme comes to reflect external reality through the operation of natural selection, such correspondence is functionally subordinate to the needs of the organism—or to put it in another way, realism and objectivity are instrumental, not absolute, values for sensory systems. Thus, even if the sensory process comes to represent the world in terms of externally definable categories, it would be wrong to build this into our very conception of sensory activity right from the start. The terminology of classification enables us to investigate the activity of sensory systems without making powerful assumptions about their conformity with external kinds.

For the moment, let us put the testing of such questions aside. The Sensory Classification Thesis is non-committal about whether there is a perceiver-independent basis for sensory classification, apart from the stipulation that it should be 'consistent'—a stipulation that is explained further in Chapter 8. Are distal stimuli classed together because they share some physical property? Or on the basis of some environmentally useful response that they evoke in sensory systems? These questions are left unanswered at this stage.

No further characterization of sensory classes is implied by the Sensory Classification Thesis. The Thesis simply claims that sensory activity groups some stimuli together and differentiates others. How are sensory classes constructed? What is the relationship between two things that are properly assigned to the same class? How are these classes presented subjectively, and what is their objective significance? What, in short, are the characteristics that purportedly unite the things that a sensory system declares to be the same as one another, and what is the mode of their being so presented? Parts II–IV of this book are devoted to discussing these questions. In Part I, the goal is simply to elucidate, elaborate, and defend the Sensory Classification Thesis.

5. In one respect, the Sensory Classification Thesis *is* realist from the very outset: it insists that sensory systems classify *distal* stimuli—objects or happenings in the external world. Thus, it gives the senses an essentially outward-looking role. In this respect, it is sharply different from traditional Sense Datum Theory, which makes inner sensory events the objects of classification: according to this traditional perspective, *red* is a feature shared by the private and inner 'direct objects' of sensory events.

The outward-looking perspective of the Sensory Classification Thesis may remind some readers of the claim that every sensory state attributes some quality to an external object—a thesis forcefully advanced by Gilbert Harman (1990), and taken over by many contemporary philosophers. Indeed, the Thesis *is* compatible with Harman's idea (which has antecedents in G. E. Moore 1903 as well as in Rudolf Carnap and Hans Reichenbach—see Firth 1949, 441n—and David Armstrong 1967), for the Thesis claims that every sensory state possesses attributive significance with regard to a stimulus, namely, that it assigns this stimulus to a sensory class. Both theses emphasize that sensory experiences are not insulated inner events that must be decoded or diagnosed by us before they can be put to use, but rather inherently *meaningful* states with representational significance beyond themselves.[2]

However, the Sensory Classification Thesis goes considerably further than the Distal Attributivism just outlined—the thesis that a sensory state attributes a feature to a distal object. Distal Attributivism touches only on two of the issues we identified above as touchstones for the perspective being introduced here, namely, the distality of stimuli and the propositional form of sensory states. It does not insist that categories like *red* are the products of sensory activity. It is thus compatible with the idea that sense-features are organism-independent natural kinds, and also with the idea that sense-features

---

[2] It should be clear that Harman's position, and the Sensory Classification Thesis itself, is meant to apply only to the small number of sense-features processed by the sensory systems: objections such as those advanced by Charles Travis (2004) seem to turn entirely on neglecting this restriction, and dealing with examples such as whether Sid looks drunk or Pia as if she is having an affair with Luc.

are passive records or traces of external reality. Indeed, Attributivism is even compatible with the notion that sense-features are subjective properties of sense-data—so long as it is held that we somehow project these properties on to external objects. Distal Attributivism says nothing about the nature of sensory classes; in particular, it says nothing about the active process by which sensory systems assign stimuli to these classes.

The difference between Distal Attributivism and the Sensory Classification Thesis, then, is that the latter is a theory about the construction of sense-features. The Sensory Classification Thesis maintains that sensory systems create classificatory categories for the use of the organism of which they are a part; sense-features are not simply patterns in the ambient energy record. Harman's theory can serve as a structural framework for the Sensory Classification Thesis, but the latter attempts to get at the workings and origins of sensory attributions as a means of understanding their significance and content.

6. The bald statement of the Sensory Classification Thesis offered above needs to be elaborated in an important way. The Sensory Classification Thesis suggests that co-classification is a yes or no thing: either two stimuli belong in the same category or they do not; either they drop into the same receptacle of Hayek's sorting machine or they do not. It suggests further that sense-features are fixed categories with predetermined boundaries.

In fact, things are more complicated. Stimuli are in fact united by *resemblance*, which is a matter of degree. Thus, it is somewhat misleading to say *tout court* that the senses assign stimuli to classes. Consider a map, in which any two locations are determinately distant from one another. One can construct regions in such a map in cross-cutting ways: the class of things that are one mile away from point A may overlap with the things that are one mile away from point B. There may be no absolute boundaries in such a map corresponding to the discrete sensory classes of Hayek's ball-sorting machine. Moreover, classes may be hierarchically arranged. Two things may belong in different categories inasmuch as one is crimson and the other scarlet, but at the same time belong in the same category inasmuch as both are red. The degree of difference permitted between two crimson things is smaller than that permitted between two red things. The best way to accommodate such hierarchical or cross-cutting categories is to arrange stimuli into overlapping classes by means of a similarity ordering.

This reflection leads to a more encompassing, that is, a more broadly applicable version of condition Ia of the Sensory Classification Thesis:

> *The Sensory Ordering Thesis*
> Sensory systems create *ordered* relations of similarity and dissimilarity among stimuli, relations which grade the degree of similarity that one sensed object bears to another.

Sensory Ordering permits the construction of more and less inclusive classes: the more inclusive classes comprise stimuli that may be less similar to one another than those in the less inclusive classes. It also allows the formation of many different cross-cutting sensory classes as the context dictates: for it may well be that what is relevant in a given situation is not some category delineated in advance, but rather the class of things similar to a given stimulus. We may, that is, be focusing on *things similar up to a certain degree to **that** colour or **that** tone*, and the latter classification may correspond to no predefined class such as *scarlet* or *middle C*.

The Sensory Ordering Thesis is the subject of Part II. (It is also prefigured in Chapter 3, section IV.) In the rest of this book, we stick with the simpler Sensory Classification Thesis. The aim in Part I is to show how the activity of sensory systems is responsible for the attributive content of sensory states.

7. Constrained Nominalism implies that it is possible for a perceptual system to misclassify a stimulus. An organism may adopt a classificatory scheme that does not well serve the purposes for which this scheme is used. It may also misapply its classificatory scheme by assigning a stimulus to a class on a particular occasion when, relative to its consistent basis of assigning objects to this class, it should not have done so. This distinguishes Constrained Nominalism from many classic approaches to defining sensory classes.

In his *Aufbau*, Rudolf Carnap (1928, §§78–81) constructed a 'phenomenalistic' system in which sensory classes are classes of *experiences*. He stipulated that these classes can be defined by means of a relationship of *sensed* similarity—a relation of similarity that holds on the domain of sensations.[3] Simplifying greatly, *red* turns out to be, on Carnap's approach, a class united by sensed similarity. If you isolate one experience as a paradigm case of red, then other experiences similar enough to the paradigm will get into the class as well. On the face of it, one cannot misclassify things on such a scheme, at least not if one assumes that it is impossible to be wrong about the character of one's own experiences. Since Carnap constructed sensory classes out of *experiences*, and since he conceives of similarity as *sensed* similarity, it seems that the appearance–reality dichotomy cannot be captured in his system—at least not without major surgery. If something *looks* similar to something else, then it *is* so; consequently, if something is classed together with red things because it looks similar to them, then it *is* red, and there can be no question of error.

---

[3] In order to accommodate past experiences, Carnap used a relationship of *remembered* similarity. This brings complications of its own—the relation is temporally asymmetric, for instance—but it is still an internally available, i.e. experienced, relationship. He also assumes that one's sensory state at a given moment is indivisible. This is simply mistaken—see Chapter 2, section II.

What happens if one thinks that *red* is a class of distal stimuli, say physical objects, not of experiences? Can Carnap's use of sensed similarity be transferred to distal objects. Can we define the sensory class *red* as follows?

> Pick a paradigm red object *r*. (The Canadian Maple Leaf would serve, for instance.)

> The class of red things contains all and only those things that are sensed as similar with respect to colour as *r* (up to some degree of similarity).

No: this definition fails as well. For it is possible that two physical things might *look* similar to one another in colour, even when they are not *really* so: for instance, a red thing like the Maple Leaf might in certain conditions of lighting or contrast look more similar to a white thing than it really is. When two things appear the same in some sensory respect, the relevant sensory system is assigning them to the same class, but because of the possibility of sensory error, they may not really be the same in this respect.

It follows that one cannot define the criteria for inclusion in sensory classes consisting of distal stimuli by reference *just* to appearance. This leaves us with a difficulty which cannot be resolved until later: How are we to define a sensory class like *red*? We will return to this problem in Part IV. For the moment all that we can draw from Constrained Nominalism is the idea that when two things appear the same in some sensory respect, it is because they have been co-classified by the relevant sensory system—perhaps disrupting certain organismic functions thereby and, in this sense, erroneously.

II. Classification and Sensory Consciousness

1. In section I.1, it was suggested that sensory classification and sensory bodily guidance operate in different ways. In human beings, and presumably in many other animals as well, sensory classification is essentially tied up with consciousness. By contrast, bodily orientation is *not* controlled by means of conscious sensation, even though we may be conscious of how our bodies and limbs are oriented.

Endel Tulving (2000) puts the point this way:

An outfielder catching the near-home-run ball near the top of the high back fence . . . can talk about his feat . . . but such a verbal description is secondary (epiphenomenal) and plays no role in the execution of the highly skillful behaviour. On the other hand, two masters can play chess without the board and pieces, entirely within their own minds. (37)

The outfielder's consciousness of his athletic feat helps him talk about it, but it does not guide his motions—conscious awareness of the ball turns out, surprisingly enough, to be 'epiphenomenal' in this regard. (There is a great deal of conscious orienting activity which accompanies the outfielder's activity—lining up with the ball, keeping its elevation steady, and so on—and so this is not the best example to use here. Tulving is presumably referring to the jump and grab at the last moment (see Clark 2001, Goodale 2002, Campbell 2002, and Chapter 13 below for further details and discussion). By contrast, the chess master's conscious images of future possible positions are essential determinants of his actions when he opens his mouth to say 'Pawn to QB4' in a game of blindfold chess. In much the same way, conscious awareness is often an indispensable intermediary when we use sensory classes to make inferences, distinguish objects from one another, infer that an object has an unsensed property on the grounds that it has an associated sensed property, and so on. When I realize that a particular Honda in the parking lot is not my own, on the grounds that it is different from mine in colour, the conscious awareness of the car's colour played an essential role in my 'inference'.

Here is a simple account of how consciousness operates in these cases. The sensory systems are, we proposed, automatic sorting machines and assign objects to various categories or classes. We become aware of relations of sensory co-classification because the stimuli that are co-classified *appear* the same in some sensory respect. Suppose, for example, that two objects look crimson: this is the means by which the colour vision system delivers to us, or our epistemic organs, the news that it has co-classified them. Conversely, suppose that one object looks crimson and another scarlet. This is how colour vision informs us that it has differentiated them and assigned them to different classes. The information so delivered is then available to be used in inferences. I remember that my Honda is green; I am able to summon a conscious remembered image of it as green; this is the continuing record of a past act of classification. The car in the parking lot looks red: this is how I know that my visual system has assigned it to the class of red things. Assuming that I accept my visual system's determination that the car is red— and I need not do this, since I am free to doubt or reject the evidence of my senses—this leads me to the conclusion that the car is not mine.

What sort of sign of classification is experience? Chapter 10 argues that sensory experience acquires its meaning by a kind of internal *convention* (in the sense of David Lewis 1969). There we shall propose:

The Sensory Signalling Thesis
A sensory experience is a *signal* issued in accordance with an internal convention. It means that the sensory system has assigned a stimulus to a certain category—the same category as when other tokens of the same signal are issue.

The nature of these action-categories will be discussed further in Part IV; in accordance with section I.2 above, the actions in question are mainly epistemic in character (not motor). In the remainder of this chapter, I develop further the idea that sensory experience betokens how a stimulus has been classified.

2. Note the three stages of the sensory process as described above.

> A. Stimuli: material objects and the packets of energy that they send to our sensory receptors.
> B. Sensory classes: the groups that the system makes of the stimuli, and sense-features, the properties that stimuli in a given sensory class share in virtue of belonging to that class.
> C. Sensations: events in sensory consciousness with a particular subjective 'feel'. These events are like labels that the system attaches to stimuli in order that we may know that they have been assigned to a particular class.

This, in outline, is the framework within which it will be argued that sensations, and relations of sensory similarity among stimuli, are the products of active data-processing.

Sensation, or sensory awareness, is, we have been saying, the consciously available record of sensory classification, a label that identifies an object as belonging to a particular class. (We are not aware of the label independently of the object: the label is, rather, part of how we experience the object.) It follows that classification must *precede* awareness of classification, much as in Hayek's ball-sorting machine (section I.3 above), the sorting of balls precedes their ending up in labelled receptacles. The importance and implications of this point are often overlooked. Many philosophers claim, for example, that sense-features are 'response-dependent', meaning thereby that it is constitutive of *red* that it evokes a certain sensation in us. If the Sensory Classification Thesis is correct, this is an inversion: things are not classified as red because they look red (under normal circumstances); instead, they look red because the visual system has determined that they are so. Yet, the characteristics of sensation are often projected backwards on to sense-features. In order to avoid such confusions, it is important to be clear on the order of the sensory process as outlined above. Let us, therefore, review some of the empirical reasons why the sensations must be sharply dissociated from the sense-features they betoken.

There are three bodies of evidence that indicate the dissociation of classification and awareness. (This evidence indicates that classification is observed without sensation. Sensation is never observed without classification, correct or mistaken. This is not what psychologists call a double dissociation.)

(A) 'Blindsight'—see Lawrence Weiskrantz 1997—is a famous case of dissociation between sensory classification and conscious awareness thereof.

Blindsight is the neurological condition in which patients are able to *use* visual information accurately for certain purposes even while they strongly deny that they are conscious of this information, typically ascribing their visual prescience to 'guessing', or the like. For instance, Weiskrantz recounts an experiment conducted by John Marshall and Peter Halligan, in which a blindsighted patient was shown two pictures of identical houses, one of which was on fire, but with the flames occurring wholly in a 'blind' part of her visual field, i.e. a part in which she had no phenomenal experience. 'When asked which house she would prefer to live in she retorted that it was a silly question, because they were the *same*, but nevertheless she reliably chose the house not on fire' Weiskrantz, (24–5). Since the houses were schematic cartoons, much as would be drawn by a child in kindergarten, there was no reason to like one and dislike the other—except for the fact that one was shown burning. Clearly, then, the patient was able to use visual information contained in her blind field though she was not conscious of it. This seems to show that the visual system has performed at least some of its classificatory functions on the picture—the classificatory functions relevant to identifying flames, or at least to disliking the house that happens to be burning—and is able to make use of this classification for certain purposes, but does not deliver news of the results to phenomenal experience.

In fact, the classificatory work done in the blind field can be quite extensive. In a recent study, Anthony Marcel (1998) reports that two blindsighted patients he has studied are able to recognize letters, shapes, and illusory contours in their blind fields. These patients were tested not only by asking them to identify stimuli presented in their blind fields, but by what Marcel calls 'indirect measures' of visual function, i.e. measures on the effects of visual information on *other* discriminatory tasks—this is significant because these measures 'are often much more sensitive than direct measures' (1566). Thus, Marcel tried to find out whether words presented in a blind field would influence the disambiguation of words presented in the sighted field (just as consciously seen words do). He found that blindsighted visual performance was reasonably good in this regard. For example, 'race' presented in the sighted field is disambiguated one way by the occurrence of 'speed' in the blind spot, and in another way by 'negro'; 'bank' by 'money' and 'river'. Such cases of 'priming' occur without *explicit* visual consciousness. (As Marcel explains, there is *some* awareness of events in the blind field, but not of the words themselves.)

(B) Something like what is true of Marcel's blindsighted subjects is also true of normally sighted individuals, as his own earlier work on 'visual masking' shows (1983*a*, *b*). ('Visual masking' is the term Marcel uses: several disparate phenomena fall under this description, however, and the term 'metacontrast' would have been more specific to the actual phenomenon studied. We'll ignore this in what follows.) In visual masking experiments, normally sighted people are presented with a stimulus, and then after a brief interval, with another stimulus of non-overlapping complementary shape, for example a disc followed by a surrounding annulus. Experimenters find that the second stimulus *masks*, or blocks recall of, the first: the experimental subjects simply cannot recall what was presented before the mask as a separate figure, though if the mask had not been presented, they would have had no difficulty doing so. The effect of metacontrast is, in other words, similar to the effect of the two stimuli presented together: when a disc and complementary annulus are presented together, they are difficult or impossible to discern as two separate objects. In the metacontrast situations, a subject's conscious awareness of the first stimulus, the *target*, is suppressed by the second stimulus, the *mask*. Marcel found that despite the suppression of conscious sensation, masking did not disrupt all visual functions with respect to the target. When asked to guess which of several stimuli had been presented before the mask, normally sighted subjects were influenced by semantic and orthographic similarities, much as the blindsighted patients described in the preceding paragraph were, even though they were unable directly to describe what had gone before. Others had discovered earlier, that subjects are able to localize the target, but not to describe it (cf. Ogmen et al. 2003). Here too we have a dissociation between sensory classification and phenomenal awareness of such classification.

(C) Finally, the hiatus between sensory classification and sensory experience is illustrated by lower organisms that possess sensory systems but lack consciousness. These organisms react predictably to stimuli of a certain type, but are not conscious of the stimulus being assigned to that type by their sensory systems. The sea hare, *Aplysia californica*, can be predictably conditioned (Squire and Kandel 1999, 16–19), but possessing only 20,000 neurons in total, it is presumably too simple to possess consciousness. This organism is another example of dissociation between classification and sensory experience. Sensory consciousness must be a later development, a new and different way of making sensory classes available to an organism.

We may summarize these observations as follows. Sensory experience is the *normal* means by which an observer (belonging to a species capable of sensory consciousness) gains access to the results of sensory classification for the formation of beliefs. In Ned Block's (1995) terminology: the function of *phenomenal* consciousness, i.e. of sensory experience, is to provide us *access* to sensory classification for purposes of reasoning. Phenomenal consciousness is, in other words, consciousness *of* sensory classification. On the other hand, the results of classification are available to many of the organism's other systems without being routed through consciousness. Sensory experience is not the *only* route by which the results of sensory data-processing are able to effect an organism's behaviour, though it may well be that *some* mental functions can *only* be exercised through conscious awareness.

3. It is extremely important to note that in the above delineation of sensory processes *sensatious* are not normally objects of our awareness. The claim is not that we are aware of our own sensations, but that by being in particular sensory states, i.e. by being subject to particular sensations, we come to know of a distal object that it has been classified a certain way.

Donald Laming (1997) attributes to the psychophysicist, S. S. Stevens, a point similar to that made when we were noting the three stages of the sensory process. In Laming's words: 'Physical stimulus magnitude is one thing and what an observer says about it may be quite another. There has to be some distinct intermediary.' (13). So far, so good: sensory states represent the magnitudes of physical stimuli, and are distinct from both the stimuli and their magnitudes. Laming goes on, however, to draw a misleading inference (again on Stevens's behalf): 'Since asking subjects the direct question "How loud does this tone sound?" gave systematic answers, those answers must be [a] direct measure *of sensation*.' Surely not. These subjects are telling us about the loudness *of the tones*, not about the loudness of their auditory sensations: they are not measuring their sensations. It may be harmless in certain circumstances to transfer these reports from tones to the sensations thereof: by saying, for instance, that one sensation is twice as large as another if the magnitude represented by the first is twice as large as that reported by the second. This would be a bit like saying that the proposition 'The room is 100 feet long' is twice as large as the proposition 'The room is 50 feet long'— harmless if used with an explicit indication of the ellipsis, but (at the very least) puzzling and misleading if taken literally.

Here is a parallel that illustrates the difference between the above-mentioned claims. When I tell you that Leon is a cat, I am not telling you something about my beliefs; rather, I am telling you something about Leon. Of course, I would not (normally) tell you this except for my belief that Leon is a cat, and in this sense, I *evince* or *express* my belief. Nevertheless, I do not in any sense, *refer* to myself or my beliefs when I say 'Leon is a cat'. Similarly in the case of sensation. Though I am aware of the blueness of a particular external object *through* my sensory experience (or sensation) of it, this sensation is not self-referential—I am aware of the external object, not of the sensation. In other words, conscious sensory experience is (normally) awareness of objects outside ourselves and of the sense-features they possess.

On occasion, one can become aware of the characteristics of a particular state of sensory awareness. Suppose, for instance, that as you are looking at something, your contact lens shifts and your vision becomes blurry. Call the second state *S*. *S* may well involve *direct awareness* of its own blurriness.

In such a case, the object of awareness is, as Alex Byrne (2001*b*, 212) rightly says, 'not the scene before the eyes', but rather 'the experience itself': that is, it is visually obvious that the distal object is not blurry, and that this is merely a condition of the eye. Thus, one might express my visual state S in something like the following way: 'That thing is blue and I am seeing it in a blurry fashion.' However, sensory states do not present information about their objects in a form that it mediated by an additional reflexive state of introspective awareness of the state itself. That is, it is never the case that in order to be aware of either the blueness of the thing seen in S or of the blurriness of how the thing is seen, one needs an *additional* experience E that is of S.

This said, it must also be emphasized that any adequate account of sensory experience will involve a description of non-representational characteristics of the perceiver's own sensory states. One cannot always exhaustively describe a sensation by giving details of the features it attributes to distal stimuli. Consider the proposition:

(1) X has a visual sensation as of a round thing three feet away.

Our experience of *visual* qualities has a particular conscious 'feel'. So (1) implies

(2) X has a sensation as of a round thing three feet away; X's sensation has a characteristically visual feel.

(1) is thus not equivalent to the sparser claim that:

(3) X is aware of a round thing three feet away.

X is *aware* of the round thing three feet away both when she has a *tactile* sensation of it and when she has a *visual* sensation of it, and a representationally equivalent, though non-commital, experience even when she closes her eyes and imagines it. So the claim in (2) that she is *visually* aware of it is not otiose; it tells us something about the *mode* of awareness.

Here again, the linguistic parallel is useful. To say that English speakers speak about cats *using the word 'cat'* is not otiose; it is not equivalent to the sparser claim that they speak about cats (period). For the French designate the same objects using quite another word, i.e. *'chat'*. Since there is this variety in vehicles of designation, mention of the vehicle or manner of presentation is not redundant.[4]

---

[4] Michael Tye 2000 protests that the *entire content* of visual consciousness contains awareness of features that can only be presented visually. For example, in the case of (1), he says, it must be the case that X's visual sensation must be as of a thing of some colour. Thus, the sensation referred to in (1) is simultaneously a sensation of a coloured thing. This, says Tye, is what makes it a visual sensation. So without claiming that it is redundant to specify that the sensation is

Daniel Dennett's (1991) discussion of 'prosthetic vision' provides us with another kind of dissociation between sensory classification and sensory experience that is relevant at this point.

Prosthetic devices have been designed to provide 'vision' to the blind, and some of them raise just the right issues. [Around 1970] Paul Bach-y-Rita developed several devices that involved small, ultralow-resolution video cameras that could be mounted on eyeglass frames. The low-resolution signal from these cameras, a 16-by-16 or 20-by-20 array of 'black and white' pixels was spread over the back or belly of the subject in a grid of either electrical or mechanical vibrating tinglers called tactors.

After only a few hours of training, blind subjects wearing this device could learn to interpret the patterns of tingles on their skin, much as you can interpret letters traced on your skin by someone's finger . . . . The result was certainly prosthetically produced conscious perceptual experience, but since the input was spread over the subject's backs or bellies instead of their retina, was it *vision*? Did it have the 'phenomenal qualities' of vision, or just of tactile sensation? (339–40)

Dennett argues, quite cogently, that many of the reasons for saying that these 'phenomenal qualities' are non-visual are founded on confusion. But then he draws a startling conclusion: these blind subjects are *seeing* by means of their prostheses, he says, and if their experience is different from ours, it is only because they don't see things in all the detail available to normally sighted people.

A detailed argument with Dennett would take us too far afield. But it is of at least expository value to redescribe prosthetic vision in the terms introduced in the present section. 'Phenomenal qualities', as Dennett calls them, are qualities of which we normally become aware through sensory experience; for example, 'visual qualities' are those of which we normally become aware by means of experiences with a characteristically visual feel. It is perfectly comprehensible to hold that Bach-y-Rita enabled blind people to become consciously aware of *visual features* or *visual classes*. This is just to say that he enabled them to become tactually (and hence consciously) aware of features that are *normally* made known to perceivers by means of experiences with a characteristically visual feel, features like shape, position, and brightness. Again, one could look to the *process*, and say that they became aware of these features but not through the eyes. (Note that these two ways of diagnosing what is happening here diverge on whether Bach-y-Rita's

---

visual, Tye insists that this specification is itself one of representational content. Tye treats one's visual consciousness at a moment as an indivisible whole: the experience of something as round is indissolubly a part of the same whole as the experience of it as coloured. This overlooks the fact that colour and shape are represented in separate acts of awareness that are bound together when we attend to something (see Chapter 3, section II). In any case, it is unclear how Tye will account for blurriness: it isn't the distal object that is represented as blurry when I take my contact lenses out.

patients would be 'seeing' if their visual cortices had been directly stimulated by his prosthetic device: this would produce visual phenomenology, but not by the normal process.) This allows us to say that they become aware of these features non-visually, and thus non-normally. (This use of 'normal' is not invidious: video cameras and 'tactors' are not, in a historical-evolutionary sense, 'normal' devices for sensing the world.) The Bach-y-Rita phenomenon can then be seen as an instance of a more general one: colour-blind individuals come to know of colours through the colour-impoverished information available to them (Chapter 3, section VI), deaf people encode phonemes in sign language, visual qualities can be conveyed to blind people through texture (cf. Lopes 1997), and so on.

We can agree with Dennett that these people come to know of these visual features by means of sensory experience. That is, they come to be aware of them by means of tactile experience. The features they come to know are visual, but the experience by which they come to know these features is not. Dennett, however, denies the dissociation between visual features and visual experience: he claims, in effect, that the *feeling* produced on the backs or bellies of these people is visual experience simply in virtue of it being experience of visual features. By distinguishing sensory classes and sensation, we are able to give a smoother account of this matter, but one which preserves much of what Dennett wants to say about it.

4. We have been saying that when a stimulus S looks different (i.e. is discriminable) from another S', it is because the visual system has assigned S and S' to different classes. That one surface looks scarlet and another looks crimson—this is news that the colour vision system has differentiated them. If two stimuli are qualitatively distinguishable, then, it is because they have been differentiated, i.e. assigned to different classes. Conversely, if they are indistinguishable in some respect—in colour, in shape, etc.—it is because they have been assigned to the same class.

The direction of the 'because' in the claims just made is crucial. Some philosophers argue that two stimuli should be assigned to the same sensory class because they are similar or indistinguishable, or to different sensory classes because they are discriminable. As we have seen, this gets it backwards. The discriminability or indiscriminability of stimuli in our sensory experience of them is a consequence of how sensory systems classify them. Sensation is how we come to know that our sensory systems have assigned a stimulus to a particular class. Sensation is the indicator, not the constitutive characteristic, of sensory classification.

Thus we have:

The Posteriority of Appearance Thesis
Appearance follows sensory classification as the record thereof. It is not the basis or ground for sensory classification.

Posteriority of Appearance implies that there is no unclassified remnant in sensation, no variation simply left over from the energy pattern incident on the sensory receptors, and hence lacking in classificatory significance. In the last section, it was argued that sensory states have non-representational aspects. Here, we note the equally important point that everything that a sensory state attributes to its external object is significant.

On the traditional view, found for example in the *Aufbau* of Rudolf Carnap (1928), *we* as epistemic agents assign sensory qualia to classes like *red* on the basis of their similarity to one another—first sensory appearance and similarity among appearances, subsequently sensory classes. On this theory, it would be quite plausible that we might allow a certain variability within classes: we might gather two or more slightly different shades of red under the classification *burgundy*, for instance, and neglect to subdivide this category into classes within which the members were indistinguishable from one another—each of these classes would correspond to a shade of colour. In other words, our classificatory scheme might simply disregard the difference between shades of red: these different shades are simply left over from differences of retinal stimulation, but unimportant to us. This is the sense in which a sensed difference might remain an 'unclassified remnant'.

On the assumption that sensation signals classification—that is, on the Posteriority of Appearance Thesis—this supposition makes no sense. Two stimuli are distinguishable because they are tagged with the labels of different sensory classes; thus they have *already* been assigned to different classes. First classification, then sensory appearance as label: since it makes no sense to suppose that the same class would have two labels, discriminable shades indicate distinct classes. Similarly, if two stimuli are indiscriminable, it is because they have been assigned to the same sensory class.

This argument leads to the following corollary of the Sensory Signalling and Posteriority of Appearance Theses:

The Classificatory Equivalence Thesis
Two stimuli present the same appearance in some respect if and only if they have been assigned to the same sensory class.

There is no *non-representational* richness or nuance in how distal objects appear to the senses.

Two clarificatory notes are required here:

a. Sensory consciousness is often quite indeterminate. That is, there are differences and changes in a sensory image that escape our notice most of the time. The point being made here is not that we are always aware of what sensory class a stimulus has been assigned to, just that sensation has the function of giving us this information.

b. It is possible for two stimuli to present the same appearance even though the experience they occasion is different in non-representational ways: for instance, two objects might look exactly the same colour, though one looks a bit blurry because of a tear in one's eye. Here, as noted before, the blurriness is not a feature attributed to the object, but to one's own vision.

5. The Posteriority of Appearance Thesis opens up a revealing perspective on sensory experience. Philosophers traditionally define sensory properties like *red* in terms of the experience of red: a thing is red if and only if it has the causal disposition to *look* red in normal circumstances. In the light of the Posteriority of Appearance Thesis, the perspective that this Dispositionalist theory offers us is lopsided. Sensory experience is the end-product of the visual process; something looks red because the visual system has assigned it to the class of red things; the experience of red is simply the visual system's *label* for that class, the way we know how the thing has been classified. As we have been saying, it is an inversion to say that something is red because it produces in us the experience of red.[5]

The difference between Posteriority of Appearance and the Dispositionalist theory can be made more stark by considering how each treats of *sensory variation*. This occurs when the sensation that one person has when looking at a stimulus is different from that of another person looking at the same stimulus. One instance of this is *spectral inversion*: that is, when I systematically have the experience of *green* while looking at stimuli that cause you to have the experience of *red*.

Now, Dispositionalism is, presumably, not just a theory about what the colours are—i.e. that they are dispositions of the sort specified earlier—but also a theory about the significance of colour experience—colour-appearances are, according to this theory, paired with the dispositions we have been talking about. For as Howard Langsam (2000), a defender of Dispositionalism, says, an appearance of red 'is the way that [a] red physical object appears to the subject' (74). So considering the above case of spectral inversion, the Dispositionalist has, it seems, two options. He can hold:

*Dispositionalist Theory of Spectral Inversion A
No physical object can have both a disposition to create a red appearance normally and also a green appearance normally. Thus, since things that seem green to me simultaneously look red to you, at most one of

---

[5] A number of theories are closely allied to Dispositionalism by their commitment to the proposition that something is red because it produces in us the experience as of red. Among them are John Campbell's (1997/1993) 'Simple Theory of Colour', which holds that colour is the ground of the disposition, and Colin McGinn's (1996) 'impressionism', according to which colour supervenes on the disposition. These theories are equally subject to the criticisms to follow.

us can be right. To at least one of us things look wrong—i.e. they look to be something that they are not.

But on reflection, he might decide that there is no good reason to prefer you to me on this matter, or vice versa. After all, we do seem to be in symmetrical positions as far as this matter goes. Putting aside the tyranny of greater numbers, no possible evidence could break the impasse regarding which of us is right about *red*. So the Dispositionalist might allow that contrary to Theory A above, both of us can, after all, be right. How can he accommodate this? By a move that is sometimes known as relationalization. Here it is:

> *Dispositionalist Theory of Spectral Inversion B.*
> Both you and I are normal observers. Thus a physical object *can* have both a disposition to create a red appearance normally and also a green appearance normally. To accommodate this, we need to relativize the predicate 'is red'. We do this by stipulating that the same object might be green *to me* while it is red to *you*.

On both versions of the Dispositionalist theory, the attribution of redness to a thing depends on identifying the experience it occasions in a normal perceiver as an experience with a certain phenomenal quality.

The Posteriority of Appearance Thesis takes a very different approach to sensory variation. First, it insists that sensory classification precedes sensory experience, and denies that the latter determines the meaning of the former. As a consequence, second, it distinguishes two sources of sensory variation.

Difference of Convention

One way sensory variation could occur is if the sensory experience by which my colour vision system signals a certain classification is different from the experience by which your system signals the *same* classification. A linguistic parallel: the English call a feline creature 'cat', the French call it 'chat': this does not mean that they are employing different classifications; all it means is that they have different words for the same classification. Analogously in sensation. Different sensations can betoken the same sense-feature.

Difference of Classification

Another way sensory variation could occur is if our two systems classified things differently, and signalled these different classifications by the same experiences. In English, the word *etiquette* designates certain actions thought to be correct in certain contexts of social interaction, while in French it more commonly refers to a label such as one affixed to an object by a store-keeper to indicate its price. Here, the *word* is the same, but what it means is different. This could happen in the case of sensory variation. The reason why you and I have different experiences when we are looking at a leaf or a tomato *might* be that our sensory systems disagree about how to classify these objects.

Dispositionalists take the view that spectrally inverted people attribute different properties to external things, since the property 'has the disposition to create a red appearance' is different from the property 'has the disposition to create a green appearance'. Thus, they take it that spectral inversion marks a difference of classification (even if only a difference relativized to an observer). However, as I shall now argue, spectral inversion is a merely conventional difference as it is normally described.

Consider an argument for the existence of undetected spectral inversion cited by Stephen Palmer (1999). Palmer points out that red-green colour blindness comes in two varieties: some people (*protanopes*) are red-green colour blind because they have a gene that causes their long-wavelength cones to have the same pigment as normal medium-wavelength cones, and others (*deuteranopes*) because they have the opposite deficiency. Palmer invites us to 'suppose that someone had the genes for *both* forms of red-green color blindness simultaneously,'

Such people would . . . not be red-green color blind at all, but simply red-green-reversed trichromats. They should exist. Assuming they do, they are proof that this color transformation is either undetectable or very difficult to detect by purely behavioural means, because no one has ever managed to identify such a person (926)

The fact that such an inversion is hard to detect suggests that these people would be making the *same* classifications as everyone else: for instance, they arrive at an equivalent set of inductive beliefs concerning colour, and they apply exactly the same colour-words to exactly the same things, though their colour-experiences are always systematically different. In other words, they would be spectrally inverted in exactly the same way as this condition is usually described in the philosophical literature. The Dispositionalist's position is unattractive in this case. What reason do we have to say that red-green reversed trichromats are *mistaken* about the colours, or even that we need to relativize colour-attribution to accommodate them? The Sensory Classification Thesis takes a more natural stand: their acts of colour classification are the same as everybody else's, though they come to be aware of these by means of different experiences.

The Dispositionalist's stance concerning the second kind of inversion is even more unintuitive. As we shall see in Chapter 6, section II, it is possible that there could be a person who experiences light in the ultraviolet part of the spectrum in phenomenally the same way as we experience violet. Here the natural thing to say, and what the Sensory Classification Thesis *does* say, is that this person is sensitive to sense-features different from those that we are sensitive to, but by means of qualia that are quite familiar to us. Unlike the red-green reversed trichromats, this individual sees things that we do not: she can warn us of excessive ultraviolet radiation and the like, and on such occasions she might even say 'The light has an excessively bluish cast today.' Perhaps this is analogous to the case of dogs, who are auditorily sensitive to ultrasonic frequencies. The Dispositionalist makes this too into an error, for according to him, these are cases where blueness is attributed to something that is not blue (i.e. which does not cause experiences as of blue in normal observers), high C to something that is considerably higher in wavelength. Surely this is the wrong line to take. It is not a mistake to detect things that normal humans fail to detect, even if one's access to these things is through qualia that normal humans attach to something different. The person simply has a slightly different classificatory scheme: she carves the world up differently. There is no error in that.

2

Sensory Classification: The View from Psychology

We turn now to defending the Sensory Classification Thesis. The present chapter presents an overview of the scientific evidence. Here, I argue that this thesis accords better with current conceptions of sensory processing than the competing 'image' view, which takes sensory consciousness to be a passive record of energy patterns that are incident upon the outer sensory receptors (Prelude, section I).

I. Descartes and the Discovery of Transduction

Until the middle of the twentieth century, psychological and philosophical paradigms of sensory systems did not encourage the view that classification was, implicitly or explicitly, an activity that could be ascribed to these systems.

In ancient times, sensory awareness was thought to result from the direct transfer of a property from an external thing to the sensorium. Aristotle, for instance, proposed that perception consisted in receiving the perceptual forms of external things without their matter. The notion was that the receptive matter of the eye—the eye-jelly, according to Aristotle—literally takes on the colour (which is an example of a sensible form) of external objects without taking in the matter of these things. Thus, my seeing something, say a piece of paper, as blue results, according to Aristotle, from a two-part process that consists *first* in the 'form' of *blue* present in the paper travelling from the paper to my eye-jelly through the transparent air that intervenes, and *second* in its being transferred thence to the sensorium, i.e. to visual awareness. As a result of the first part of this process, Aristotle suggests, *the eye comes literally to resemble the object of perception,* to share a property with that object—initially, the paper was blue, and when I sense it, my eye-jelly becomes blue as well, even though the paper itself, the matter of the perceptible thing, remains outside my eye. (It is not entirely clear what 'literally being blue' amounts to as far as Aristotle is concerned: it could be that the eye-jelly does not *look* blue, even though it shares the property *blue* with the paper.) Since my epistemic access to the blueness in my eye—the result of the second part of the process—was thought to be direct and unproblematic, so also was my access to the colour of the object itself—they are one and the same thing. In this paradigm, the sensory organ and the sensorium contribute nothing by way of their own activity to the perceptual event. They are completely passive. Assuming that nothing goes wrong with the natural processes underlying perception something blue will naturally strike me as blue. Similarly, I perceive two things as possessing the same property because they *are* objectively similar: sharing the same perceptible form, they transfer the same effect to my sensorium. This is all that there is to it.

Descartes laid the foundation for what we may entitle the 'classic theory' of perception—the theory that held sway before the Sensory Classification Thesis—by criticizing Aristotle's direct-transference theory of sensory awareness. Right at the beginning of the posthumous treatise, *The World*, he writes:

The first point I want to draw to your attention is that there may be a difference between the sensation we have of light (i.e. the idea of light which is formed in our imagination by the mediation of our eyes) and what it is in the objects that produce this sensation within us (i.e. what it is in a flame or the sun that we call by the name 'light'). For although everyone is commonly convinced that the ideas we have in our mind are wholly similar to the objects from which they proceed, nevertheless I cannot see any reason which assures us that this is so. (AT XI, 3)

Descartes expresses himself cautiously on the question of resemblance of sensation and object: 'I cannot see any reason which assures us that this is so'; 'there *may* be a difference between the sensation we have of light' and that which 'produces this sensation within us'. Similarly, in the *Sixth Meditation*, he says: 'the bodies which are the source of these various sensory perceptions possess differences corresponding to them, though *perhaps* not resembling them.'

Descartes's empiricist successors were more strident in their way of putting this point. Berkeley points out that our 'idea' of *orange* is a *mental* particular. As such it *cannot* resemble or share any attribute of material things; it cannot have, in Hume's words, that kind of 'double existence' (*Treatise of Human Nature*, I, 42). Thus having a sensation of *orange* does not amount, as Aristotle thought, to possessing direct awareness of an intrinsic characteristic of an external thing. Our having this sensation is nothing more than our being, ourselves, in a sensory state with a certain characteristic. *Orange* is a characteristic of our sensation, a modification of our sensory consciousness— here Aristotle was correct, Descartes would have allowed—but not a characteristic of external things. All that we can infer about the external object of our senses is that it produces this kind of sensation in us. Descartes and Locke supposed that we call external objects 'orange' because they have the power to produce orange sensations in us, not because they possess the *same* feature as orange sensations. Note that the direction of the 'because' in this thesis is the opposite to that asserted by the Posteriority of Appearance Thesis (Chapter 1, section II.3).

Descartes's achievement, to put the matter in modern terms, was to realize that the image focused on the retina by the cornea and lens has to be *transduced* into a different form before it can function in the mind or, for that matter, in the brain. According to him, the retinal image, which is a pattern of light and colour, is translated into a 'movement of the brain, which is common to us and the brutes'. This movement of the brain is not a mental event; it is not accompanied by awareness or consciousness. In the 'brutes', the 'movement of the brain' accounts, by itself, for behaviour. But in humans, it results in a mental act that consists of the 'mere perception of the colour and light' (*Replies to the Sixth Set of Objections*, AT VII, 437). Each of these transductive transformations preserves the topography of the energy pattern incident upon the retina and mirrors the energy incident at each point in a new form: the visual consciousness that humans enjoy is, according to the Cartesian conception, an image of the image cast by the lens of the eye, a picture of a picture of the world.

Descartes thought that perceptions of light and colour are mental entities in a full and robust sense of the term. And he insists that when we view a stick, 'it should not be supposed that certain "intentional forms" fly off the stick towards the eye' (ibid). This implies that even at the stage of perceptions of light and colour, the mind and its innate ideas have already played a role. Nonetheless, the perceptions that are first occasioned by an external object do not represent three-dimensional material objects; they are merely perceptions of colour and light. Descartes thought that the sensory image was *raw*—in close correspondence with the physical image projected on the retina, and not yet sorted by the similarity and difference relations that create classes. Neither of these transformations—retinal image to movement of the brain, movement of the brain to perception—involves classification; the concreteness of the retinal image is preserved, albeit in different forms. Classification comes, in the case of humans, from the operations of the mind on these movements of the brain.

This turned out to be an influential idea. Traces of the Cartesian theory can be found in philosophies of very different motivation. It is present in Rudolf Carnap's (1928) idea that sensation is a temporal succession of momentary indivisible wholes, and that qualities such as *red* are not literally present as separable parts of sensation but abstracted from it by means of relations of similarity and indiscriminability which we impose on it. It is found also in the phenomenology of Edmund Husserl (1931/1913), who holds that sensation provides only the material (*hyle*) out of which the mind constructs descriptive forms (*noemata*). In both of these philosophical systems, sensation lacks all attributive significance. It has no semantic value; it is not true or false, correct or incorrect. It is rather the material from which the epistemic faculties draw classifications or beliefs; the latter have semantic value, but not sensation itself.

II. How Can Sensation Function without Classification?

According to Descartes, the proper function of sensation is to guide motivation.

> The proper purpose of the sensory perceptions given me by nature is simply to inform the mind of what is beneficial or harmful for the composite of which the mind is a part; and to this extent they are sufficiently clear and distinct. But I misuse them by treating them as reliable touchstones for immediate judgements about the essential nature of the bodies located outside us; yet this is an area where they provide only very obscure information. (*Sixth Meditation*, AT VII, 83)

Since sensation is, at best, a source of 'very obscure information', it cannot be used as a 'reliable touchstone for immediate judgements', at least not judgements about the intrinsic character of bodies in the external world. What then does it do? In animals, presumably, the output of sensory organs leads directly to behaviour. When a dog is in the presence of water, its eye sets up a movement of the brain that leads it to drink if it is thirsty. In humans, Descartes says, action is—or ought to be—initiated by the soul. But in making decisions concerning action, the soul is, or ought to be, aided by sense perception, which conveys information about what is beneficial and what is harmful. In humans, a movement of the brain analogous to that which occurs in the dog, leads, by a process implanted in us by God, to the perception of the water as beneficial (when we are thirsty), and this idea is 'sufficiently clear and distinct'. This is how perception figures in practical decision-making. Its use for other epistemic purposes is not well grounded, Descartes suggests.

This account of sensation suggests that I am not justified, on the basis of perception, to attribute thirst-quenching properties to bodies of water that may be present in the environment, if one conceives of such properties as belonging to the water independently of the existence of any organism. I am nevertheless able, on the basis of perception, to choose the beneficial action in these circumstances; I can even attribute to the water a relationally specified property, namely that it can quench my thirst and thus do me some good. However, this seems to imply, at the very least, that I am able to sort my perceptions into two kinds: those which indicate that it is beneficial for me to drink a particular body of water, and those that indicate that it is not. This in turn implies a classificatory capacity in sensation itself; for it divides things into two kinds, those that quench my thirst and those that do not. And since the dog too does the same thing, it too seems to possess a classificatory capacity, though in its case, the capacity is not guided by mental entities, i.e. conscious sensations. But this seems to contradict the thrust of the Cartesian conception of sensation, at least as it was understood by generations of empiricists. They seem to assume that sensation is nothing but an image, that it is not informed by any such classificatory structure as might differentiate beneficial-to-drink things from harmful-to-drink ones.

Here, then, is a problem for the classic theory. How can vision guide behaviour if it does not possess a classificatory capacity? Let's consider this question first in the domain of the brutes. According to Descartes, animals possess neither the powers of conceptualization nor the conscious states of awareness that lie within the proper domain of souls. How then are they to act in ways appropriate to circumstances—to drink water when they are thirsty, but not a liquid previously found to have been noxious? How do they manage the discrimination necessary for this task? Must this sameness of response not be based on classificatory activity?

W. V. O. Quine took this argument one step further. The argument just presented concentrates on bodily responses to situations. Let us consider another kind of response, namely learning. Animals learn on the basis of sensation to respond in a certain way to situations of a certain type: for example, when a substance of a certain sort once proves to be sick-making, they learn to avoid it. Learning too depends on classification, for the change in an animal's dispositions with respect to a particular substance presupposes a pre-existing capacity to differentiate that substance from others. Quine's important observation was that since learning presupposes classification in this way, at least some classifications must be innate.

There could be no induction, no habit formation, no conditioning, without prior dispositions on the subject's part to treat one stimulation as more nearly similar to a second than to a third. The subject's 'quality space', in this sense, can even be explored and plotted by behavioural tests in the differential conditioning and extinction of his responses. Also there are experimental ways of separating, to some degree, the innate features of his quality space from the acquired ones. (1969*b*, 306. Quality spaces are discussed in Part II.)

Quine's point is simple: animal and human conditioning and learning needs some innate jumping-off point if it is ever to get going—an innate classification scheme. According to Quine, the 'subject's "quality space" ', or 'similarity space' as we will call it in Part II, serves in this role. Innate pre-existing features of the similarity space anchor conditioning, Quine argues. (As we noted in Chapter 1, section I.6, sensory ordering is a more elaborate version of sensory classification.)

Some complications arise here. In insisting that sensory *similarity* is the innate basis for learning, rather than sense-features themselves, Quine is relying on a construction offered by Rudolf Carnap (1928), in which sense-features are reductively defined in terms of similarity. Quine says:

There is no reason to suppose that the stimulations for which the child thus learns his uniform verbal response were originally unified for him under any one idea, whatever that might mean. If the child is to be amenable to such training, however, what he must have is a prior tendency to weight qualitative differences unequally. He must, so to speak, sense more resemblance between some stimulations than between others. Otherwise a dozen reinforcements of his response 'Red', on occasions where red things were presented, would no more encourage the same response to a thirteenth red thing than to a blue one. (1959, 83)

In the absence of Carnap's construction of sense-features in terms of similarity, the sense-features themselves would have to be 'given': the child would have to sense blue things under one idea in order to be able to learn the meaning of a word like 'blue'.

That *blue* and the like are antecedently given seems, indeed, to be the position of empiricist philosophers like Berkeley, who says that ideas furnished by the senses 'come to be marked by one name, and so to be reputed as one *thing*' (*Principles of Human Knowledge* §1; the 'so' is inferential perhaps), and Hume, who believed that 'simple ideas' are a direct consequence of sensory experience ('impressions'): the simple ideas of distinct colours 'enter by the eyes', he says, and are derived from a simple impression, and exactly correspondent with it (*Treatise* I, 1, 1). Given Carnap's construction, Quine does not have to insist on *features* or *classes* being given as Berkeley and Hume do, but this is because an innate conception of similarity is doing the same work for him by constructing these. Quine's argument is, in short, that learning depends on the more general Sensory Ordering Thesis rather than on the Sensory Classification Thesis. But the difference between ordering and classification need not concern us here.

Quine's argument seems to lead Descartes into trouble. For if Descartes were to have acknowledged that learning to respond consistently to environmental objects implies an innate similarity space, then he would have had to accept that animal conditioning demonstrates that animal sensory systems would have to engage in what I have been calling 'classification'. And this would have implied in turn that human sensory systems, which operate in the same way as their animal counterparts, also perform classificatory functions, and deliver the results of this classification to consciousness. But this is precisely what Descartes denies—for him, sensory systems are devices for transduction only, while classification is a mental activity. He holds that there are innate ideas in the soul—the ideas of mathematics, the idea of God, and even certain ideas which operate on the raw sensory image, yielding the notion of material objects, for instance—but he does not allow that the senses are a source of any such ideas.

How then can Descartes account for the regularities and appropriateness of *animal* behaviour—keeping in mind that such behaviour is unmediated by ideas? Here is how. Very likely, he thought that animal behaviour depends on properties that the retinal image itself has as distinct from those that it, or some object in the world, is *represented as having*. Let's reconstruct his position. Animals react to 'brain movements' alone, and these brain movements result from the image on the retina. Let's suppose that in the retinal image, TL and BR are both a certain way—they are both green in this instance. This leads to certain brain movements, TL^* and BR^*, and each of these leads in turn to a certain behaviour. Since TL and BR are the same in some respect, TL^* and BR^* are also the same in some respect—when causes are similar, so also are the effects. So, further downstream, the behaviour to which each leads is the same. Similarities in the world, and derivatively in the image, account for the sameness of the animal's reaction, without the need for it, or its sensory system, to record or represent this sameness.

This suggests the condition under which the property of the retinal or visual image can bear the explanatory burden of responses dependent on that property:

> *Same-Cause, Same-Effect Principle
> There are similarities and dissimilarities present in the retinal images of various situations that are sufficient to account for similarities and dissimilarities in an organism's response to those situations

If this condition were satisfied, there would be no need to posit a state that *represents* the greenness of both TL and BR, or of the corresponding objects, or their sameness in colour. The similarity of TL and BR and of the internal states caused by these retinal spots would do the work. Probably, this is how Descartes envisaged animals getting by without sensory or mental classification.

Now, in the case of humans, Descartes held that TL^* and BR^* lead to further 'perceptions of light and colour'. Call these perceptions TL' and BR'. He maintains that insofar as we can be aware of such perceptions, or arrive at judgements on their basis, they must somehow be informed by ideas innate in the soul.

We judge that this or that idea which we now have immediately before our mind refers to a certain thing situated outside us. We make such a judgement not because these things transmit the ideas to our mind through the sense organs, but because they transmit something which, at exactly that moment, gives the mind occasion to form these ideas by means of the faculty innate to it. Nothing reaches our mind from external objects through the sense organs except certain corporeal motions . . . . But neither the motions themselves nor the figures arising from them are conceived by us exactly as they occur in the sense organs . . . . The ideas of pain, colours, sounds and the like must be all the more innate if, on the occasion of certain corporeal motions, our mind is to be capable of representing them to itself. (*Comments on a Certain Broadsheet*, AT VIIIB, 358–9)

The point is that *TL'* and *BR'* are occasions for the initiation of mental processes of representation, calculation, and inference, 'because they transmit something which, at exactly that moment, gives the mind occasion to form . . . ideas by means of the faculty innate to it'. *TL'* and *BR'* are different from the brain movements that led to them, because they are somehow infused, structured, and identified by ideas, as a consequence of which 'our mind is . . . capable of representing them to itself'. In an animal, the brain movements lead directly to behaviour, but in the case of humans they 'inform the mind of what is beneficial or harmful'. (See the quotation from the *Sixth Meditation* at the start of this section.) With such conceptually informed sensory information—*perception*, in short, since it tells us of external *things* and their features—humans are able to exercise the facility of reasoned action. This intrusion of mental representation notwithstanding, Descartes is committed to the idea that the identity and difference of judgements occasioned by sensation is fully explained by the Same-Cause, Same-Effect Principle. 'Every time this part of the brain (i.e. the pineal gland) is in a given state, it presents the same signals to the mind,' he says (*Sixth Meditation*, AT VII, 86).

Descartes ends up with a position which is, in certain respects, recapitulated by John McDowell (1994). Both he and McDowell think that the causal chain between the retina and human sensory experience passes through an intermediate stage that we share with the animals. Both suppose that this intermediate stage consists of physical events—'movements of the brain', as Descartes puts it: these correspond to 'feelings' in McDowell's scheme of things. Of course, there are differences between Descartes and McDowell that concern this intermediate realm. McDowell does not agree with Descartes that animals have no consciousness: he supposes that they have conscious 'feelings' which are the conceptually unarticulated counterparts of human 'experiences'. But now consider Descartes's thesis that sensory brain movements get transformed by the human soul into something more conceptual, and that this more conceptual notion of benefit or harm is capable of figuring in rational decision-making. McDowell makes a similar claim: his idea is that animal feelings become 'experiences' in humans because they are infused with concepts. The counterparts of animal brain movements in human souls are action-relevant according to Descartes, but in other ways they do not go beyond the retinal images: they are still 'perceptions of light and colour', and not much more. McDowell presumably allows for a greater degree of conceptualization. (We will return to a further consideration of McDowell's position in Chapter 3; its main thrust is anti-Cartesian.)

Descartes believes that the sensory process *preserves details* of the receptoral image, and that the soul, at least when playing it safe and sticking with clear and distinct ideas, inserts content only to the extent compatible with such preservation. Let's call this the *Principle of Passive Fidelity*. In the case of animals, similarities of response are going to be explained in terms of similarities in the images, or parts of images, that lead to these responses. To ensure the same degree of environmentally appropriate response in humans, the similarities and difference of these images have to be preserved downstream, through to their perceptual counterparts.

Passive Fidelity is a fragile basis on which to construct reliable behavioural responses to environmental contingencies. It is not designed for particular similarities; rather, it preserves all. But, as any camera or hi-fi enthusiast knows, this is an easily disrupted project. Information tends to decay as it is transmitted. The retinal image is already a distorted picture of the world: the imperfections of lenses and irregularities in the image plane create all sorts of aberrations. When this image is transduced into 'movements of the brain', further distortions will occur, and these will be magnified as they pass through long fibres; in addition, the nervous system's own activity will introduce 'noise' into the message.

A more reliable system would seek to enhance similarities that are relevant to its operations. More to the point, it will record these similarities explicitly— it will create an internal symbol scheme to record features of interest to itself, rather than leaving these features implicit in the transmitted record, where they can decay and become illegible. As we shall now see, this is precisely what sensory systems actually do.

III. Visual Processing

Passive Fidelity is insufficient to account for what sensory systems in fact do. Animal behaviour is not sufficiently explained by the action of concrete images acting individually or together, but—as we shall now explain and argue—the result of the system processing, detecting, and recording certain facts about an image.

In addition to the deficiencies of Passive Fidelity, Descartes's use of the Same-Cause, Same-Effect Principle is deficient because it overlooks the fact that all sorts of similarities can be found amongst and within retinal images, and not all of these can be linked up to similarities of subsequent behaviour. We shall see in a moment that sensory systems are so organized as to detect and record the presence of specific patterns in retinal images, and only the similarities so recorded end up influencing behaviour. The sensory system acts as a filter, so to speak, among the myriad retinal patterns and similarities. The Same-Cause, Same-Effect Principle fails as an explanation because it does not introduce this filtering as a separate term in the explanation of behaviour, extending as it does to any and every similarity. This deficiency is of more than trivial importance. We shall see that the patterns which the sensory system detects may be, as one might say, non-evident—the system has to extract these patterns from the outputs of retinal receptors; it is not simply reacting to these outputs. So the question of why the system reacts to some patterns and not to others has real bite. What is needed in the explanation of even simple reflex behaviour is explicit notice of the classificatory activity of sensory systems.

The fundamental point to be made here has to do with the neuronal organization of the retina. Descartes saw, and saw clearly, that the light that impacts the retina has to be transduced, i.e. changed in form, before it can make an impact on visual consciousness. Indeed, it has to be transduced twice in humans, according to his proposal—first, environmental energy patterns have to be translated into movements of the brain, and then these movements have to be translated into sensory 'ideas', or perceptions of light and colour. The first of these transductions occurs, as we now know, by the activity of neurons which emit electrochemical impulses when irradiated by light. What has become clear by means of recent investigation is that the neurons in the retina are organized in a way that Descartes did not know, and could not have known, given that he had neither the microscopes nor the knowledge of electricity needed to investigate these matters. This organization is clearly not designed for passivity, nor literally for fidelity either. It is organized for the detection of specific kinds of events.

When light falls on the retina, its *first* impact is on 'receptors', i.e. *rod* and *cone* cells. Such cells are sensitive to the quantity of light energy in selected spectral wavebands: they fire at a rate that is proportionate to the number of photons they absorb within these wavebands. Let us call the totality of rod and cone *outputs* the 'retinal array'. It could be argued that this array corresponds in a rough and ready way to Descartes's transduced image of light and colour. For the output of each such receptor cell is proportionate to the energy incident on it (i.e. light intensity) within a waveband of sensitivity (i.e. colour). This needs to be qualified.

> In the eye, the receptors do not faithfully record incident energy, but rather *sample* it: they are sensitive to specific portions of incident energy—particular wavebands, for instance—and this already implies that the image is *shaped* to a certain degree. Moreover, the output of each receptor cell is somewhat transformed by its own previous activity and by the simultaneous activity of other receptor cells. That is, (a) it becomes fatigued when subject to a strong stimulus for a long period of time, and thus ceases to react: this is known as 'adaptation'. And also (b) its activity is modulated by the activity of adjacent cells ('lateral inhibition'). Adaptation and lateral inhibition can be regarded as adjustments to the activity and output of each receptor cell because of spatially and temporally extended features of the energy pattern incident upon the entire

retina over a period of time. These adjustments play an important role in shaping visual processing, and ultimately visual consciousness.

The non-correspondence of receptor output and incident energy is even more evident in audition. The transduction of sound is effected by a complicated apparatus culminating in an organ known as the basilar membrane. This membrane is narrower and thicker at one end, and wider and thinner at the other. Because it is so constructed, sounds of different frequencies cause different parts of the basilar membrane to vibrate. The apparatus downstream of the basilar membrane transduces the vibration of the different parts of the membrane into signals transmitted to the auditory cortex by the auditory nerve. The basilar membrane is, in effect, a spectral analyser, delivering output that breaks a complex sound into its spectral components.

It is strictly speaking false that, even at the level of receptors, there exists a counterpart of Descartes's retinal image, a mere picture of the world. Let us, however, ignore this point for the moment. The important point that we must now note is that even if we generously grant that the retinal array is a point by point record of light and colour, this record is destroyed before it reaches visual consciousness, and much the same holds for audition. Descartes assumed, as did empiricist philosophers right down to the twentieth century, that the retinal array corresponds point by point to sensation. As we will now see, this assumption is false.

Immediately after the first impact of external energy patterns on retinal receptors, the information gathered by adjacent groups of rods and cones is transmitted to other neurons in another layer of the retina—a layer 'downstream' of the rods and cones in the 'data stream'. Let's call the group of cells from which a downstream neuron receives input its *receptive field*. To a first approximation (which will be amended shortly) the downstream cell is sensitive to a specific pattern of activity in its receptive field—this is experimentally determined by varying the stimulus and recording the activity of the cell.

For instance, one of these 'downstream' cells E might be activated by a sharp *change* of light intensity across its receptive field—an *edge* as such a pattern is called. E is silent when the light across its receptive field is uniform, whether that light be bright or dim. It will speak up—emit an electrochemical pulse different from its normal activity—when it detects an edge, regardless of whether the light level is bright on the left side of this edge and dim on the right, or bright on the right side and dim on the left, and regardless of the colour and exact position of the edge. All such individual differences of input are discarded, or suppressed, by the cell—that is, they make no difference to its activity. The cell's response is *not* proportionate to firing rate of the cells from which it receives input. In particular, its response is not proportionate to the energy incident upon the rods and cones in the retina. All that we can gather from its silence is that the light intensity changes smoothly across its receptive field; all that we can infer from its speaking up is that this field is divided by an illumination edge. The downstream cell is sensitive to a *type* of energy array; it does not record the details of a particular array.

We'll call a pattern that elicits a cell to respond in this way its 'response condition'. Thus:

> The *response condition* of a cell *C* is a proposition *p* such that *C* **normally** responds positively (i.e. evinces a firing rate higher than its resting state) when *p* is true within *C*'s receptive field.

The crucial point to note here is that the response condition of a cell does not simply record the *level* of activity in its receptive field. *p* may demand a very different kind of connection between receptors and responders than simple energy measurement. Nor does it simply reproduce some 'pictorial' aspect of the retinal image.

The theoretical framework within which we now understand this kind of activity was constructed in the 1940s by Warren McCulloch, Walter Pitts, Arthur Rosenblueth, Norbert Wiener, and Jerome Lettvin at the Massachusetts Institute of Technology, and by Donald Hebb and co-workers at McGill University.[1] This extraordinary group of scientists proposed that individual neurons are 'computing machines', and that these are organized into networks which analyse incident light energy in ways that amount to detecting the presence of particular patterns in that input. McCulloch and Pitts (1943) gave a general mathematical description of a neuron that could take various inputs, and deliver various different logical and mathematical functions of the component values as output. Hebb mathematically modelled how these outputs might be involved in learning and behavioural control. In the 1950s and 1960s, the organization of these functions in the visual system was mapped out by means of the emergent technology of single neuron recordings by such pioneers as Horace Barlow at Cambridge University and Stephen Kuffler, David Hubel, and Thorsten Wiesel at Harvard. The 1970s marked the emergence of a full-fledged computational theory of visual processing in the work of such pioneers as Marvin Minsky, Seymour Papert, and notably the young Cambridge (England) mathematician, David Marr, who had moved to MIT to work in Minsky and Papert's Artificial Intelligence lab. (Marr died at the tragically early age of 35, just before his brilliant work *Vision* [1982] was published.)

---

[1] For further information, a good starting point is Wilson and Keil (1999)—see the entries on Hebb, Marr, McCulloch, Pitts, Wiener, and the cross-references and bibliographies contained therein.

The picture that emerged from these and subsequent investigations is one of layered processing—a multiple iteration of the upstream-downstream layering described above—in which the outputs of each layer are fed to the next downstream layer and subjected to a new process of pattern–detection. Marr, in particular, insisted that these processes were most appropriately described in terms of transformations of mathematical propositions, rather than in physical or neurological terms. The paradigm of Passive Fidelity was shattered; the visual system now became known as a calculator.

With this historical information as background, let us now examine how this layered computational activity forces us to abandon the Passive Fidelity view of sensation introduced by Descartes. Consider a neuron that computes a *logical* function: it fires when the following response-condition is met, and is silent otherwise.

(G) There is a green spot in the top-left quadrant of the retinal array (*TL*) *or* in the bottom-right (*BR*).

The state of affairs to which this neuron responds is significantly different from the concrete images on which Descartes relied in his account—images like the retinal green spots which we discussed in the previous section. G's firing does not correspond point by point to the pattern to which it responds: it reports on a state of affairs, but does not depict it.

Here are some of the characteristics of G that lead us to the conclusion that it represents without depicting.

Non-concreteness. The condition *There is a green spot in TL* is already non-concrete and inclusive. It is satisfied by a variety of green spots, not just the concrete one that happens to be present, but also, for example, by a larger one, of a different shape, slightly displaced from it, but still in the top left quadrant. G will respond when any such spot is present.

Altered Topology. Moreover, G does not preserve retinal scale—the area of the retina it surveys is larger than the individual concrete images in virtue of which its response condition is satisfied—or topography—the shape of the area it surveys is different from these concrete images too.

Many-one mapping. G can be activated or deactivated by retinal images that are specifically different from one another. It is activated by *Green-spot-in-top left-and-no-green-in-bottom right, No-green-in-top-left-and-green-spot-in-bottom-right, Green-spot-in-top-left-and-Green-spot-in-bottom-right, Two-green-spots-in-top-left-and-no-green-in-bottom right*, . . . , etc., etc.

Loss of information. The precise condition of the retina is generally not recoverable from such states. When G fires, we can infer (with some degree of confidence) that there is at least one green spot on the retina; we have no idea how many, or of what size or shape or shade.

Abstractness. G is activated on occasion by two concrete green spots. It is activated on other occasions by a single green spot. So it would be wrong to subsume two instances of its firing to the Similar-Causes, Similar-Effect principle: from the point of view of *physical* variables and their numerical values, these causes are not similar.

Rather than transmitting pictorial records of retinal activity, the visual system actually does something much more like constructing a propositional record of retinal patterns. According to the 'computing machine' conception of neural functioning, neural networks can be so constructed as to respond to *any* logical and arithmetic transformation of rod and cone activation levels. The similarities preserved by such functions may not be *physically* relevant. Consider a neuron that fires when either the left portion of its field is much brighter than the right or when the right is much brighter than the left. This neuron's response-condition is a mathematical transform of physical quantities, but the range of physical conditions to which it responds is not united by physical similarity: the physically intermediate conditions of equal luminosity are excluded from this range (cf. Lewis 1999/1971, 161–3).

Classification is commonly defined as a process by which distinct entities are treated as equivalent. *Many-one mapping* and *loss of information* show that G responds equivalently to distinct entities. As Zenon Pylyshyn (1986, ch. 6) emphasizes, conditions like G gather physically disparate conditions into psychologically relevant equivalence classes: that is, G does not simply gather together physically similar conditions of the retina, but conditions that are equivalent in that they betoken a particular condition (of the retina, in this case) that happens to be relevant to the organism. *Non-concreteness* shows that the distinct entities to which it responds are patterns present in the retinal area that reports to it, i.e. its receptive field. *Abstractness* shows that this equivalency of response cannot be explained by Descartes's principle of Passive Fidelity: G is searching for a similarity that was not explicitly represented in earlier layers. In short, then, G is engaged in classificatory activity.

Let's call units like G *feature-detectors*. The layering of feature-detectors in the visual system is well illustrated by visual object recognition. Information flows from the retina to a number of discrete processing pathways, each consisting of layers of feature-detectors. Consider, for example, how we recognize the character 'A'. We encounter this character written in many fonts, in many hands. The shapes of these instances of 'A' differ substantially from one another. It is therefore clear that 'A' cannot be recognized by matching a given instance with a template: most instances of 'A' will be different from the template even when resized and rotated. The variation in the appearance of 'A's can, however, be reduced by parcelling it out to its various parts. An 'A' standardly consists of a right-sloping line intersecting at the top with a left-sloping line, with a bar joining them in the middle.[2] Considerable latitude is possible about how exactly these are made and joined together (Barlow 1999). Character recognition proceeds in two stages. The first identifies letter-parts. Character-part recognition occurs at a specific stage of visual process-ing. The output of this stage is a signal selectively sensitive to the presence of specific character-parts in specific orientations. (Presumably, the detection of character parts depends in turn on the detection of lines and their orienta-tions.) This output is received by a second stage, which assembles the charac-ters out of the character-parts. The signal that passes from the first to the second stage has lost its pictorial specificity. For instance, the signal that a horizontal bar is present has lost information about the thickness and colour of the bar. All that is important, from the system's point of view, is the same-ness of these bars in the relevant respect, the sameness that enables them to stand in for the horizontal bar of an 'A'. The process that recognizes the 'A' is insensitive to information about the orientation and thickness of its elements.

Single neuron recordings suggest that much of sensory processing occurs in a similar hierarchical fashion. In the visual system in particular, feature-detectors respond selectively when a certain pattern occurs in their receptive fields. Some retinal cells will respond when a movement in one direction occurs in its receptive field, others when a sharp change in illumination level (an edge) is present, and so on. The activity of such neurons is quite specific. Consider a neuron that fires when there is rightward movement in its field. We find that it will fire even when the luminance of the scene is increased or reduced, when the contrast of the moving thing is reversed from light against dark to dark against light, when the shape of the moving thing is changed, and so on. It is sensitive to *rightward movement*; its activity is invariant with, and gives us no information about, other characteristics of the image in which it detects such movement. Such neurons feed into another layer of processors, and cells in this layer will respond in turn to a specific pattern in *their* receptive fields. Each of these steps from layer to layer involves 'throwing away information': if I, II, and III are three stages of the process, the neurons in stage III have no access *through neurons in stage II* to the precise description of the activation-pattern of neurons in stage I. (They might have direct access to these activation-patterns, however, by means of a shunt from I to III.) Supposing that stage II neurons are sensitive to right-moving edges in their stage I recept-ive fields, and insensitive to luminance changes in stage I, stage III neurons will not have access *through stage II neurons* to luminance variations at stage I. (The italicized qualifications reiterate the point that information thrown away by a particular stage of visual processing may still be available elsewhere

---

[2] It is character recognition that is at issue here, not alphabetic letter-recognition. The cursive 𝔄 is presumably a different character, or visual shape, linked to the same letter by a separate convention.

in the system.) In traditional models of visual processing, the entire process was 'feed-forward' as described in this paragraph; recently, it has been increasingly more emphasized that the activity of upstream layers may be influenced by results of computation downstream by means of feed-back loops.

Horace Barlow (1972) describes the functioning of the retina this way:

[It] transmits a map not of light intensities at each point of the image, but of the trigger features in the world before the eye, and its main function is not to transduce different luminance levels into different impulse frequencies, but to continue responding invariantly to the same external patterns despite changes of average luminance. (373)

Barlow's statement directly contradicts the claim Descartes made more than 300 years earlier. The output of a neuron in the visual processing pathway indicates that its receptive field belongs (or fails to belong) to a certain class, the class of those that contain a certain retinal pattern, and suppresses additional information about its input. This discarding of information is characteristic of classification; a sensory feature-detector responds to the presence of a feature, but having responded to this feature, it does not store or pass on other information about receptive field.

There is a big difference between what feature-detectors do in Barlow's statement above, and what 'brain movements' do in Descartes's paradigm. In Descartes's paradigm (which was more or less universally accepted until roughly the middle of the twentieth century) brain movements reflect the continuous variation in the energy pattern that excite the outer sensory receptors. This is consistent with the idea that the retina transmits 'a map of light intensities at each point of the image' thrown by the lens. In this classic paradigm, the two retinal arrays are combined and passed on to later stages of visual processing: the consolidated binocular array forms the sensory core of visual consciousness. This was the conception of visual data-streams that led nineteenth-century physiologists to call the primary visual cortex a 'cortical retina'. In this paradigm articulated by Barlow, there is no such simple correspondence between the value of a physical variable like light intensity and the activity of neurons beyond the rods and cones. Rather, each neuron in a visual data-stream 'respond[s] invariantly' to the presence of a certain pattern or feature in its receptive field. This is a bit exaggerated, as we shall see in a moment. Not all neurons downstream of the retina are feature-detectors in exactly the sense here delineated. Nevertheless, the idea of feature-detectors is extremely important, and deserves further exploration.

Think of a lookout who is supposed to shout 'Ship ahoy!' when he sees a ship, but cannot be queried about the size, direction, and type of ship that elicited his call. This observer's message simply sorts observed situations into two kinds, those in which ships are present and those in which they are absent. The lookout is assigning a Boolean value to the proposition 'A ship is in visual range': True when he shouts 'Ship ahoy!', False when he is silent. He discards all information redundant to this assignment. The captain is not loaded up with information about the colour of the sky or sea, or about the miserable condition of the man in the crow's nest. *To a first approximation*, we can think of feature-detectors similarly as assigning a Boolean-value to their response condition: True when they fire or come on, False when they are silent or go off. They discard information redundant to the assignment of this value, and thus they are able to reduce the amount of information flowing from the retina. Since information is progressively thrown away, 'channel capacity' gets smaller as visual information gets more processed. The computational model of visual processing assumes that the whole layered organization of feature-detectors constitutes a system of inference in which response conditions represented by information-heavy units in earlier layers of the process provide 'premises' for, and get replaced by, information-light 'conclusions' drawn by fixed 'rules of inference'—these premises and rules of inference can also be modified by feed-back ('re-entrant') fibres. Since these response conditions are *propositions*, visual processing can be functionally represented by propositional attitudes, and their transformation by inferential patterns (cf. Pylyshyn 1986, ch. 6; Matthen 1988).

Now, the truth is actually a good deal more complicated than this. (A reader not interested in complications can skip ahead to the next section at this point.) For as Barlow goes on to acknowledge, feature-detecting neurons have varying rates of firing: they are not On-Off units. Thus, one cannot say simply that they assign Boolean values to their response conditions. What then do the different values of these neurons say about their response conditions? Before dealing directly with this question, let us note first that variable firing rates are *not* a good reason to revert to the idea that neurons in the visual process simply encode the energy levels incident upon the retina. That is, they are not a good reason to revert to the 'image' paradigm of visual sensation. For as Davida Teller (2002/1984, 310) points out, 'the set of stimuli that makes any appreciable response in the cell is small and homogeneous', and this is especially true with respect to cells that correlate with events in sensory consciousness. Thus, it is a fundamental constraint on interpreting variable firing rates of neurons that contribute to sensory consciousness, that their silence does not correspond to zero energy levels at the corresponding point of the outer sensory receptors. Rather, we must interpret their silence in much the same way as before, namely as assigning the value False to some proposition.

Very well: with this understood, let us suppose that a particular neuron responds to a horizontal bar in its receptive field. Silence indicates that no horizontal bar is present. But what does a fast-firing rate indicate by contrast with a slow-firing rate? Barlow's own answer is to suggest that the faster a neuron fires, the stronger is its 'confidence level' with regard to the response condition: 'The frequency of neural impulses codes subjective certainty,' he says in this 'Fifth Dogma' (1972, 381). This suggests that these neurons assign a Bayesian value (i.e. a 'subjective probability') to a proposition, rather than Boolean value (True/False). This, of course, implies that each data-processing neuron is many-valued, or even continuous in value, and not bivalent, as we have been suggesting. Nevertheless, this value is attributed to a proposition, or 'event', that consists of a feature attributed to a material object (see Chapter 12).

Now it may well be that this is an adequate conception for cells that detect discrete conditions such as the presence of a horizontal bar. But what about a colour-detecting cell that responds most strongly to a particular wavelength, λ, and less strongly to neighbouring wavelengths? (This is an oversimplified example, since colour-detecting cells are not tuned to wavelengths as such—see Chapter 6, section I—but let this go for the moment.) One *could* say that the response condition of this cell is simply the presence of light of wavelength λ, and that weaker values indicate a lack of confidence occasioned by the small discrepancy between the response condition and the actual state of affairs. But it would be equally natural to say that the cell in question was *measuring* the wavelength of light within a certain interval. (Here, I am indebted to David Hilbert.) The question is: why should we insist on the response-condition/feature-detector way of looking at sensory neurons at the expense of the measuring instrument model of at least some neurons? Should we not, at least in the case of neurons such as those that measure colour or brightness (etc.), restrict the domain of the idea that 'a neuron's role in the neural code is to signal the presence of the stimulus which makes that neuron respond most vigorously'? (cf. Teller 2002/1984, 308–11).

It is not important that we should settle this issue here. What is more important is that we should note that even if we admit the measurement conception of sensory neuron activity—a conception that is quite at home in the context of the Sensory Ordering Thesis offered in Part II—we should recognize that this non-propositional attitude should not lead us back to the 'image' conception of sensory consciousness. And here, it is crucial that the following propositions should be clearly recognized.

1. The silence of a sensory neuron that contributes to sensory consciousness does not correspond to a zero-energy state of the receptors; rather, it corresponds to the absence of a 'small and homogeneous' set of conditions, and as such, silence is its normal condition.

2. The quantity measured by a non-propositional neuron will not correspond to the state of a receptor neuron such as a rod or cone cell. Rather it represents a quantity that has been computed by comparing the outputs of several different receptors, a quantity that is specifically of utility in the guidance of the organism's innate activities, and thus not a passive record of the environment's impact on the receptors.

With these provisos, we will now put the question of measurement to one side, and continue as if all neurons that contribute to sensory consciousness are feature-detectors. For a more detailed treatment of non-Boolean sensory concepts, see Chapter 3, section IV and Part II.

IV. Feature Maps and Feature Integration

The feature-detection conception of the outputs of sensory processing requires a major revision to the way that Cartesians conceive of sensation. In the early part of visual processing, sensory processing produces maps of features which retain the spatial layout of the retina.[3] For example, colour is represented by a map in which the various colour spots present on the retina are represented in map-like correspondence: if the retina contains a red spot in the top-left quadrant, then the brain's colour map will contain a representation of red in its top-left quadrant. So the classic paradigm is correct in the supposition that a map of the retinal image is conveyed to the brain. It must be emphasized, however, that what we find in these maps is symbols not pictures. Suppose that there is a horizontal bar in the retinal image. It is easy to fall into the mistake of thinking that in the map of line-orientations, we will find something like this—an image, in short—in the corresponding location:

========================

Not so. What we actually find is a horizontal array of neurons, each responding to the presence of a horizontal edge in its receptive field, and silent when there is no such edge. Representing the on-state of each of these by an 'H' and the off-state by '0'—recall that we are treating these as Boolean-valued symbols—what we find is something more like:

0	0	0	0	0	0	0	0	0	0	0	0	0	0	0	0	0	0	0	0	0	0	0	0	0	0	0	0	0	0	0	0	0
0	0	0	0	H	H	H	H	H	H	H	H	H	H	H	H	H	H	H	H	H	H	H	H	H	H	H	H	H	0	0	0	0
0	0	0	0	0	0	0	0	0	0	0	0	0	0	0	0	0	0	0	0	0	0	0	0	0	0	0	0	0	0	0	0	0

where the zeros at each end of the row of H's indicate H-cells that are silent.

---

[3] The retinotopic organization of feature maps starts to disappear in stages of processing downstream of the primary visual cortex, where it is increasingly replaced by maps of real three-dimensional space.

Another example: consider a cross on the retina. Neglecting the zeros, and letting 'V' stand for a vertical line-element, this will be represented in the map of line-orientations as follows:

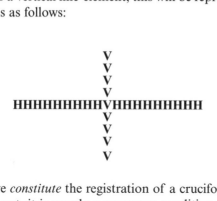

Nor does the above *constitute* the registration of a cruciform pattern. As we shall see in a moment, it is merely a necessary condition for such a pattern being registered.

The point being made here may remind some readers of a point made by Daniel Dennett (1991, 347–52). Dennett is discussing the internal storage of images in digital computers. He points out that these computers operate on strings of 0s and 1s. Consequently, an image (taken from a camera, for instance) must be converted into 0s and 1s before it can be stored in a digital computer. The brain for its part is a computer that operates on strings of neural activation levels. So the retinal image must be stored in the form of neural activation levels. This is an important and insightful point, but different from the one being made above. Dennett is emphasizing that the retinal image can be reproduced in digital form. Dennett's point is about transduction: the retinal image has to be recoded in digital form in order to be stored inside a digital computer. The point being made here—the point of the Sensory Classification Thesis—is that what is sent downstream from the retina is *not* the retinal image, however coded, but a record of various features present there. This has to do with classification, not merely transduction. As the discussion of condition G in section III shows, classification does a lot more than simply change the form in which the retinal image is stored. In Dennett's form of storage, two green spots would be stored as two green spots, though the record would use digital symbols for green (for example, 'g'), rather than green pixels, as on a video display, and might also be digitally compressed, so that three green pixels in a row might be represented as 3g (instead of ggg). The G-neuron, on the other hand, detects a feature which occurs discontinuously across the whole retina, and throws away retinal topography in the process.

Let us return now to sense-feature maps. The map for colour is separate from the one discussed above, namely the map of line-elements. Suppose that the bar we have been speaking of is red. Phenomenology might lead us to expect, naïvely, that we would find a red line in some map created by the visual system, or, less naïvely, that the Hs above would somehow be tagged as red. Not so. The redness (R) of the bar would be represented not in the map of shapes, but in a *separate* map of colours. Thus there would be an entry in the separate colour map that looked like this:

RRRRRRRRRRRRRRRRRRRR

How is it then that the horizontal bar is seen as red? In order for this to be the case, the Rs in the colour-map have to 'bound' to, or integrated with, the Hs in the line-orientation map.

The empiricists, for example Hume, thought that this string of red-representations *is* the bar that we see: this is the content of Hume's claim 'If we see it, it is a colour'; this claim is vividly captured in David Lewis's (1999/1966) term 'colour mosaic'. But modern studies show that Hume was wrong about this. There are two empirical reasons for rejecting Hume's theory. The first is that when, for any reason, the conscious effect of the string of Hs is blocked, we still consciously detect red in the specified area, but do not see it as a bar. Similarly, when the Rs are disrupted, we are still visually aware that a bar is present, though not that a red one is. The second reason for rejecting the colour mosaic theory is that in situations in which observers are attending to some other part of the scene, they sometimes report that the red is conjoined to some other shape. Both these experimental determinations show that our conscious visual representation of the red is separate, at some level, from that of the bar. As we shall see, it is only when we pay attention to particular locations in the visual field that these features get bound together.

Feature binding is necessary for a surprisingly large number of different operations of the visual system. For instance, let us return to our example above of the Hs and Vs created in a map of line-orientations by a cruciform image focused on the retina. The array presented above does not sufficiently account for our conscious awareness of a cross. The line orientation map is dedicated to detecting the *directions* of lines, not shapes. It registers the occurrence of several conjoined vertical and horizontal line elements. Together these elements constitute a cross, but it is one thing for such a pattern to be present in an array, and quite another thing for it to be recognized as such (cf. Dretske 1981, 144). It takes a different operation to determine that together these constitute a cross, and a different map to register this fact. This map might look like this:

CROSS

There has to be a further feature detector that responds to the presence of this particular pattern.

This is an extremely important point for the argument of this book. To detect a cross in the retinal array requires a special feature-detector. Such a feature-detector will occur in a biological organism only if it emerges during the course of evolution. So it is entirely possible that some organisms will have cross-detectors, while others lack them. This is the simple reason why different organisms may see different things: they may have different feature-detectors.

Another point to appreciate is that not all of the feature maps present in the visual system have the same resolution. For example, the colour map may well have a coarser grain than the shape map, and have gaps in it. So the red bar discussed above might actually look more like this:

$$\textbf{R} \quad \textbf{R} \quad \textbf{R} \quad \textbf{R} \quad \textbf{R}$$

There is no obvious way that these representations of red can be exactly and precisely equivalent to the finer-grained representations of the continuous horizontal edge. How, then, do we see the horizontal bar as red? This shows that the binding of Hs and Rs alluded to above is not a trivial overlay operation: the visual system has to guess at boundaries and fill them in in order to provide consciousness with a smooth picture. Thus, binding is somewhat like a conjunction of symbols—H at location l, and R at some cruder location in the vicinity of l. Moreover, binding is active: its contours and boundaries are determined by data-processing, not just retinal topography.

V. Classification and Realism

One important lesson to be taken from the present discussion is that at each stage of the visual process, the results of classificatory activity up to that point are recorded as a state of one or more neurons constituting that layer. The input to these neurons is a pattern in their receptive fields. This input is transformed by the activity of the neurons, and the output is a Boolean value (True or False) attached to a propositional function characteristic of that neuron (its response condition), or a Bayesian value (a confidence level between zero and one) attached to a set of propositions, or a numerical value attached to some variable. The model of layered, sequential processing does not, perhaps, generalize smoothly to all other modalities. What does seem clear, however, is that whenever we have a unified experience of a sensory feature that we are *innately* able to generalize over, that feature is discretely represented somewhere in the system.

For example, the loudness of sounds has a characteristic phenomenology, and animals are able to learn that certain events occasion loud noises. This is an indication that loudness is separately represented somewhere in the auditory system, independently of pitch and timbre. On the other hand, many musical sounds contain an overtone of C ♮. This can be recognized by a suitably trained and sensitive ear, but there is probably no one experience that attaches to all such sounds, and it is improbable that one could condition animals or humans to respond to this feature in a consistent way. Again, many verbal messages contain a threat. There need be no unified *auditory* experience attached to these messages, a sign that they too do not activate some discrete sensory symbol. The latter features are not explicitly processed by the auditory system, though they may fall out of processing for other characteristics. Dretske (1981, 151) reports a similar phenomenon: monkeys can be trained to respond to the larger of two rectangles, but not to the intermediate-sized one of three. Yet the information corresponding to both of these conditions is present in the visual array. The difference between the two conditions is that one is discretely represented by the monkey's visual system and thus available as a key for conditioning, and the other is not.

What are the classes that visual processing yields? Some feature-detectors respond to retinal occurrences, regardless of whether they are caused by distal objects or not. For example, a colour-sensitive retinal receptor might respond to there being more red than blue in its field: it would make no difference whether this condition traces back to oddities in the illumination, or to stable features in the distant object projected onto this retinal area. But even as early in visual processing as the retina, certain neurons respond only to distal occurrences. For example, there are retinal cells that respond to motion in the receptive field centre, but only if the wider surround moves with a different trajectory, a condition normally met only when the movement in the receptive field centre is distal (Ölveczky et al. 2003). Later in the process, as more refined processing takes place and as information from other sense-modalities get incorporated into the message, we find that neurons respond to events and states of affairs in the distal environment. For instance, comparison of retinal colours across the whole array might reveal that though a particular spot is reddish, it is less red than the average for the whole array: this might lead to a discounting of the reddish appearance.[4] Or propriocentric information about body movements might be used to arrive at ever more refined and reliable separations of moving patterns due to the body's own movement from those due to external movement. As a result of processes like these, a particular object might appear white, even though it is sending a reddish message to the eye; it might appear stationary though its image jiggles across the retina.

The result of such computational processes is that in many cases the simplest way of defining the response conditions of some feature-detectors is

---

[4] These are examples only. It is not entirely clear where the transition from retinal feature classification to distal feature classification occurs, and the suggestion is not intended that all such transitions occur deep into the visual process.

in terms of distal conditions. In other words, it is natural and reasonable to say that some feature-detectors are responding to distal objects and events. (This is not to imply that there is any simple way of identifying exactly which features of the distal environment sensory experience tells us about.) The response conditions of (at least some of) these neurons can be specified in two different ways. They can, of course, be specified as some kind of condition that holds of the retinal image; after all, that is where they come from in the end. But they can also be specified in terms of a distal condition. These two specifications are not exactly, but only approximately, coextensive. To the degree that they are coextensive, they explain why the organism is successful in navigating the external world.

These observations lead us to the realism question concerning sense-features. Do these features correspond to physical characteristics of the external things that we sense? What is the commonality that the visual system latches on to when it informs us that two things are blue? Is there a distal feature that this message indicates? We will go into this question in more detail in later chapters; it was parenthetically conceded in the preceding paragraph that there is no simple or authoritative way to capture the distal response condition. The point that needs to be emphasized *here* is that visual processing cannot be analysed solely in terms of external significance. When I see something as blue, I may conclude, as Descartes recommended, that *there is something in the object, whatever it may turn out to be, which produces in me the sensation as of a blue thing.* But this detour through an object's power to produce sensations in me, while commendable as a counter to Aristotle's direct-transmission theory, is incomplete. A more complete statement would take account of the activity of the sensory system itself as an indispensable term in the explanation. To amend Descartes: there is something in the object, whatever it may turn out to be, *which my visual system classifies together with other things that look blue (and which for this reason produces in me the sensation as of a blue thing).*

Some realists reject the need for such an addition. My visual system classifies things as yellow because they are yellow, they insist. We gain nothing of significance by mentioning intervening stages between external object and internal representation. From the opposite viewpoint, phenomenalists, who insist on the priority of sensory experience over physical properties, and Dispositionalists, who hold that external qualities are defined in terms of the sensory experiences they produce in normal observers, might also suspect that this addition has no effect: they hold that things are yellow because they appear so, or because they appear so in 'normal' or 'ideal' circumstances. According to them, the *appearance* of similarity screens off and renders irrelevant the explanatory value of the real quality. Both parties have made a decision on the significance of the presentation, and so they feel entitled to eliminate all reference to the activity of the system that delivers the presentation of things as yellow.

These shortcuts are misleading. Whether or not we adopt a realist attitude towards colour and other sensory properties—and in Chapter 8, a certain form of realism will be recommended—the contribution of the visual system is not a constant that can simply be 'crossed out' or normalized away. For even if objects are yellow in virtue of their power to produce in us a sensation as of yellow, that sensation is, nevertheless, the product of the visual system treating such objects as belonging to a certain class. Discounting the activity of the visual system assumes, wrongly, that it either receives causal input from objects and passes it down to the sensorium with minimal distortion, much as a fine camera would, or that its activity is confined to reconstructing external reality from the impoverished projection found on the retina. But sensory systems are not faithful recorders of the retinal array. Nor are they like forensic historians ferreting out the objective truth, scrupulously avoiding all intrusions of subjective interest. As Kathleen Akins (1996) argues, they assess environmental events from a self-interested point of view: if a sensory system co-classifies two things, it is because these two things are comparable from the point of view of the organism they serve, not because anything else would so regard them, much less because *nature* would so regard them, whatever this might mean.

3

Sensory Concepts

We argued in Chapter 2 that visual sensation does not merely reproduce the retinal image; it is not anything like a picture of a picture of the world. Rather, it is the result of the visual system's extracting and representing relevant information from the retinal array and discarding what the organism does not need. The present chapter is devoted to a discussion of three philosophical positions—those of Fred Dretske, Gareth Evans, and Richard Heck—that seem to undercut the idea that sensory systems have a classificatory function. All rely, as we shall see, on powerful versions of the Cartesian intuition that the sensory image is raw and unprocessed, and that we as epistemic agents extract concepts from it. The aim is to diagnose these intuitions, and to work towards a positive account that corrects or replaces them.

I. Analogue vs. Digital

Fred Dretske (1981, ch. 6) famously holds that sensation is analogue in its representational form (cf. Peacocke 1989), while judgements and beliefs are digital. From this, he concludes that sensation is unprocessed, in a manner which contradicts the Sensory Classification Thesis. We will therefore need to examine and rebut the argument. In preparation for this, we now embark on an explanation in intuitive terms of the various terms— 'sensation', 'perception', 'digital', 'analogue'—used in the debate.

Traditionally, the term 'sensation' refers to conscious sensory experience, which is supposed to consist of a succession of concrete holistic images, in which there is no immediate awareness of distinct objects, or of such classificatory categories as *red* or *green*. Sensation might thus correspond to the feature mosaics of traditional sense-datum theory, or to what Roderick Firth (1949/50) calls the 'sensory core' of perceptual states (though he himself doubts that there is such a thing). It is something like a TV screen viewed very close up, which occupies your entire visual field: colour spots in every visual location, but no discernible contours, objects, or features (other than particular colour shades). 'Sensation' thus understood is usually contrasted with 'perception'. The latter traditionally denotes a cognitive state that is the product of organizing, segmenting, and classifying sensory images, thereby yielding awareness of objects and the qualities they possess, at least to the point where one is able to make classificatory judgements like 'That thing is red'. More recently, the contrast between sensation and perception has been drawn in a slightly different way, namely to differentiate relatively unprocessed sensory states, which reflect states of the sensory receptors, and more processed states, which reflect distal conditions. In vision, for example, a state that retains retinotopic spatial relations might be classified as sensation, while one that presents the world in three-dimensional real space might be classified as perception. In either case, sensation is thought of as less processed, perception as more. (Dretske does not use the term 'perception' in exactly this way, i.e. to denote more processed states, he contrasts sensation with *perceptual belief*, but this does not matter for present purposes, since his distinction between sensation and perceptual belief corresponds reasonably closely to the traditional one between sensation and perception.)

What does Dretske mean when he says that sensation is *analogue*? Usually, when people talk about 'analogue' and 'digital', they are talking about the medium in which something is represented—the language or 'notational scheme' (as Nelson Goodman 1976 calls it). In an analogue medium, the representational units or 'characters' (Goodman's term again) are continuously ordered.[1] For example, an analogue instrument such as a thermometer uses points on a dial as characters: when the pointer is at any one of these continuously ordered positions, the instrument is in a representational state distinct from those constituted by its being at neighbouring points. With respect to sensory experience, *qualia* are the 'characters' in question. As we shall see, these characters are indeed analogue, or at least approximately so. When I enjoy the experience as of a blue thing, I am in a sensory state that is barely distinguishable from that of experiencing a closely similar but distinct shade of blue, but easily distinguishable from experiences as of most shades of green, and utterly different from experiences as of yellow. In this way, sensory qualia are structured much like pointer positions. Thus, they form a notational scheme that is, roughly speaking, analogue in Goodman's sense. If one understands 'analogue' in this way, one would gather that Dretske means to draw attention to the quasi-continuous ordering of sense-features.

This, however, does *not* go to the heart of the thesis that Dretske means to argue for when he says that sensation is analogue. For he defines the terms 'digital' and 'analogue' in a way that is not obviously connected to continuous ordering.

A signal carries the information that s is F in *digital* form if and only if it contains no information about s other than that which is nested in s being F.

---

[1] Goodman's condition calls for dense, not continuous, ordering, but this is unimportant here. See section IV below.

A signal carries the information that *s* is *F* in *analogue* form if and only if it carries additional information about *s* that is not nested in *s* being *F*. (ibid., 137, paraphrased).

Suppose that I say:

(1) There is a capital 'A' written on the blackboard.

By uttering (1), I do not say anything about the font, colour, size, and so on, of the character written on the blackboard. True, if you get my message over the telephone, you can deduce from (1) something that I did not explicitly say: that is, you can deduce (ignoring cursive script) that there is a horizontal bar on the blackboard. But this information is 'nested' in the definition of capital 'A'; it is part of what a capital 'A' is: this is what enables you to deduce it from my message. My message gives you no information about the character on the blackboard other than that which is strictly implied by its being a capital 'A'. Thus, by the above definition, (1) conveys its message in digital form.

Dretske is concerned with two things here. They are, first, the *information* carried by a signal, i.e. what one can infer about the source of the signal from characteristics of the signal itself, and, second, the *usability* of this information. His insight is that in order to *use* the information present in a signal, a perceiver has to *extract* bits of data from it by analysing its properties. When such information is extracted it is separated out from other information present in a signal. Extracted information is in digital form, according to Dretske—how this connects to Goodman's sense of the term is something we'll worry about in a moment. This is why a digitized message contains no other information.

The following example illustrates the distinction and the concern about usability.

[Consider] a young child, one whose receptor systems are fully matured and in normal working order, learning to recognize and identify [daffodils] . . . Given the child's keen eyesight, she may already (before learning) be receiving more information from daffodils than her more experienced, but nearsighted, teacher. Still, the teacher *knows* that the flower is a daffodil and the child does not. . . . What the pupil needs is not more information . . . . The requisite information . . . is getting in. What is lacking is an ability to extract this information, and ability to decode or interpret the sensory messages . . . Until this information (viz. that they are daffodils) is recoded in digital form, the child *sees* daffodils, but neither knows nor believes that they are daffodils. (ibid., 144)

When the information about the daffodil is extracted from the sensory message, it is encoded in an explicit way: 'Daffodil there'. When it is encoded in this way, it is not mixed together with non-nested information about the particular daffodil that is in view.

Dretske's model of data-extraction is congruent with our discussion of sensory classification in Chapters 1 and 2. Oversimplifying greatly, the essential idea is that in order to use the information carried by a signal, you have to develop a procedure that will allow you to answer a yes-no question about its source. For instance, consider the question, 'Is there anything in the vicinity that is going to collide with me unless I change course?' Data-extraction consists of a procedure capable of querying each of the vast variety of visual images, and getting a 'yes' or 'no' from every one. An *unprocessed* visual signal is an analogue mess: it contains the answer to this question and lots of irrelevant information besides, but none of this information is available to be used. The processed signal, on the other hand, contains the answer to the above question, and nothing else. The processed signal is clean, distinct, and legible; its representational scheme consists of just two values, 'Collision impending' and 'Collision not impending'. This gives us the connection with Goodman: since the state corresponding to 'Collision impending' is not one of a continuously ordered series of states, it is in digital form by his definition; on the other hand, the unprocessed signal is analogue because it is subject to continuous variation. In any event, the essence of digitization, according to Dretske, is that all information other than that which is being used is discarded.

Now, Dretske's definition of 'digital' is not absolute; it is relativized to a particular message. So when he says that some message is in digital form, one should not conclude that it carries only a small amount of information, compared to an analogue signal. Thus, one cannot say *tout court* that a picture, for instance, is analogue because of the great quantity of information it carries: one has to say of some message *m*—for example, the message contained in (1)—that the picture carries *m* in analogue form. Dretske acknowledges that if *p* is a proposition that expresses *all* the information contained in a picture, then the picture carries the information given by *p in digital form*. Consider the sentence:

(2) There is an exact copy of the Mona Lisa on the easel.

Or imagine a pattern recognition system that sounds a bell when and only when an exact copy of the Mona Lisa is exhibited. The sentence (2), the sound of the bell, and the Mona Lisa itself carry the same information, all in digital form (ibid., 138). Thus, Dretske's point is *not* that sensation is pictorial, hence analogue, perceptual belief propositional, hence digital.

This leads us to a problem. The distinction between *digital* and *analogue* is relative to a message, but Dretske's thesis about *sensation* is not: he does not say that sensation is analogue relative to this or that message, but that it is analogue period. It does not seem as if his thesis is about the *information* carried by sensation. It is not true, for instance, that the sensation contains *no* information in digital form. For consider the proposition *I* that is *equivalent* to the sum of all the information contained by a sensation. The sensation carries the information that I and no further non-nested information. Thus, it carries the information that I in digital form.

It seems clear therefore that Dretske must have intended to make a point about *extracted* information. His point must have been that, considered on its own, sensation contains *no* extracted information.

Our perceptual experience (what we ordinarily refer to as the look, sound, and feel of things) is being identified with an information-carrying structure—a structure in which information about a source is coded in analog form and made available to something like a digital converter ... until information has been *extracted from* this sensory structure (digitalization), nothing corresponding to recognition, classification, identification, or judgment has occurred. (ibid., 153)

Dretske is here implying that sensation (which in the above quotation is referred to as 'perceptual experience') does not answer any yes-no questions; it does not divide the world into two sorts of occurrence, one of which it certifies as true: in a word, it does not contain or convey the results of classification. Thus, while the 'A' I visually sense *is* of a certain font, colour, size, etc., and though my sensation contains this information, Dretske holds that having the sensation does not suffice for me to know this—that is, the sensation does not present it as such, or as possessing any other characteristic for that matter. There is, as we have argued, a proposition I that expresses all the information carried by a sensation, but this proposition is not available to us simply in virtue of experiencing the sensation. I have to *extract* information from the sensation before I can use it. All such information-extraction results from post-sensory perceptual processing. 'Seeing, hearing, and smelling are different ways we have of getting information ... to a digital-conversion unit whose purpose is to extract pertinent information from the sensory representation for purposes of modifying output' (ibid., 143).

In short, Dretske is really telling us that sensation carries information, but not information that has been chiselled into a determinate message. The essential point he wants to convey is this: one may sense something without being able to articulate any coherent description of that thing. Put in a form that extends to non-linguistic animals, his point would be this: one can sense a thing of a certain kind without thereby finding oneself in any determinate dispositional state with regard to responding to things of that kind (ibid., 151–2). For example, it may be that whenever a certain animal sees a daffodil, it eats it. But if it has not recognized something as a daffodil, then it won't do this—even though it may well be the case that it has *seen* it. Sensation is totally inarticulate in this sense: it is not sufficient for the mobilization of *any* response that has a consistent basis.

As observed before, Dretske's characterization of the digital conforms closely to the conception of a classificatory state in Chapter 2, section III: a proposition like (1) is non-concrete, and stands to retinal input in a one–many relation. It sorts the input array into types, signals when a particular type of array is present, and throws away all the more specific retinal information that relates to differences among the individual instances that fall under the type—it treats distinct things as equivalent. As Dretske says:

Until information has been lost, or discarded, an information-processing system has failed to treat *different* things as essentially the *same*. It has failed to classify or categorize, failed to generalize, failed to 'recognize' the input as being an instance (token) of a more general type. (ibid., 141)

Consider a number of different occasions on which I might issue the utterance (1). On each occasion, my visual image is of a multi-coloured field. In that coloured field, I discern a certain pattern. The patterns I see vary with respect to font, colour, size, etc. Suppressing these individualities—not merely 'losing' them inadvertently because the message has been degraded, but purposely discarding them for purposes of classification—I simply convey the information that the character is an 'A'. In this way, I divide all visual patterns into two kinds—those that conform to (1) and those that do not. The representational vehicle that conveys the information, in this case (1), is Boolean-valued—*true* if the visual pattern is indeed of the requisite type, *false* if it is not. (The state could also, as noted earlier, divide visual patterns into two kinds and express some level of confidence that the present state falls into a particular one of these kinds.) This is why my uttering (1) contains no information about the character other than that which is nested in its being a capital 'A'—all such information marks irrelevant differences amongst visual images in which a capital 'A' is present. Classificatory states are similar in this respect—they too throw away irrelevant detail—and so they are digital in the sense defined by Dretske.

Dretske's insistence that sensation is analogue seems to be based on a remnant of the Cartesian notion of sensory concreteness, the idea that the visual image is unclassified, a raw image that results from just (a) a map of light intensities created by the laws of optics, and (b) a transduction of this projection into neural forms (cf. 'movements of the brain') by biochemical laws. (Dretske allows [ibid., 146] that cross-modal information influences sensation, but this is at most a minor correction to the Cartesian paradigm.) Sensation does not, in this conception, divide some class into two subclasses, one consisting of those members of the class that satisfy some condition, and those that do not. Each sensory state is a concrete individual, an occurrence from which Boolean-valued messages can be extracted, but not a classificatory state in itself. This conception allows that sensory processes may be subject to what we might call 'entropic' loss of information—degradation of the signal through the process of transmission. Such loss of information may lead to gaps in the representation—coarseness of grain, diminution of the colour palette, blurring of outlines, and aberrations of various sorts. But this loss and distortion of information is random; it is not the systematic and purposeful discarding of information as a consequence of having sorted the input into particular types or patterns.

Dretske's notion of sensation as an entropic transform of receptor states is precisely what Barlow (1972) contests (see section III of Chapter 2). Barlow's thesis is, we saw earlier, that the retina transmits feature-maps, rather than light-intensity maps. Barlow points out that a cell that registers a rightward-moving edge transmits no *other* information—nothing about the illumination level, nothing about whether the edge is dark on a light background or light on dark, nothing about whether it is moving fast or slow, etc. By Dretske's definition, therefore, it carries the information that there is a rightward-moving edge in its receptive field *in digital form*. True, there may be *something* in the system that corresponds to Dretske's description. The retinal image, the outputs of all the rod and cone cells carries the information about a rightward-moving edge in analogue form. But visual consciousness, or 'perceptual experience'—i.e. sensation—has no access to this image. It corresponds to a state of processing considerably beyond anything found in the retina. Sensory consciousness contains *extracted* information.

In fact, as mentioned above, Barlow's thesis and the Sensory Classification Thesis are antithetical to this kind of distinction between sensation and perceptual belief. There is no reason to think that sensory consciousness is of some unarticulated substrate of perception in which we are unable to distinguish objects and their properties.

II. The Phenomenology of Concreteness in a Digital Medium

Barlow's article (1972) was meant to be a distillation of an emerging consensus; that consensus is now the dominant paradigm of sensory processing (see, for example, Masland 2003). Psychologists now believe that visual processing consists of the parallel construction of a large number of separate 'feature maps', each carrying information about the way that a different feature is distributed in space. A great deal of processing occurs in the retina itself, where as many as fifty-five different types of neuron have now been identified (Masland 2001), each most likely corresponding to a different computational function, some of considerable sophistication. By the time retinal information gets to the primary visual cortex of a macaque monkey, it already represents a large number of stimulus dimensions independently of one another: spatial frequency of gratings, length and orientation of lines and gratings, direction and speed of movement of lines and other shapes, colour (represented in terms of hue, brightness, and saturation), and so on. Each of these maps is separate. Information regarding the length of various lines is stored separately from that of various colours present in the scene, and so on. The maps available to visual awareness record the presence and location of colours, shapes, the speed and direction of movements, and so on. These maps, too, are separate. Shape information is recorded independently of the colours we see; colour information is not present in the shape map. A cell that responds to the presence of a square in a certain part of the visual field has no information about the colour of that square. (This is somewhat exaggerated: many cells respond to more than one feature.) As Austen Clark (2000, 45) has said,

In vertebrate sensory psychology [feature maps] seem to be everywhere. You will not go far wrong if you summarize the neuroscience in a series of headlines: Layered Topographical Distributed Feature Maps.

What moves Dretske to such a mistaken view? Presumably, it is intuition based on introspection of visual states. He thinks, rightly, that one *cannot* look at an 'A' without seeing what colour it is—call this the phenomenology of concreteness. This phenomenology is puzzling in the light of the scientific evidence. If colour and shape are stored independently, why is it that it seems impossible to see an 'A' without seeing its colour, font, and size? What accounts for the phenomenology of concreteness?

The answer is to be found in the theory of visual perception known as *feature integration theory*—the essential points of this theory were presented in Chapter 2, section IV. When a perceiver pays attention to a particular location, the features present at that location (or thereabouts) get 'bound' together or 'integrated', and she then sees a single image with a number of distinct characteristics. Anne Treisman (1996, 172) describes this process as follows:

A 'window of attention' scans a 'master map' of locations, selecting the features currently active in corresponding locations of various specialized feature maps.

These 'active' features are then represented as a conjunction occurring at the attended location. When the perceiver is *not* attending to a particular location, however, these characteristics are not bound together; she is aware of colours, shapes, etc., but not of colours together with shapes or colours in particular places. Thus, when asked to describe a briefly presented scene, subjects report 'illusory conjunctions': as Treisman puts it, 'the presentation of a green X and a red O might yield the illusory percept of a red X and a green O.' Conversely, 'directing attention in advance to the location of a target improves identification more for conjunctions than for simple features.'

Returning to the maritime metaphor of Chapter 2, section IV, let's imagine that we have three separate lookouts on board our ship, not one—all are in windy crow's nests high above the bridge and must speak and be spoken to laconically. The first is supposed to shout out 'Friend' or 'Foe' whenever he sees a ship. The second is supposed to indicate the direction of any ship motion he detects as he scans the scene: 'Approaching' or 'Receding'. The third is supposed to yell the size of any ship he sees: 'Big', 'Small'. Each of these look-outs is a digital converter producing Boolean-valued output; each sorts scenes into two types, and two types only—each need only shout 'Yes' or 'No' or hold up a card '1' or '0', and provided one kept track of which classification goes with which, that would be sufficient. (Actually, there is a third value, i.e. silence, representing the absence of shipping. But let's ignore this and assume heavy traffic.) For the most part, we get an uninformative cacophony from these informants in random and unpredictable order: 'Foe', 'Approaching', 'Big', they might yell in sequence, but since these may describe different objects, no count or description can be drawn from the sequence, except that there is in the vicinity something unfriendly, something that is approaching, and something big. There is no effective way of repairing this deficiency given the detachment of the messengers from one another. There is no point in asking the direction man, for instance, 'Is the *foe* approaching?'—he has not been trained to sort friend from foe.

Now, suppose that a convention is introduced by which all the messengers converge their gaze on the same ship-relative location when commanded by the captain to do so. At these coordinated moments, their yells convey much more useful information. Suppose the captain (or her crier) booms out 'Straight ahead' and *then* the above sequence is heard: 'Foe', 'Approaching', 'Big'. The joint message now amounts to: 'Big-foe-approaching-straight ahead'. (Of course, it could happen that there are two ships straight ahead, one of which is a big friend, and the other an approaching foe: this is a limitation of the system, let us ignore it.) This is precisely how Treisman's 'window of attention' operates. In response to a demand for reports about a specified 'master location', reports are taken from various maps, and bound together, or integrated, into a single conjunctive message. The 'window of attention' is not necessarily *initiated* by a query about a location: it may some-times be activated by a message. Imagine a ship sailing along in comparative silence when suddenly a distant boom of cannon-fire is heard. The captain might not be sure where the sound came from. She cannot, however, say 'Where?' (There is no 'where' lookout.) She has to 'scan the scene'. She would do this by reciting the possible locations one by one: 'Straight ahead', 'One o'clock', and so on, until she gets a positive reading. Alternatively, she may know where the sound came from, and investigate this location. This corres-ponds to what happens when our visual attention is attracted by a sudden event. A sudden movement or a shout causes the window of attention to scan and locate, or investigate a particular location.

It is true, then, that one cannot *attentively* see an 'A' without seeing an 'A' of a certain size, colour, and font. This is why the attentive 'A' message seems to be analogue in the sense defined by Dretske: it comes inextricably bound up with information about size, font, and location. However, it would be wrong to conclude that the visual 'A' message has not yet been processed by 'a digital-conversion unit whose purpose is to extract pertinent information from the sensory representation'. What has happened is that the message has been assembled from digitized components in a prescribed form. The attended image seems, from the point of view of the perceiver, to be pictorial in character, to resemble the image projected on the retina. (Not surprising: *looking* at the image projected on somebody else's retina yields a visual image digitized in exactly the same way as looking at the scene itself.) Consequently, the attended image appears, from a subjective point of view, to be concrete and fully specified, and not to have been subjected to a process of categorization. Visual attention creates this illusion by reassembling the messages it has separately devised.

III. Analogue Conversion and Quantitative Information-Extraction

There is another question that must still be resolved with respect to whether sensory messages are in digital form. Consider a visual representation of something as red. Nothing is seen as red without being seen thereby as some particular shade of red. A digital signal that something is red—for example, the sentence 'That is red'—does not convey this additional information about shades. This is a pervasive phenomenon—a consequence of Sensory Ordering, which is the subject of Part II. When the senses group several things together under capacious classes like *red*, or *high-pitched*, or *to the left*, we still see each of these things as belonging to a more specific kind within that range: *scarlet*, *high C*, or *three feet to the left*. Thus, it maybe thought that any sensory state that carries the information that something is red also carries *non-nested* information about what shade of red the thing is. Is *this* an indication of some non-digitized remnant in sensation? Though this problem cannot be fully resolved until Part II, we will embark now on a preliminary treatment. The important point that we will seek to establish in this section is that extracted information *need not consist of a simple yes-no answer to a single question*. There are several reasons why it might contain several messages inextricably tied up with one another, and hence appear less clean and discrete than Dretske anticipated.

First, let us consider Goodman's (1976) sense of 'analogue' in greater detail. Let us first define a *mark* or *inscription* as any pattern—visual, auditory, experiential—that can be considered to belong to a class known as a *character*. A character is, for present purposes, a class of marks with equivalent *orthographic value* in some system of signs. A chalk-mark made on a blackboard is such a mark: it may belong, or fail to belong, to the class of marks which are instances of the character 'A'. I want here to treat sensory qualia as marks. For instance, an occurrent colour experience is such a mark: it may belong or fail to belong to the class of experiences of a particular shade or colour—for present purposes, we treat the latter class of experiences as a character.

Goodman stipulates that a notational scheme is *syntactically dense* if the scheme 'provides for infinitely many characters so ordered that between each two there is a third' (136). When a character scheme is ordered by the experienced similarity of the characters themselves (or some other ordering relation defined on the domain of characters rather than on the domain of what they represent), it is not possible to determine whether a mark is an instance of a particular type, because for every symbol there will exist another so slightly different from the first that it is impossible to determine which of the two a particular mark instantiates. A syntactically dense scheme ordered by similarity in this way is *analogue* in Goodman's sense. Note that syntactic density is a property of the representational medium, that is, of the characters used to represent things, not of the representational domain.

Here is an example. Consider a map of a city drawn to a 1:50,000 scale. In this map, lines of any length are characters—they represent distances between geographical locations in the city—and lines of distinct lengths are distinct characters—they represent different distances. Between any two distinct characters in this scheme, there is another one, intermediate between them with respect to length. All the lines 1.5 cm long belong to a character, and this character represents a distance of 7.5 km. All lines 2.0 cm long similarly belong to a character, which represents a distance of 10 km. Between these are other characters: lines 1.8, 1.9 cm long, and so on; between these in turn are yet other characters intermediate in length between them, and so on. This scheme is syntactically dense. Since marks belong to these characters simply in virtue of their length, and since it is syntactically dense, this is an analogue scheme. Such a scheme is not, as Goodman says, 'differentiated' or 'articulate': for any given fineness of discrimination, there will be lines close enough together that it will be impossible to resolve which character they instantiate. In Goodman's system, a digital scheme would have clearly differentiated characters, such that one can, at least in principle, determine, for every mark or inscription, to which character it belongs.

Now, consider colour experiences as the marks in a similarity-ordered scheme. We suppose (a) that every colour experience is a mark that belongs to a colour character—the experience of a shade or of a colour. We suppose further (b) that y is closer to x than z if y is (experienced as) more similar to x than it is to z. Such a scheme is not syntactically dense—there are only finitely many type-different colour experiences, sensorily differentiable shapes, and so on, and density demands an infinite number of experiences. Nevertheless, it is closely packed. This means that the colours are, strictly speaking, articulate—it is always at least theoretically possible to tell what colour something looks, and to differentiate it from things that look different. Nevertheless, the colours are *practically* inarticulate, since given their close packing, it is operationally *difficult* to distinguish neighbouring colours—the closer together two colours are the more time-consuming it is to tell them apart, and the more difficult to discriminate them consistently in repeated tests. One might say then that experience within a given sub-modality—the colour experiences, the shape experiences, and so on—constitute, in Goodman's sense of 'analogue' at least, a *nearly* analogue scheme—that is, a representational scheme in which the characters are *closely packed* and *similarity ordered*. (Haugeland 1998/1981 is an interesting study of what I am calling nearly analogue schemes.)

According to Goodman, 'Where the task is gauging or measuring, the analog instrument is likely to play its chief role in the exploratory stages, before units of measurement have been fixed; then a suitably designed digital instrument takes over.' Any instrument that is directly affected by the physical variables it is measuring is analogue. Such an instrument yields analogue output because the effects that these physical variables have on the instrument are continuous in their mathematical form. A weighing machine, for instance, might contain a fine metal wire that gets progressively longer (i.e. more strained) as things of greater weight are placed on it. With the increase in weight placed on the machine, the electrical resistance of the wire increases (since it becomes thinner and longer); thus a read-out of current strength resulting from a fixed voltage applied across the wire is an inverse indication of the weight of the object placed on it. The various current strengths constitute a syntactically dense scheme of characters denoting weight.

Every measuring instrument contains some such progressively affected environmental interface. In some cases, a group of transducers is affected monotonically by impinging energy or force. As we have seen, the rods and cones in the eye play this role in the visual system; in the auditory system, it is the basilar membrane; in other systems, other such devices. In other cases, as in the chemical sensors employed by olfaction, the transducers themselves release energy in response to other kinds of interaction with objects. So Goodman is right at least to this extent: the early stages of measurement are analogue.

In the present context, however, it is the converse implication that is in question. We observed that collectively, shades of colour constitute a nearly analogue—a practically inarticulate—scheme of characters. Are we justified in assuming for this reason that they are produced by an analogue measuring device? This seems to be Dretske's train of thought: for as we saw in the previous section, he seems to think that sensation, including colour experience, carries information but no articulate message—nothing corresponding to classification, as he says explicitly. Sensation is, according to him, the underlay of the perceptual process, the substrate from which digitized messages are extracted. This, presumably, is what he has in mind when he says that 'seeing, hearing, and smelling are different ways we have of getting information . . . to a digital-conversion unit *whose purpose is to extract pertinent information*' therefrom (1981, 143, emphasis added: notice the parallel with Goodman). This line of reasoning is deeply misguided. There is no reason to think that a more closely packed character scheme always contains less extracted information than a more clearly differentiated one.

Dretske makes much of 'digital conversion', which entails the removal of continuous variation from a signal. But there is such a thing as analogue conversion too. A spreadsheet programme takes year-by-year income data and converts it into a graph; a curve-fitting programme draws a smooth curve through a number of discrete data-points—these are examples of analogue conversion. Goodman (1976, 164) uses the term 'supplementation' in this context. He has in mind cases where the intermediate values *exist*, but are unknown, and have to be provided by extrapolation or interpolation. Analogue conversion encompasses supplementation, but also cases in which the intermediate values simply don't exist. In the year-by-year graph generated from a spreadsheet, the graph makes it look as if there is such a thing as annual income for 2003½, but in fact there is no such thing.

We present information in graphical, i.e. analogue, form because it is easier for humans to grasp certain kinds of information when it is expressed in this way, or because the graph displays certain relationships within the data-set that are invisible in a digital display, or just because it is convenient to display it in this way for reasons related to the nature of the medium. Such representations are misleadingly information-rich. It seems as if there is information about points in between discrete data points, but this is simply an artefact of the process of drawing a curve. This manufactured information stems from a process of classification-and-representation, not necessarily from the 'front end'—the analogue sampling device in the environmental interface. Not every analogue or near-analogue scheme results from analogue sampling. The question we have to ask, therefore, is whether the near-analogue character of the colours (and other sensory qualities) is the result of analogue sampling devices at the outer periphery of the sensory system, or of analogue conversion. We cannot simply assume the former.

We shall see in Chapter 5, section III, that the notational scheme of colour experience, and of other sense-features, has been subjected to a form of analogue conversion. That is, colour information is represented in a three-dimensional graph-like scheme of representation. So at least some close packing is introduced *after* information has been extracted.

There is another important source of analogue concepts (and here I am indebted to David Hilbert for insightful discussion). *Not all information-extraction queries the data about the truth or falsity of a proposition.* Some information-extraction procedures involve the calculation of the *quantitative* value of some variable. The retinal array *contains* information about such quantitative values, much as it contains information about the truth and falsity of various propositions. However, just as a computational process has to be conducted before the truth or falsity of a given proposition is determined, a determination that can then be transmitted to other units, so also the value of quantitative variables has to be calculated before it can be separately recorded and transmitted. Sensory systems perform a number of such quantitative calculations. For example, there are many situations in which a sensory system computes the *difference* between the outputs of two receptor cells. This happens in the case of the opponent processing of colour. The output of such operations are in analogue form in the sense defined by Goodman, but this is not merely a remnant of the output of the measuring device. These quantitative values constitute extracted and usable information every bit as much as a digital signal does.

The closely packed ordering of the colours does not simply reproduce the continuous variation of wavelength and brightness present in light. In fact, the ordering is produced by the sensory system itself, in three stages.

Analogue Measurement. In colour vision, the analogue measuring device posited by Goodman is found in the three kinds of cone-cell in the retina.

Extraction of Quantitative Data. The output of these cells is subjected to comparison and subtraction—i.e. opponent processing—the results of which are transmitted onwards in separate channels. The content contained in these channels is quantitative but not unprocessed.

Analogue Redeployment. The information available in these discrete channels is then recombined into a vector, or ordered triple; each separate value becoming a distinct coordinate in the combined representation. This combination of independent information can be compared to a graphical representation in which several discrete variables are plotted together as the independent axes of a graph.

The vectors that emerge from this third stage are experienced as the closely packed colours. This recombination is a process that goes from one analogue medium to another; the colours are experienced as shading into one another in two dimensions because they are so arrayed.

To summarize, then, it is true that colour is represented in analogue form, according to Goodman's criterion. However, as we shall see more fully in Part II, this does not imply that colour-experience is the product of analogue interaction with the environment. The important point to remember here is that the analogue concepts of sensation are the product of quantitative data-extraction and analogue conversion; they are not merely remnants of analogue measurement.

IV. Discrete Colours

With the distraction of analogue conversion out of the way, we can now return to the phenomenology of specificity in sensation: we never see something as red without seeing it as a specific shade of red. Should we take this as evidence that the origin of discrete colour concepts such as *red* are imposed post-perceptually on an underlying continuum given us in sensation?

Another illustrative example will help us understand this phenomenon. Consider a tachometer which combines a traditional rotary pointer with the numbers up to 5000 rpm highlighted in green, those between 5000 and 6000 in orange, and the numbers above 6000 'red-lined'. The colour coding constitutes a kind of classification device, the green-outlined numbers are meant to indicate engine speeds that are safe for the engine, the red ones unsafe, and the orange ones borderline. The message conveyed by the pointer being in the green zone discards information about the actual speed of the engine: thus it is a classificatory state. But this does not mean that the latter information is unavailable. In fact, it is simultaneously available. The message conveyed by the colour coding of the tachometer *could* have been presented separately—for instance, by means of a light that glowed red, or orange, or green—but in fact it was not. So the simultaneity of presentation here had more to do with a design choice than with the representational form of the message.

Colour vision involves, in much the same way, a hierarchy of classificatory levels. At the finest level, it gives us information about shades of colour. This information is presented, as we shall see in Part II, by means of relational three-dimensional coordinates. In addition to this, there is a much coarser level of colour categorization. For it seems the semantics of our colour words derives from certain basic colour categories that are cross-culturally salient for sensory reasons (Brent Berlin and Paul Kay 1969; Rosch Heider 1972; Hardin and Maffi 1997: Figure 1 below shows these colours). These broad categories are, in other words, products of the colour vision system's classificatory activities. (There is an issue in the literature about whether language plays a role in forming these categories: this is beside the point being made here. See, however, the discussion towards the end of the next section.)

Now, there is no reason why the coarser categories corresponding to the colour words cannot be presented simultaneously with the finer categories that derive from the graphical combination of colour information—just as the coarser categories corresponding to the colour codes on the tachometer are presented alongside the finer categories corresponding to the numbers on the dial. We cannot see blue without seeing a particular shade of blue. This does not imply that *blue* is a category assembled from shades of blue. It just means that *blue* is a sensory class presented to us simultaneously with more specific information about shades of blue. In certain circumstances, this dual

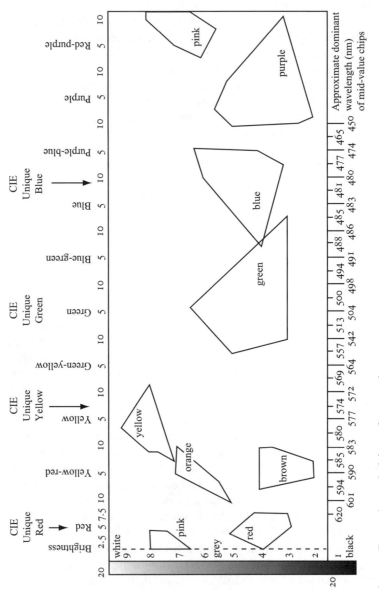

FIG. 1. Discrete Categories underlying colour words.

Source: Adapted from Berlin and Kay (1969, 9) with authors' permission.

presentation may be pried apart or dissociated. For example, a person remembering a scene may be able to say that something in it was red, but not remember what shade it was. Conversely, she might be able accurately to match the shade of what she saw to a colour sample, but not immediately be able to say whether it was orange or brown.

Two kinds of phenomenology have been presented in the last two sections as putative counter-examples to the thesis that sensory consciousness is digital representation—that one cannot see a capital 'A' without seeing its colour, font, size, etc., and that one cannot see red without seeing a specific shade of red. The same strategy was used to defeat both supposed counter-examples: both were said to involve the redeployment of extracted information (some of which is in analogue form). In fact this is a common strategy employed by sensory systems: first, they analyse the input array feature by feature and then they recombine all the results in a composite map. This accounts for our being presented with non-nested pieces of information simultaneously. Dretske's definition of 'analogue' and 'digital' neglects the possibility that digitized messages could be recombined. Further, his insistence that sensation is free of extracted information, seemingly on the grounds that it is nearly analogue, neglects the importance of quantitative information-extraction and analogue conversion. This is how his analysis of sensation takes a wrong turn. He assumes that when a message contains mutually non-nested bits of information, these bits of information have not been extracted. We have shown that things may be more complicated.

V. Is Sensation 'Conceptual'?

It is sometimes claimed that the classifications that the visual system gives us are not what one might call *concepts*, where the latter are supposed to be components of logically structured units. Let us make a distinction here between *linguistic* structures—words, phrases, sentences, and so forth—and the entities they refer to or denote—individuals, concepts, propositions. Language uses *syntactic* structure to build up complex linguistic structures from simple ones: sentences from words, for instance. Understanding a sentence demands that we correctly identify the words it contains and the syntactic type of these words. Moving to the semantic level, we find a similar and parallel sort of structure. The entities expressed by words combine to produce propositions. Identifying a proposition expressed by a syntactically complex sentence demands that one identify the concepts and individuals expressed by the parts of the sentence.

Now, one might want to distinguish between the kind of structure that propositions exhibit and the kind of structure that sentences do. It seems reasonable to say that sentences exhibit *syntactic* structure, while propositions exhibit *logical* structure—after all, propositions are not linguistic entities, and syntax is *linguistic* structure. If this is accepted, one should be careful *not* to claim that only syntactic entities can be used to express propositions. The Sensory Classification Thesis implies that sensory states express propositions: they convey to the perceiver that some distal object belongs to a particular class, or in other words, that this distal object possesses some feature. Yet it does not seem, for the very reason given above, that sensory states are *syntactically* structured: we are trying to avoid saying of any non-linguistic entity that it is syntactically structured, and sensory states are non-linguistic entities. The appropriate stance would be to hold that sensations exhibit a kind of structure that parallels the logical structure of propositions, and derivatively parallels also the syntactic structure of language, but lacks some of the distinguishing features of language.

So though one should be cautious about imputing syntax to sensory states, one can comfortably hold that these states have a certain combinatory structure, and that it is through this structure that they express propositions. This is precisely what will be argued, here and in Part V. The 'message' that sensory states convey to the perceiver is assembled from (a) sensory referential components, which identify objects, and (b) descriptive components, which dentify sense-features. This compositional structure is essential to how we grasp sensory content. To understand 'red' is to understand how it contributes to the sensory content expressed by the sentence: 'That round thing is red' and to understand propositional sensory content is to understand components like *red*. It is a consequence of the theses advanced in Chapters 1 and 2 that in such sensory states, *red* is a concept and has an extension—this is implied by the thesis that it is a 'sense-feature', and corresponds to a sensory class. It will be argued, further, that such sensory concepts are intimately related to those used in language: the sense-feature *red* has an intimate relation to the semantic concept 'red', which is expressed by the word, 'red'. (Bermúdez 1995 has a similar thesis, but stops short of identifying sense-features as a kind of concept: however, the intimate connection just posited between sense-features and linguistically expressible concepts provides the motivation for going this extra step.)

The claim that must now be examined is that sensory states possess *no* compositional structure, and that hence sense-features are not concepts. Gareth Evans (1982, 100–5) makes something like this claim, and says that the absence of compositional structure differentiates *thought*, which is conceptual according to him, from sensory states, which are not.

Here is Evans's claim about *thought*:

If we hold that the subject's understanding of *Fa* and his understanding of *Gb* are structured, we are committed to the view that the subject will also be able to understand the sentences *Fb* and *Ga*. And we are committed, in addition, to holding that there is a common explanation for the subject's understanding of '*Fa*' and '*Ga*', and a common explanation for his understanding of '*Fa*' and '*Fb*'. Each common explanation will centre on a state—the subject's understanding of '*a*', or his understanding of '*F*'. (101–2)

Sensory states do not partake of this kind of structural recombination, he says. Richard Heck (2000) echoes this:

To entertain the Thought that John is tall . . . a thinker would have to exercise a capacity to think of John and a capacity to think of a thing as being tall . . . [B]eing in a perceptual state with a given content need not require one to grasp certain concepts . . . of which its content is composed. (487–8)

It would be premature to deal here with the example of singular sentences, since sensory reference will not be dealt with until Part V. Let us therefore substitute another test, also related to the compositionality of Thought, but more directly applicable to the questions of sensory classification we have been dealing with in Part I. In fully generalized form, Evans's compositionality test implies that in order to entertain the Thought that something is blue *and* a disc and something else is red *and* a square, one should also be able to entertain the Thought that something is blue *and* a square and something else is red *and* a disc. (The logical connective 'and' is italicized in order to emphasize compositionality: there is a difference between being able to recognize blue discs, holistically as it were, and being able to sensually combine the separate visual concepts *blue* and *disc* into a logical whole. Evans is asserting the impossibility of the latter, not the former.) Evans's claim, as applied to perception, is that if one is to be taken as sensing something as blue *and* a disc and something else as red *and* a square, one should possess in virtue of some common factors, the capacity to sense something as blue *and* a square and something else as red *and* a disc. The Evans–Heck thesis is that such combination and recombination makes no sense with respect to sensation.

On its most natural reading, the Evans–Heck claim is false. What does it mean in a perceptual context to 'grasp' a concept—for instance a visual idea? Presumably, at the very least to respond occurrences of the idea in different presentations. Thus:

Perceptual Grasp
An organism perceptually grasps a sense-feature *F* if and only if there is some (learned or innate) behaviour pattern *B* that it executes in the presence of things that are *F*, but not in the presence of things that differ from the former only insofar as they are not *F*. (This is a minimal test: we shall see in Chapter 6, section IV, and Chapter 11, section I.2 that there is more to perceptual grasp.)

Suppose that a bird can be trained to perform some action in the presence of blue squares—to peck at these objects, for example. Now what happens if it is presented with a blue disc? If its experience of the blue squares were decomposable, then it should show some tendency to peck at it—at the very least a tendency to do so, or a hesitation. If, on the other hand, its experience of *blue square* was holistic, then it should not be tempted—the separate presence of *blue* will not confuse or tempt it. Note that if the former case obtained, there would be some common explanation of the bird's behaviour in the presence of a blue disc and the blue square. It is precisely this common factor that I am entitling 'perceptual grasp' of *blue*. Thus, it certainly makes sense to claim that perceptual grasp can be decomposed—one should not assert a priori that it cannot.[2]

Feature Integration Theory (section II above) suggests that perceptual grasp *is* compositional. A human's visual state when it attends to a blue disc is the result of 'binding' *blue* in a colour map to the co-located *disc* in a separate map of shapes. These two classifications are independent of one another. This implication of Feature Integration Theory accords with everyday experience: if one is able to entertain, in visual imagination for instance, images of a blue circle and of a red square, then one is able to entertain visual images of a blue square and a red circle. (Just try it!) What is more, my grasping the *blue* of both a blue disc and a blue circle—as evinced by my being trainable to respond to the *blue* in them by saying 'Blue'—has a single common explanation, namely a certain aspect of my experience that is repeated when I look at the blue disc and at the blue square. So it seems that *pace* Evans and Heck visual features *are* subject to composition and decomposition, and further that the visual grasp of complex visual features leans on the visual grasp of their components. *Blue* does occur in combination with other sensory features. The mode of combination might not be the *same* as occurs in thought or language—but then neither Evans nor Heck insist that it must be.

Further, like the concepts that we use in linguistic communication, sense-features have extension. *Blue* is repeatable; more than one thing can visually seem to be blue; more than one thing can seem visually to be any given shade of *blue*. Indeed, one generally does not see *blue* all by itself; rather, one sees it as belonging to some thing (see Part V). Thus, most visual states have combinatorial structure: they present a feature as belonging to a thing. But it is precisely in virtue of the complementary roles that concepts and individuals play in logically structured entities that one recognizes them as concepts and individuals. This, once again, is strong reason for thinking that the deliverances of the senses, particularly vision, are compositional entities. This is implied by the Sensory Classification Thesis.

These observations seem to bring our view in line with the requirements on sensory representation expressed by Wilfrid Sellars (1963/1956) and John McDowell (1994). Sellars and McDowell demand that sensation must furnish

---

[2] I am very much indebted to Paul Bartha and Ori Simchen for discussion of responses to Evans's Generality Constraint.

us with *reasons* to believe, and that it must be conceptually articulated if it is to do this. If the concept *red*—the concept that is expressed by the English word 'red'—is not somehow related to something in the visual sensation by which something looks red, then how can that sensation serve as a reason for us to believe that the thing is red, or to believe that it *looks* red for that matter? How would the sensation be *relevant* if it did not contain a concept related to the one that occurs in the belief? The Sensory Classification Thesis holds that sensation is propositional, and thus it seems to meet these worries—provided that a reasonably intimate connection can be established between the sense-feature presented to us by sensory experience and the concept that figures in the resultant belief.

McDowell *might* be inclined to deny that there is a sufficiently intimate connection—or at least that sensory classification as it has been described in Chapters 1 and 2 is sufficient to establish such a connection. For he demands that genuine concepts should be freely or spontaneously constructed under the influence of conscious decisions, and he suspects that 'cognitive psychology' is unable to accommodate such spontaneous construction. '[T]he contentfulness of our thoughts and conscious experiences [cannot] be understood as a welling-up to the surface of some of the content that a good psychological theory would attribute to goings-on in our cognitive machinery', he says (1994, 55).

Now, the account on offer here does indeed suggest that the content of certain concepts in thought wells up from the operation of sub-personal systems outside the perceiver's 'spontaneous' control. The principles for co-classifying things by colour are, according to the Sensory Classification Thesis, outside the conscious control of the perceiver, and the perceiver's beliefs that things are of a certain colour involves concepts that are subject to these sub-personally imposed criteria. This lack of spontaneity seems to conflict with McDowell's philosophical principles. (Or perhaps not, for McDowell only requires that 'observational concepts are *partly* constituted by their role in something that is indeed appropriately conceived in terms of spontaneity' [ibid., 13]: he makes it an example of such partial constitution that colour concepts must include a background belief that these are attributed to external things. So he may allow that whatever there is in the concept *red* that exceeds the terms of this background belief and differentiates it from *blue*—both of which are attributed to external things—need not be attributed to spontaneity. But let's continue as if the claim is more extreme.)

This apparent conflict between cognitive psychology and spontaneity does not survive scrutiny. It might well be true that the sensory concepts we use in language and thought are heavily determined by sensory classification, and also that the latter is not subject to our control. But this does not imply that we lack the freedom to *modify* the sense-derived categories we use in language. Indeed, there is ample empirical evidence that we *do* in fact exercise a degree of freedom in the construction of categories derived from sense-features.

The evidence is of two kinds. First, there are cultures in which colour categories are somewhat different from those—see Fig. 1 in the previous section—that we employ in English, even though the practitioners of these cultures (presumably) sense the world in precisely the same way as English-speakers do (Roberson, Davies, and Davidoff 2000; Jameson and Alvarado 2003). In these cultures, the same perception will lead to different beliefs. Seeing the sky, *speakers of Indo-European languages* (and many others) are led to the belief that it is blue; seeing grass, *these speakers* are led to the belief that it is green. These two perceptions lead IE-speakers to different beliefs concerning these types of things. However, members of the Berinmo tribe in Papua, New Guinea, apparently do not linguistically distinguish between *blue* and *green*. Consequently, the Berinmo are led by precisely the same pair of perceptions to the *same* belief concerning both sky and grass. Since there is every reason to think that the Berinmo sense colours the same way as other humans, it is reasonable to think that the difference between the Berinmo language and English can be traced to a degree of freedom in constructing colour categories in language.

Second, there are many human beings who have enhanced or reduced colour perception—tetrachromats, who see more colours than normal, dichromats, who see fewer, and even rod monochromats, who see no colour at all—but who still use the colour-categories of the majority, under the pressures of living in linguistic communities dominated by trichromats (Jameson unpublished). These individuals are in quite different perceptual states than normal trichromats when they look at many everyday things, yet under the pressure of the majority culture, they are able to learn and use the concepts that the majority use. Again, this shows that they are able, by means of some epistemic facility, to construct linguistic categories that do not agree with their perceptual sensory classifications. This is more evidence of the operation of spontaneity. Presumably, 'normal' trichromats, if immersed in a culture shaped by the colour-deprived would be able to adapt to the colour vocabulary of the dominant culture.

What then are we to make of the strong interpersonal and intercultural convergence of sensory categories referred to towards the end of section V above (notwithstanding the differences just alluded to)? Perhaps just that sensory classification exerts strong pressure on linguistic categories, pressure that can be evaluated by the operations of 'spontaneity', and resisted on some occasions, but generally conformity-inducing. Conformity should not be taken as evidence that we lack freedom. What McDowell refers to as 'cognitive psychology' does affirm, and with good reason, that sensory content is not modified by our 'conceptual capacities', but this does not put the sense-derived concepts that we employ in language and thought beyond the reach of spontaneity.[3] What it shows is that the concepts we employ in language are closely related to those that we get from perception, although not necessarily the same in intension or extension.

There are other characterizations of concepts in the literature, but I shall not consider them here, as they seem not to match our concerns in this context. For instance, Michael Tye contends (2000, 62) that concepts must come associated with theoretical 'correctness' conditions. Since the exercise of our perceptual capacities is compatible with our being ignorant of such conditions, this may indicate that perception is non-conceptual. However, this seems to be a question-begging definition. Why should our *intellectual* or *theoretical* grasp of correctness conditions be relevant to our *perceptual* grasp of sensory concepts? Tye might argue that we possess a *theoretical* grasp of sensory concepts and their correctness conditions, and that since our perceptual capacities do not presuppose knowledge of these, the concepts that figure in our theories of colour and the like cannot be exactly the same as those that figure in perception. This is quite plausible; indeed, it is supported by the cases of colour-abnormal perceivers and Berinmo people just discussed. This much granted, we do not have to concede further that perception is *non*-conceptual.

There is, however, good reason for supposing that sensory concepts are different in kind from those that we typically use in language and thought. Christopher Peacocke (1989) gives us a directly relevant example of this.

Anyone who has bought a house . . . knows that there are two quite different ways in which you can be ignorant of the size of a room. From the agent's handout, you can learn that the sitting room of a prospective purchase is 25 feet long: but this is consistent with your not knowing in another sense how long it is. . . . What you fail to know about the length of the room is precisely what someone who is in the room is in a position to know: . . . he can see how long it is. Equally this is consistent with his *not* knowing what you know when you read the handout: he may not know the length of the room in feet. (298)

Now, this difference between perspectives is sometimes conceived as merely a difference between modes of representation and not a difference concerning what is represented: that is, it is sometimes thought that in a case like the above, the *same* thing—length—is being represented both by the real estate agent and by vision, but in different ways. (See indexical theories such as Perry 2001 and physicalist theories such as Byrne and Hilbert 2003 for different versions of this idea.) Peacocke wishes to argue that this is wrong.

---

[3] Roberson et al. (2000) found that there was more variance among the Berinmo as to the focal examples of their five 'basic colours', and a lesser ability to remember colours in the short term, than with English subjects. Does this suggest that the English categories, which are shared by most peoples and linguistic groups in the post-industrial world, are more 'natural'? Perhaps, and this conclusion is encouraged by the fact that the Berinmo apparently don't speak about colour much. This would strengthen the case for spontaneity.

He holds that the difference between the real estate agent and vision is not notational, but a difference of the *concepts* that each brings to the scene.

When you look at a room, you subsume it under a *visual* length concept. The agent's handout subsumes the same room under a different length concept—let's call it *physical* length—that of being 25 feet long. Both are in some sense measures of length, but the visual idea is not just an idiosyncratic presentation of physical length. For as far as the perceiver is concerned, the meaning of the two presentations is different. The perceiver has an intuitive grasp of the visual feature: it enables her to make certain comparisons and estimates concerning the length of the room—how long it would take her to walk across it, whether her furniture would fit properly, how large a cocktail party would be comfortably accommodated, and so on. But she does not automatically calibrate the length in terms of *feet*, or in any other physical measure. This is not just because her knowledge of the latter measure is imperfect. The point is rather that the visual presentation of length is essentially perspectival, essentially related to the perceiver's own position and potential actions. Physical length, on the other hand, is not immediately applicable to actions, and is insensitive to changes in position and orientation. That a room is 25 feet long implies nothing about where the perceiver is relative to it, or about how it stretches away from her. Thus, the two representations bring the room under two different kinds of abstraction. The difference between these abstractions is akin to that between saying that the airport is *twenty minutes away*, and saying that it is *five kilometres away*. This difference is *not* like that between saying that the airport is 3.1 miles away and saying that it is five kilometres away. The mile-measure and the kilometre-measure are inter-translatable: much like 'cat' in English and 'chat' in French (see Chapter 4, section III.1). These are different ways of expressing the same concept. The time-measure of distance is not, however, inter-translatable with any length measure: to say that something is twenty minutes away is essentially situational and perspectival; while physical descriptions are not. On the other hand, the time-measure *is* a measure of length. (The foregoing is not Peacocke's argument, though it is a related line of thought.)

Let us say that a *domain of representation* includes the set of concrete *individuals* referred to by a particular representational vehicle—for example, the individuals into which vision breaks up a scene—*and*, in a sense that recalls the Sensory Classification Thesis of Chapter 1, the *features* under which these individuals are presented. Following this usage, one might say that vision presents us with a domain of representation which consists of at least some perspectival features, and this is different from a description in physical terms. If this is so, then the solution to the Sellars–McDowell conundrum is not quite as straightforward as they assume. Recall that these philosophers argue that if sensation were not conceptually articulated, it could not give us *reasons* for forming beliefs about the world. True, but this is not the end of the story. If some or all sensory concepts are fundamentally different in kind from some or all theoretical concepts, there is still a problem about how we get from one to another in a reasoned way. If we grant that many of our sensory concepts are perspectival in character, and many of our beliefs are non-perspectival, there is still a problem about how there can be rational communication from one to the other. We will not be pursuing this problem here, but it is worth observing that a major part of Heck's paper is devoted to epistemic procedures that could be useful in this regard.

VI. Describing Sense-Features

The Cartesian idea that sensation is raw, a transduction of a photographic image formed on the retina, retained in sensory consciousness but unfit for epistemological service, continues to have a remarkably tenacious hold on philosophers. Richard Heck Jr. (2000) agrees that sensations have content, but seemingly because he is impressed with the classic paradigm of visual sensation as photographic, he finds it problematic to hold that sensation contains extracted information (though this is not the way he puts it). Heck insists that when we draw beliefs from such content, we engage in a reasoned process of 'conceptualization'.

Here is what Heck says about sensory images:

Before me now . . . are arranged various objects with various shapes and colours, of which it might seem, I have no concept. My desk exhibits a whole host of shades of brown, for which I have no names. The speakers to the sides of my computer are not quite flat, but I cannot begin to describe their shape in anything like adequate terms. The leaves on the trees outside my window are fluttering back and forth, randomly, as it seems to me. . . . Yet my experience of these things represents them far more precisely than . . . any characterization I could hope to formulate. The problem is not lack of time, but *lack of descriptive resources, that is, lack of the appropriate concepts.* (489–90, emphasis added)

Heck says that this phenomenological report 'challenges anyone . . . to explain how experience provides us with a grasp of *all* the various concepts that would figure in a conceptual report of its content' (498, my emphasis). His claim, in short, is that the peculiar pattern of fluttering is information that has not been extracted from the sensory image. This amounts to a new challenge to the Sensory Classification Thesis as it has been articulated so far. The claims made in the previous section were that the senses present sense-features as possessing extension, and that sensory classification constrains the extension of concepts like *red, blue,* etc. Heck counters this with the proposition that if we could indeed decompose sensory states into concept and object, then we would possess a grasp of the bare features that are components of these states. But visual phenomenology shows that we do not possess all of the concepts that enter into sensory images, he argues. He calls this the 'Richness Argument'. (Bermúdez 1995 endorses a similar argument, which is also to be found in Evans 1982.)

It is not entirely clear what positive conclusion Heck would like us to draw from this argument. Does he think that a sensory state is an *un*articulated message, much like the pattern recognition system we discussed earlier, which sounds a bell when the Mona Lisa is displayed? This is extremely implausible, for the reasons considered in the previous section. We *do* react to features of a scene. Nor is this a matter of extracting concepts from experience: we have totally unconditioned, i.e. instinctive, reactions to many features. Besides, the Richness Argument itself tells against it in spades: how many such unarticulated messages would it take to deliver the range of sensory experiences we are capable of having—whole-scene experiences such as that Heck describes above?

Or consider this. I draw two straight vertical lines on a blackboard or tablet, and say, pointing to these lines:

(3) John and James are related thus in height.

This way of talking could potentially invoke all of the 'richness' present in Heck's scene. Yet, it is conceptually 'articulated': it says of two people that they partake of a certain relationship. To prove this, consider the following, also pointing to the above-mentioned lines:

(4) Martha and Dorothy are also related thus in height.

This explicitly relates two other individuals to each other in the same way, and proves that the image of the lines on the blackboard is compositional.

(Heck objects to such demonstratively ostended concepts because he thinks that this method of specifying concepts cannot accommodate perceptual error. We need not go into his reasoning in detail here. It suffices to say that if error is an issue with respect to how concepts are specified, then instead of drawing lines on the board and pointing to them, one can just mentally visualize two lines, or say 'Martha and Dorothy are related in height as those two lines *look*'—imagine doing that with a Müller–Lyer diagram. Actually, it is possible to dispense with demonstrative concepts altogether: in Chapter 11, section III.2, we introduce the notion of an 'autocalibrated sign', which does the same work, but without ostension.)

The Richness Argument may be taken as a challenge to the following proposition:

(5) There is no unclassified remnant in the visual image (or more generally, in any sensory image).

The Sensory Classification Thesis is committed to (7) (cf. the Classificatory Equivalence Thesis in section II.4 of Chapter 1), and, as we saw in Chapter 2, section III, it is supported by the fact that classification (including quantitative data-extraction) starts at the layer immediately downstream of the front-end transducers. From this layer onwards every neural state is representational. But (7) seems to be challenged by the visual phenomenology Heck describes; his claim is that our alleged inability to describe every shade and every shape that we see challenges the thesis that we grasp every such shade and shape. And if we *don't* grasp every such shade and shape, then it seems that we can take in or grasp scenes such as that of Heck's office while at the same time lacking an independent grasp of some of the sense-features they comprise.

Now, as we have just argued, Heck's argument does not rule out the possibility that the visual system classifies. In his example, there are two speakers on each side of his computer, and they look as if they have the same shape. The visual system seems, therefore, to be co-classifying them. So far Heck could well agree. The problem he poses is that of identifying the traces of this classification *in our conceptual vocabulary*. It seems to him that there are just too many shapes, and too many colours, for us to have discrete concepts for every single one. The fact that the speaker has a particular shape *could* be something we grasp; it could be a reason for doing or saying something. Yet, it does not seem to Heck that we possess, by virtue of the sensation alone, a concept corresponding to that particular shape. The detail of the sensory image, its richness, seems to transcend the possibility of verbal or conceptual description. Heck takes this to be a reason for supposing that there is something like a pictorial residue in visual experience, and that *we* (acting as epistemic agents) find similarities of various kinds in the detritus of icons.

So interpreted, the crucial point to notice in rebutting the Richness Argument is that even if we grant Heck his description of the phenomenology of visual experience, it does not follow that visual experience lacks the resources to describe every shade and every shape. True, visual experience is highly nuanced: it does not provide us with discrete classes or categories ready to be attached to discrete *names*; there are far too many sensory categories for us to be able to name each one. Nevertheless, vision provides us with the tools by which to *describe* each and every feature it presents to us. For as we shall see in Part II, vision gives us the capacity to compare and order features within certain domains. This ordering provides us, in fact, with what Heck contends we lack— 'a grasp of *all* the various concepts that would figure in a conceptual report of its content'.

The colours are a good example. As we saw in the previous section, certain basic colours are salient to us without instruction, this salience enables us to give them discrete names. Now, the basic colours that we name are not shades, but broader, more inclusive features like *red* or *brown*. Does vision provide us with some way of describing every shade included within a category of *red* or *brown*? Yes, it does! For within the broader sense-features to which we give names, we sense a certain variation and order. A particular shade of brown may be different from another in that it is redder, or yellower, or lighter. To quote C. L. Hardin (1997):

Sternheim and Boynton (1966) . . . required their experimental subjects to use only a restricted set of hue terms to describe light samples drawn from the longwave end of the spectrum. If the subjects were permitted only the names 'red', 'yellow', and 'green', they were able to describe all of the samples in the longwave range . . . . *The Hering primaries are necessary and sufficient for naming all of the colors.* (291–2; my emphasis)

There is nothing peculiar about the longwave end of the spectrum as far as this goes (see Werner and Wooten 1979): it merely illustrates the fact that sensation helps us 'grasp', the whole range of sense features, and that this intuitive understanding is an important determinant of the conceptual vocabulary we use to *describe* (not 'name', as Sternheim and Boynton say) the scenes we face. Indeed, the descriptions that sensation gives us may not be merely relational. That is, they may not be restricted to the description of a particular shade of brown as darker, redder, or more yellow than another. For it appears that normal observers may, with only a little training, become adept and consistent at describing various shades in terms of *percentages* of the Hering primaries contained by them. In fact, Alex Byrne and David Hilbert (Byrne 2003; Byrne and Hilbert 2003) take the Sternheim and Boynton result alluded to by Hardin above as the basis for describing the subjective content of colour vision. They take it that a particular shade of brown might be described, for instance, as 50 per cent red, 50 per cent yellow, and halfway between neutral grey and black—much as it is in the Swedish Natural Colour System.

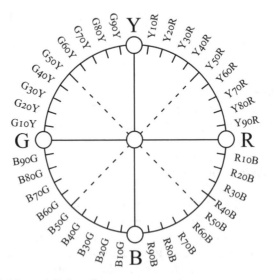

Fig. 2. Swedish Natural Colour System.

Intuitively, one might be inclined to think that Byrne and Hilbert go too far—it might seem introspectively false that one is able instinctively to quantify the colours in this way. And indeed reliable percentage estimates of colour components in a sample are good to only about 10 per cent—the Swedish Natural Colour System does not match the discriminations made by any one observer on every occasion, but is a statistical composite. (I am grateful to Larry Hardin for pointing this out to me.) However this may be, the point that emerges from such studies as Sternheim and Boynton (1966) and Werner and Wooten (1979) is that sensation *does, pace* Heck, contain the means by which to grasp and describe individual shades of colour, at least to discriminate them in terms of intensive relations like 'darker', 'redder', and so on. Such relations do not arise from the free employment of 'conceptualization', which would entail much larger individual differences in descriptive vocabulary, but are there in the sensory image itself. We do not, to be sure, possess a name-like marker for every shade of colour; nevertheless, these shades come to us in an ordering that enables us to *relationally discriminate* and *intensively describe* every shade.

This invalidates the Richness Argument. As we have noted, Heck insists that the ratio-specification of sense-features are explained by post-perceptual conceptualization of the sensory image. This will be contested in Chapter 5, where it is argued that the relational descriptions of sensory features arise directly from the way that they are coded by the brain. Putting this proposition aside for now, notice that the Richness Argument proceeds from an alleged lack of descriptive resources: the claim was that this shortcoming 'challenges anyone . . . to explain how experience provides us with a grasp of *all* the various concepts that would figure in a conceptual report of its content'. What has been shown above is that we are *not* in fact lacking in descriptive resources for this task.

Heck's own description illustrates this: his computer speakers are 'not quite flat', he says—in other words, they are somewhat *less flat* and *more rounded* than a strict rectangle. Similarly, you might describe a shade to the clerk in the paint-store—you want something a bit *more pale* than the beige in this sample here, you tell her, and her expertise enables her to mix you something more like what you want. Or one could show somebody a colour chart and ask her to pick out a shade of green that is yellower than some target (cf. Wittgenstein 1977, §§7–10). The fact that we have no name for the exact shape of the speakers or for the shade wanted for our living-room wall does not prevent us from describing the percepts present in these things using only materials available in visual sensation. Comparisons of more and less made with respect to specific sensory parameters give us the means to take in the entire range of sense-features available to us, and even to describe them to others. These scalar comparisons are the subject of the next chapter.[4]

---

[4] I am grateful to Richard Heck for useful comments on material contained in the last two sections.

Part I: Afterword

A Look Ahead: Pluralistic Realism

We have been arguing that sensory systems classify stimuli in their domain, assigning these stimuli to overlapping classes. Sensory experience conveys to us that the sensory system has made the associated classification: for example, when we experience *red* in a certain part of our visual field, we are made aware that our colour vision system has classified the thing that occupies that map location as a red thing. The argument implies that phenomenal states have attributive significance, and further, that classificatory sameness and difference are expressed as phenomenal sameness and difference. This sheds light on the link between the classificatory content of a sensory state and the experience associated with being in that state.

This Sensory Classification perspective has a surprising consequence that is worth outlining now, even though a full discussion is premature. In the Cartesian paradigm, sensation is a record of the energy pattern that impinges on the outer sensory receptors. Given that there are only minor differences among the outer sensory receptors of different kinds of organisms—at least with regard to those sense modalities they share—this leads one to expect that the sensations delivered by shared modalities are highly comparable across species. Once one takes on board the idea that the output of our sensory receptors are subject to data-processing, however, this expectation loses its appeal. Of course, there might be similarities among the ways that snakes, honey bees, and humans process visual data. These similarities may trace to common ancestry, to the nature of the data available, the constraints of the environment, and so on. However, adopting the Sensory Classification perspective, we will not be surprised to learn that there might be idiosyncrasies as well. The snake and the honeybee live very differently from us. They need access to information about very different kinds of environmental factor than we do. Consequently, they employ some classifications and some classificatory systems that are quite different from our own, i.e. they will classify things differently from us. In addition, their sensory processing streams are very differently organized: they lack cortical structures, for example. This could have the consequence that they have different sensory processing capacities. Thus, the contours of sensation cannot be specified in an organism-independent manner.

There is a link here to certain ideas in the German school of cognitive ethology, particularly the visionary (though all too often wildly fanciful) speculations of Jakob von Uexküll (1934), and his notion of an '*Umwelt*', which, as Andy Clark (1997, 24) helpfully defines it, is 'the set of environmental features to which a given type of animal is sensitized'. The *Umwelt* reflects perceptual specialization. Von Uexküll (1934,13) puts this in terms of the implausible image of 'a gourmet who picks raisins out of a cake'. (What kind of 'gourmet' would do such a thing?) Contrary to what one might be led to believe by the Cartesian paradigm, there is no sensory image common to all kinds of animals, which all of them use to guide their specialized actions. Rather, the perceptual system of each kind of animal produces a representation of 'a section carved out of the environment' (like a raisin picked out of cake). If sensation were common to all creatures, then each creature would need to devote post-sensory computational resources to figuring out what is relevant and what is not, and what each sensation signifies. Consequently, creatures with limited capacities for computation—ticks, honey bees, snakes, lobsters, and so—would have a rough time of it. We ourselves would be inundated with information which would be difficult to sort out and interpret, even given the large resources of the human brain's cortex. So it makes sense to think that perceptual systems focus on what is important for the organism's own activities, and leave out what is not. This is how the *Umwelt* is formed in evolutionary time.

It is a particular strength of von Uexküll's conception of the *Umwelt* that, though he pays lip-service to the traditional distinction between sensation and perception, he in fact supposes that sensory *experience* is a product of perceptual processing. In some cases, he takes sensory receptors to be the primary loci of environmental selectivity. For example, consider his account of the *Umwelt* of a tick. This creature hangs on to a branch until a trace of butyric acid emanating from mammalian skin loosens its grip and causes it to fall on the animal passing below. At this point, it roams around the hairy surface of the mammal until the sensation of heat alerts it to bare skin. When this happens, it bores into the skin, and feasts on its host's blood. 'The whole rich world around the tick shrinks and changes into a scanty framework consisting, in essence, of three receptor cues and three effector cues—her *Umwelt*' (von Uexküll, 12). Similarly, a honey bee divides flowers into those that have 'broken forms, such as stars and crosses' and those that have 'compact forms, such as circles and squares' (ibid., 40). This is significant because blossoming flowers, from which bees collect pollen, have broken forms, while buds have compact forms. The human visual system does not divide the world up in this way. So what the bee sees is different from what I see.

One might ask: given that the bee sees the world differently from humans, which species is right about its contours? Is the world more like my *Umwelt* or its? We can't both be right, it might be argued, since we see the world in essentially incompatible ways. But since there is no reason to privilege either the bee or humans, both of us must be wrong. This is an argument for subjectivism. It is not very persuasive. Why not say that we are sensitized to different features of the environment? We are simply classifying things in different ways, for our own purposes. The honeybee's sensory categories may be different from mine, but both of us can be right—or at least both of us can be capturing objective truths about the world. Von Uexküll agrees with this, but asserts, nevertheless, that *some* features of a creature's *Umwelt* might be subjective. Bears recognize the territory marked by themselves and other bears; they defend their own territories and occasionally try to steal others'. This, von Uexküll contends, is 'an entirely subjective product, for even the closest knowledge of the environment does not give the slightest clue to its existence' (ibid., 54). Really? Surely, territory *does* have a basis in fact: it is a matter of fact, and something about which one can be right or wrong, i.e. that a particular region has been marked out by a bear as an area in which only he and his may roam. Equally, it is a matter of fact that bears sense what is their own territory and what 'belongs' to another by physical cues, just as bees recognize blossoming flowers by physical cues. What von Uexküll means is that if one scrutinized the environment without knowing anything about bears, *then* one would have no clue as to the existence of ursine territory. But this is beside the point. Just because ursine ownership has no significance for humans, and is not detected by human sensory systems, one should not assume that it is merely subjective and has no basis in fact. Nor should one draw such a conclusion from the fact that a concept has no meaning independently of organic life. Indeed, such an assumption is quite at odds with the thesis of the species-specific *Umwelt*.

These reflections prepare us for the thesis of Pluralistic Realism: each organism fastens by means of its sensory systems on objective features of the environment in which it has a particular interest; such features may have no interest for other species and may not be detected by them. We will engage in an examination of sensory specialization in Part III, and flesh out Pluralistic Realism in greater detail there. The main point to be made here is that the Sensory Classification Thesis is friendly to Pluralistic Realism. This Thesis is fully congruent with the idea that the sensory systems of different organisms might classify stimuli differently because of the different interests and styles of life that different species are specialized for. It is no more surprising that birds or snakes should see the world differently from us than that they have modes of locomotion different from ours.

PART TWO

Similarity

4

The Sensory Ordering Thesis

Sensory classification was the subject of discussion in Part I. Sense-features were there defined as the properties ascribed to things in virtue of their assignment to sensory classes. We turn now to the more generally applicable framework prefigured in Chapter 3, sections IV and VII, sensory similarity, and the role that it plays in enabling and systematizing our grasp of sense-features within a particular modality.

Our senses make us aware of relations of comparative similarity and dissimilarity—graded similarity relations such as $<x$ is more similar to y than to $z>$, $<x$ is as similar to y as v is to $w>$, and possibly even $<x$ exceeds y by a ratio of 2 with respect to $F>$. These relations are an essential part of our sensory classification schemes, for as Quine observed (see Chapter 2, section II), they form the basis for conditioning, induction, and learning—for perceptual grasp, in short: the more similar two stimuli are to one another, the more likely that an innate or conditioned response to one is likely to spread to the other. Moreover, it seems, as noted in Chapter 3, section VII, that such relationships give us a way of grasping and describing the wealth of sense-features with which we are acquainted. It is a part of how we identify and re-identify a particular shade of red that we know it to be yellowish or dark, less or more so than other shades we know, or even that it contains such and such quantity of yellow as opposed to blue, black as opposed to white. Generally speaking, sense-features such as *round* or *red* comprehend a range of more specific features ordered and arrayed by graded similarity. These more specific features are experientially known, described, compared, and identified by their place in this ordered array. Sensory similarity and ordering constitute, in short, a structural framework that systematizes our grasp of the sense-features constructed by each sensory modality.

In this chapter and the next, we examine the character and source of this structural framework. In the present chapter, we examine

(a) the phenomenal character of sensory similarity,
(b) how it helps us grasp sense-features (section I), and

(c) the scientific practice of measuring sensory similarity and representing it graphically (the remainder of Chapter 4).

Then in Chapter 5, we turn to

(d) how sensory similarity is to be explained.

We shall find that it arises from the representational activity of sensory
systems.

Taken as a whole, Part II is a defence of a proposition stated in Chapter 1:

The Sensory Ordering Thesis
Sensory systems create *ordered* relations of similarity and dissimilarity
among stimuli, relations which grade the degree of similarity that one
sensed object bears to another.

The principle just stated is the counterpart in the domain of similarity of
condition I(a) of the Sensory Classification Thesis defended in Chapter 1.
Consequently, much the same issues are at stake here: the active role of sensory
systems in creating relations of similarity, the propositional form of sensory
states, and the orientation of sensory systems towards distal objects.

One important caveat should be noted here. Sensory ordering is *more fine-
grained* than sensory classification. In Part IV of this book, we propose that
two objects having the same sense-feature is a matter of the system treating
them as equivalent for certain epistemic purposes. In the bulk of the book,
sense-features are presented in this manner as classes constituted by equivalence or indiscriminability. It is important to realize, however, that such
grouping is ultimately based on similarity to a certain degree. Similarity to a
degree does not, strictly speaking, give us equivalence relations, and hence
defining features in this way is a simplification. Thus, as Carnap (1928) realized, the proper accommodation of sensory similarity demands a complicated logical system. Here, for the most part, we operate with the simple logic
of discrete classes.

In Part II, we examine the nature and consequences of sensory ordering.

I. Generative Hierarchies

Sensory classifications present themselves to us in well-defined ordering
relations. In this section, we recapitulate a philosophical analysis of sense-
features due to W. E. Johnson, an influential Cambridge University logician
of the 1920s. This analysis relies on the idea that a grasp of sensory-ordering
relations is characteristically a part of our grasp of sense-features in general.
This will prepare us for a consideration of quantitative treatments of sensory
similarity in the next section.

1. *Inclusion Hierarchies*

Classification consists of sorting some domain of objects into subclasses, where 'subclass' is defined as follows:

> *X* is a subclass of *Y* relative to classification scheme *S* if there is a feature *F* significant in *S* such that *X* consists of all and only those members of *Y* that possess *F*. Here *F* is the defining property of *X* within *Y*.

For example, *footwear* (*X*) is a subclass of *apparel* (*Y*) relative to *classification schemes used by fashion designers* (*S*), because it consists of items of apparel *made to be worn on feet* (*F*). Note that not every sub*set* of apparel is a sub*class* relative to these classification schemes. For instance, the clothes on the floor of a teenager's room are not a subclass of apparel relative to the classification schemes used by fashion designers—though they constitute a subset of apparel. On the other hand, they may well be a subclass of apparel relative to the classification scheme of a parent taking an inventory of the teenager's clothes—they might be the ones that need to be taken to the laundry.

Classes *include* their subclasses. *Red* is a relatively capacious category: it includes such subclasses as *bright red, burgundy, ruby, scarlet*, and *crimson*—anything that is bright red or scarlet must also be red, and the same goes for the other subclasses named. Similarly, *mammal* is capacious: it includes *ruminant, primate, dog, rattus rattus*, and *homo sapiens*. Each of these subclasses is distinguished from the more capacious class because its members possess some relevant feature.[1] Thus, classes and their subclasses constitute what we may call an *inclusion hierarchy*. The relationship of *inclusion* should not be confused with the instantiation relation that holds between *red* and individual red things—particular pieces of red cloth, for instance—or between *homo sapiens* and individual humans, for the second members of these pairs are not classes. *Inclusion* is a relationship between a class and its subclasses, while *instantiation* is a relationship between the defining property of a class and its individual members.

2. *Determinables*

Johnson (1964/1921) noticed an important difference between inclusion hierarchies in the contrasting domains of, as he put it, 'adjectives' and 'substantives'. According to him, more inclusive adjectival classes *generate* their subclasses: for instance, 'less than 4' generates '3' and '2' and '1' in the sense that understanding 'the meaning' of 'less than 4' 'carries with it the notion' of '3', '2', and '1' (ibid., 177). In the case of 'substantives', he said, our grasp of classes does not depend on such generative relations: you can understand *mammal* without possessing the wherewithal needed to generate the notions

---

[1] As it happens, this relevant feature is relational: what distinguishes members of a biological taxon is that they share a common evolutionary origin. But this does not affect the point being made here.

of *ruminant, primate, dog*, etc. Johnson proposed that 'adjectives' such as *colour* and *red* generate subclasses that are defined and distinguished from one another by means of relations implicit in our understanding of the class *red*: thus, one's grasp of *colour* or *red* already provides one with the where-withal to generate *burgundy, crimson*, etc. The technical notion of *perceptual grasp* introduced in Chapter 3, section VI, is relevant here: Johnson's idea could be glossed by saying that one can respond differentially to capacious classes such as *red* only if one can respond differentially to some subclasses thereof. For example, one does not not grasp *red* unless one can also differ-entiate some subclasses of *red*, for instance *dark red* and *pink*. This is by no means a trivial thesis.

Johnson called classes that thus generate their subclasses *determinables*. The aim of the present discussion is to understand the nature of deter-minables, and how they relate to their subclasses. It should be said that the distinction between more inclusive classes that generate their classes and those that do not, like *mammal*, is not always respected today, and the word 'determinable' is sometimes used to cover both. This contravenes Johnson's usage, to which we revert here.

Before we embark on this discussion, we need to register two clarifying notes. Johnson was the first to make explicit the important distinction between determinables and classes like *mammal* that do not generate their subclasses. But his formulation is couched in misplaced terminology. First, the distinction cannot be applied over as large a domain as he specifies, namely, 'adjectives' vs. 'substantives'. Since we are interested here only in the domain of *sense-features*, where the notion of generative inclusion does seem to be universal, or nearly so, we may disregard the wider issues that Johnson's choice of words raises, and simply concentrate on his characterization as it applies to sense-features.

Second, Johnson suggests that these are *linguistic* or *logical* issues, since he speaks of our 'understanding' of the *meaning* of determinables like 'less than 4'. When this is applied to the colours, it suggests that our grasp of colour similarity leans on our grasp of the meaning of the *words* we use to describe the colours. In other words, Johnson seems to suggest that it is part of the meaning of the English word 'red' that it names a colour more sim-ilar to *orange* than to *blue*, and that our grasp of this similarity relation derives from the meaning of 'red'. This is wrong—though the assumption pervades many philosophical discussions of this topic. (Cf. Wittgenstein 1977, §6: 'How do I know that I mean the same by the words 'primary colours' as some other person who is also inclined to call green a primary colour? No,—here language games decide.')[2] Again, we will simply ignore

---

[2] See Jonathan Westphal 1986 for an interesting discussion and repudiation of Wittgenstein's view.

this, and confine our attention to the *perceptual* grasp of sense-features themselves, as distinct from the kind of linguistic or abstract understanding that we may possess with regard to such entities as words or concepts.

3. *Generative Hierarchies*

Now, let's look more closely at *how* determinable sense-features generate their subclasses. How exactly is *red* or *green* like 'less than 4'?

Johnson's own characterization—that an adequate understanding of a determinable like *red* 'carries with it the notion of' its subclasses—is unhelpful: even granting him the vague notion that *red* and *green* do this somehow, his definition is far too broad, and drags all sorts of irrelevancies into its purview.

To see why, think of the following example. Imagine that the term 'French colour' is introduced by pointing to a French flag and stipulating that just those shades of red, white, and blue are to be included in the meaning of the term. The relationship between *French colour* and its subclasses is contingent and circumstantial; it is so because the more capacious class was created bottom-up as it were—assembled from subclasses that were arbitrarily grouped together. We cannot 'generate' white from *French colour* by some relation constitutive of the latter in the way that we can generate 3 and 2 and 1 from the *less than* relation implicit in our grasp of 'less than 4'. Because of how it was defined, our grasp of the class *French colour* carries with it the notion of its subclasses, but seemingly not in the same way as *red* and *green* carry with them the notion of their subclasses.

Johnson was thinking of class-conceptions associated with *systematic top-down* ways of 'generating' subclasses, where the class itself cannot be grasped without knowing certain relations that generate subclasses. His example of a natural number range illustrates this well. There are certain relations constitutive of the domain of natural numbers—successor, predecessor, greater than, less than, and so on. Given a grasp of some members of this domain, these relations are sufficient to identify, in a non-contingent way, at least *some* other members. The idea is that we can generate subclasses from the more inclusive class by using relations that are essential to grasping the more inclusive class. We'll reserve the term 'generative' for this kind of systematic identification of subclasses by relations that are part of the definition of the class itself, and call an inclusion hierarchy based on such a top-down identification of subclasses a *generative hierarchy*.

The striking thing about *sensory determinables* is that their generative hierarchies seem to depend on how we *experience* sense-features. As we began to see in Chapter 3, section VII, sense-features are typically experienced as varying intensively in a number of dimensions. Every colour has a *black-white* (or *dark-light*) component, a *blue-yellow* component, and a *red-green* component; a colour can be darker or lighter, bluer or more yellow, and redder or greener

than another. Musical sound has pitch, timbre (the relative strength of overtones relative to the fundamental frequency), and loudness. Each of these
components is independently intensifiable: a sound may be higher or lower
in pitch, purer or richer in timbre, and louder or softer than another.
Similarly, every taste is a combination of fundamental tastes, *sweet, bitter,
sour*, and *salty*; a taste can be saltier or sweeter than another (or both). These
relations of intensification yield a form of graded similarity; for if one feature is generated from a paradigm by a smaller amount of intensification than
another, then the first is more similar to that paradigm than the second. If,
for example, x is only a little redder than y, and a lot redder than z, then x
is (in this respect) more similar to y than it is to z. There is, in each of these
cases, as Johnson puts it, 'a certain serial order, which develops from the idea
of what may be called "adjectival betweenness" ' (1964/1921, 182).

   Johnson was on to something important. It is, for instance, an essential part
of our experiential grasp of *green* that we can visualize, or form mental images
of, the range of shades that *green* comprises: that these vary from the bluish
(*turquoise*) to the yellowish (*lime-green*), and from those in which the green is
clothed in white (the pastels) to those in which it is obscured by black (*olive*),
with no unoccupied places. Indeed, it is possible to describe a colour to somebody who has not seen it by means of such variations: to tell somebody that
Kaffir limes are less yellow than Mexican limes is a useful form of description. Further, it is a part of grasping *green* that when we are shown several
shades we are able to recognize that they share something in common, and
even that the shades shown are shades of green. (The abstract painter, Josef
Albers, exploited such relationships among shades of colour in the series
called 'Homage to the Square'.) Still putting the matter vaguely, a full sensory
grasp of *green* entails grasping how different shades of *green* are different from
one another while still being shades of the same colour, and being able to visualize some shades by means of this variation. And the same goes, *mutatis
mutandis*, for the other sense-features mentioned above—sounds, tastes, etc.

   Hume remarked that even if one had never seen a certain shade of blue, one
could form an idea of it. In fact, this phenomenon is even more extensive
than Hume imagined. Reflect on this: until the invention of artificial dyes and
the discovery of incandescent gases, there would have been some shades that
nobody had ever seen. W. R. Webster (2002) cites scientific speculation that
naturally occurring colours in our ancestral forest environment occur in
just three ranges: 'grey-red', which includes 'tree bark, dead leaves and animal
melanin pigmentation', 'leaf green', and 'leaf contrast', 'which are spectra of
fruit and flowers that have evolved to be conspicuous to pollinators and
frugivores.' There is probably no such thing as a saturated pure red or of an
equivalent blue in nature. So in all likelihood, *nobody* had seen a focal instance
of red or blue until a few hundred years ago. Even today, it is entirely possible
that some normally sighted people have never seen certain colours. Yet, they

do not react to a new shade in the same way as a previously colour-blind person would if her colour vision were restored. Indeed, one often cannot even remember whether one has seen a particular shade before.

If our perceptual grasp of sense-features includes a grasp of relations of intensification, then this perceptual grasp gives us a notion of similarity, of 'serial order' and 'adjectival betweenness', to use Johnson's terms. Just as relations like successor, predecessor, and so on give us a 'certain serial order' constitutive of the domain of natural numbers, 'adjectival betweenness' constitutes our grasp of sense-feature domains. Clearly, this similarity is apt for defining sense-features as subclasses of determinables. Features defined in this way form generative hierarchies as defined above. The existence of generative hierarchies with their relational orderings of sense-features invalidates what Richard Heck calls the 'Richness Argument', the argument that we lack the concepts by which to express each and every sense-feature we are capable of experiencing (see Chapter 3, section VII).

4. *Determinables and Variation*

Determinables include a variety of subclasses, but there are subclasses of any given determinable that are fully specific and do not admit of variety in respect of these generative relations: in this sense, they are *fully determinate*. (Strictly speaking, the notion of a full determinate is logically defective since, as Peacocke 1987 points out, the relation of sensory indiscriminability is intransitive—we'll ignore this and stick with this convenient notion here.) The colours to which paint manufacturers give trade-mark names—'Cape Cod Blue', 'Tudor Rose', and the like—accompanied by mixing instructions for paint-stores, are fully determinate in this sense (or at least approximately so). They are guaranteed not to admit of variation (with respect to colour), even when one has to make a second trip to the store for another can—or at least that the variation will be less than a just-noticeable-difference step or two. (*X* is less than a just-noticeable-difference step away from *Y* if the average observer's ability to discriminate *X* and *Y* is at chance.) Such fully determinate colours are generally called *shades*. The instances of such fully determinate colour are all the same as one another with respect to colour, and no two are different in this respect. Shades do not have subclasses, and so it makes no sense to say that an instance of a *shade* of green is yellower or bluer than another instance of the same shade. Shades are colours, then, but not all colours are shades, since some colours consist of collections of shades ordered by some relation that is included in our grasp of the colour.

In view of this, it is natural to say that:

> *Determinables* are sensory classes the perceptual grasp of which involves grasping certain relations of intensification that can be used to generate their subclasses.

Full determinates are classes that admit of no more than a just-noticeable difference between any two members with regard to the relations of intensification by which they are generated from the determinables that include them. Full determinates are the *infimae species* of sensory classification.

Because we experience determinables like *red* as essentially involving an aspect of variation, it seems natural to say that two shades of red, say *scarlet* and *crimson*, are similar with respect to being shades of red, but also different with respect to the redness that each exemplifies. This seems just another way of saying that these shades occupy different positions within the colour range constituted by one and the same determinable. But David Armstrong (1978, 117–18) argues that to put things in this way is to suggest that one and the same thing can be both the same as and different from one another *in the same respect*, which he finds logically unacceptable: 'Nothing can agree and differ in the identical respect,' he insists; *scarlet* and *crimson* cannot both agree and differ with respect to *red*. Thus, he finds the idea that determinables are classes (or 'universals', as he calls them) logically suspect, and he insists that 'all universals must be determinate'. (Armstrong's proposal immediately founders on the fact that, strictly speaking, there are no determinates. We ignore this and concentrate on other problems.)

Armstrong claims that but determinables are experientially derivative from full determinates. Seeing something as red is just a matter of seeing it as scarlet, or as crimson, or as some other shade of *red*. He assumes that capacious sense-features like *red* have no sensory unity of their own—there is no immediately given unity that shades of red possess with regard to one another. In effect, he is claiming that these capacious classes are assembled piece by piece from the fully determinate classes that they comprise.

Armstrong's position overlooks the difference between (i) Johnsonian determinables, the grasp of which leans on a grasp of relations of matching and intensification, and (ii) classes specified bottom-up in the way of 'the French colours'. In the latter case, the class is defined by enumeration of determinate subclasses, not by some generative relationship that the subclasses bear to one another. The fact that these shades belong to the French flag gives me no grasp of how they vary from one another, and no way of generating any of them from my experience of the whole class. Thus, I need to grasp each of the French colours before I can grasp the whole concept. Contrast this with our grasp of *green*. If you happened to come across a shade of green, and had not seen it before or could not remember having seen it, you would still have no difficulty identifying it as a shade of *green*. If *green* were grasped 'bottom-up', how could this be possible? If somebody showed you the French flag, but with the red bar obscured, you would have no way of recognizing *red* as a French colour. If our grasp of colour were like our grasp of the French colours, then, the sheer extent of Hume's phenomenon of missing shades (noted above) would be very difficult to understand.[3]

These considerations reinforce the idea, noted before, that the mere fact that a term has subclasses does not suffice to mark it off as a determinable. Armstrong's position that all universals are determinate misses the peculiar use of top-down definition in sensory classes, the characteristic relationship between *red* and its subclasses. It also misses the point, made in Chapter 3, section V, that vision directly provides us with classes of different inclusiveness—determinables like *red* as well as shades like *crimson*.

5. Exclusion Ranges

The comparability of two sensory classes by relations of intensification means that they belong to the same *type*—for example, colour. Now, two different classes of the same type are always somewhat dissimilar from one another: a fully determinate colour will, for example, be somewhat redder or greener, bluer or more yellow, darker or lighter, than any other fully determinate colour. This has been taken to mean that any two fully determinate colours are mutually exclusive: to assign the same stimulus to *both* implies that it is dissimilar to itself. This is what Johnson is after when he says:

Adjectives under the same determinable are related to one another in various ways. One relational characteristic holds in all cases; namely that, if any determinate adjective characterizes a given substantive, then it is impossible that any other determinate under the same determinable should characterize the same substantive: e.g. the proposition that 'this surface is red' is incompatible with 'this (same) surface is blue'. (1964/1921, 181)

This principle requires clarification and amendment. Taken one way, *red* is not 'incompatible' with *blue*—purple things are both red and blue. Similarly: 'Nothing looks both square and round', 'Nothing tastes both sweet and bitter', etc. In these cases too, the possibility of blends and intermediates makes it difficult to state the principle in a precise way: a square with rounded corners, a cup of sweetened espresso coffee are counter-examples.

One must distinguish here between *feature-incompatibility* and *component-incompatibility*. *F* and *G* are *feature-incompatible* if no full determinate that falls under *F* also falls under *G*. *Red* and *blue* are feature-incompatible

---

[3] Boghossian and Velleman (1997/1991) object to the view that 'to see one color is, in a sense, to see them all'. It is not clear how strong the position to which they object is supposed to be. To see a colour, or perhaps a few colours, does imply an at least latent grasp of the ordering relations in the similarity space of colour, and this is enough to give one some degree of familiarity with all the colours—this is shown by the fact that seeing a new colour is nothing like seeing colour for the first time.

because no shade of red is a shade of blue. On the other hand, *blue* and *green* are feature-compatible, because there is an overlap: some shades are identified as belonging to both. (Notice that any two fully determinate features will be feature-incompatible with one another.) *F* and *G* are *component-incompatible* if they cannot be components of the same colour. *Red* and *green* are component-incompatible because no shade is both reddish and greenish. On the other hand, *red* and *blue* are component-compatible, since purples are reddish and bluish simultaneously. Johnson may have meant only to claim only that *red* and *blue* are feature-incompatible, which is true: see Figure 1, Chapter 3. However, this does not prevent them from being a component of the same colours: they are both, as noted, components of *purple*.[4]

Incorporating this refinement, let us restate Johnson's principle:

Feature Exclusion Principle
A fully determinate feature excludes other features *of the same type*. If *FD* and *FD** are distinct fully determinate features of the same type, there is some range of individuals, *x*, such that *x* cannot be both *FD* and *FD**.

It seems that this principle is true for visual features. Intuitively, there are colour shades that exclude other colour shades, but do not exclude shapes—such shades form, in Armstrong's apt phrase (1978, 112), a 'mutual detestation society', as do certain sets of shapes, sizes, and so on. But *scarlet* does not detest or exclude a cross-cutting feature like *circular*. Thus, *scarlet* excludes other *shades*, but not shapes, sizes, etc.

So understood, the Feature Exclusion Principle should be taken not as an empirical discovery, but as implicitly defining sense-feature *types* or *exclusion ranges*. We construct such types by collecting *all* sense-features that exclude some other feature in the collection. Every determinable includes mutually

---

[4] The literature contains disputes that arise from failing to distinguish between component and feature incompatibility. One of these starts with Jerry Katz's (1964, 532) claim that *blue, yellow, green, red*, and *orange* are 'antonymous', i.e. feature-incompatible—the claim is that nothing is, for instance, both red and orange. This is somewhat inaccurate—there is a small overlap between some neighbouring colours, including *red* and *orange*. There are shades that are both green and blue, some that are both orange and yellow. But Katz's claim is roughly correct, construed as a claim about feature-incompatibility. However, Paul Kay and Chad McDaniel (1997/1978) construe it as a claim about *component* incompatibility, and reject it out of hand: 'The inadequacy of [Katz's] treatment is apparent when one considers compound terms such as *yellow-green* or *blue-green* . . . .We propose instead that color categories . . . are continuous functions' (401). Kay and McDaniel's formalization of colour categories entails that *every* shade of orange, even focal orange, is also red (ibid., 427–8). Surely, this is wrong: it is shown to be wrong when you look at the diagram of basic colour terms made by Brent Berlin and (the same) Paul Kay. The right thing to say is that every orange is *reddish*, not red. Alex Byrne (2003, n. 38) makes a similar point: 'an aubergine is reddish, but not red'—*aubergine* is a mixture of *red* and *blue*, but not a *conjunction* of *red* and *blue*. (I am grateful to Martin Godwyn for forcing clarity on the difference between feature-incompatibility and component-incompatibility.)

exclusive determinates: *red*, for example, includes *scarlet* and *crimson*. *Red*, however, is not *complete*. It does not include all the features excluded by its shades—*red* includes *scarlet*, and *scarlet* excludes *azure*, but *red* does not include *azure*.

A (complete) *exclusion range* is a determinable E such that

(1) E includes at least one fully determinate feature F, and
(2) if any member of E excludes another fully determinate feature F', then E includes F', and
(3) any determinable that includes a member of E is itself a member of E.

Colour is an exclusion range. It includes *scarlet* (F) and thus satisfies clause (1) above. Since scarlet excludes *azure* (F'), azure is also a member of colour by clause (2). Every other fully determinate colour is excluded by either *scarlet* or *azure*. This brings in all the determinables that are subclasses of colour, by clause (3). However, *colour* does not include features like *round* and *high-pitched*, since *scarlet* and *azure* do not exclude them. Exclusion ranges collect together all the features that constitute sense-feature types.

There are exclusion ranges in all the sense modalities: this follows from the fact that in every modality there are fully determinate features, and that a fully determinate feature excludes some other fully determinate feature. A single sense-modality may deliver information in more than one exclusion range. Within vision, colour, shape, and size are distinct exclusion ranges. *Scarlet* and *azure* exclude each other, but both accommodate *round*. *Round* in turn excludes *square*, but both accommodate *scarlet* and *azure*. Thus *shape* and *colour* are independent exclusion ranges for visual objects. In other modalities, there may be only one exclusion range. This appears to be so with regard to olfaction, for example.

To summarize then: exclusion ranges embrace the full extent of intensive variation within a certain group of sense-features, while full determinates admit of no variation. Determinables admit of some variation. Exclusion ranges are maximal determinables.

II. Sensory Similarity Spaces

Johnson's introduction of generative hierarchies is a relatively recent application of old philosophical knowledge—nearly 2,500 years have passed since Plato assigned sense-features to the realm of the 'more and the less' in the *Philebus*, and more than 250 years since Hume observed that one can 'raise up' a never-seen shade of blue by filling in the blank in the ordering of previously seen shades of blue. But such knowledge long remained qualitative in nature, much as it is in Johnson. About 150 years ago, when sensory variation began to be examined quantitatively, initially by physical scientists in Germany and England—Ernst Weber, Hermann von Helmholtz, Ewald Hering, Charles Wheatstone, Thomas Young, and James Clerk Maxwell were some of the great names in this enterprise—these investigations gradually gave way to the new science of 'psychophysics' (see Hatfield 1991 and Turner 1994 for informative and philosophically sophisticated historical accounts). These investigations (of which Johnson was presumably well aware) give geometrical shape to sensory-ordering relations, and throw considerable light on the relations implicit in our perceptual grasp of determinables and generative hierarchies.

Experimental psychophysicists ask observers to make judgements about experienced sensory variation and correlate reported sensory variation with physical variation in the presented stimuli. The experiments immediately relevant to us are restricted to individual exclusion ranges. For example, observers might be presented with stimuli that differ from one another in colour only, or in size only; the conclusions drawn from the experiences that derive from such a set of stimuli are meant to be relevant to this special similarity only.

Here, briefly, are some examples of the judgements subjects are asked to make. In *confusability-scaling* experiments in colour vision, subjects are presented with carefully calibrated coloured lights sufficiently similar to one another that it is possible to confuse them, and are asked whether two lights are the same or different. Within a group of such lights, it is assumed that x is more like y than z if x and y are *more often* identified as indiscriminable from one another than x and z. Out of such comparisons, we get the separation of determinate sense-features within an exclusion range by the standardizing measure of the just-noticeable-difference—the difference between two stimuli just far enough apart as to reliably elicit different behaviours. This makes it possible to compare similarities: to make judgements of the form $<x$ is more similar to y than to $z>$ and $<x$ is as similar to y as v is to $w>$. It also allows us to estimate the *distance* between two stimuli in terms of just-noticeable difference steps. Note that it is possible to perform confusability scaling experiments on animals. You condition the animal to act in a certain way when it sees a stimulus of one kind: to peck at it with its beak, perhaps, in the expectation of some reward. Then you present the animal with other stimuli and estimate how often it acts in the way that it has been trained on the initial stimulus. This gives you an estimate of confusion with the initial stimulus.

In a different kind of experiment—call them *stimulus-matching* experiments—researchers measure how stimuli differ from one another. For example, they might ask observers to vary a test stimulus by using a set of controls so that it matches another target stimulus. For example, the colour of a test light might be varied by manipulating two or more rheostatic control switches attached to component colours in order to make it match a target.

Performed on a variety of stimuli, this will afford us a measure of distance: the greater the adjustment required, the more dissimilar the initially presented stimuli were. Another experiment might be to match a coloured chip presented in one context with chips presented in another. For instance, a subject might be presented with an orange surface in a light-yellow surround and asked to match it with one of several patches of the same orange presented in darker surrounds. Such coloured chips look lighter in darker surrounds, and the matching experiment provides a precise measurement of how much they shift in apparent colour. This kind of experiment too is performable on animals. For instance, you might train a bird or a fish to look for food under a yellow cover, and then you see what stimulus elicits this learned behaviour in different surrounds or conditions of illumination. This gives the experimenter an idea of sensory equivalences among stimuli and gives her a mapping from physical stimuli to experienced sense-features.

In *direct-estimation scaling* experiments, subjects are asked to make direct comparisons between stimuli. This might be confined to judging which of two presented stimuli is greater than another in some respect (e.g. painfulness), or subjects might be asked to assign ratios or magnitudes to stimuli: for instance, to judge what proportion of yellow there is in a light, and what proportion of red. These experiments are examples of what G. S. Brindley (1960) (cited by Mollon and Jordan 1997) called Class B observations: 'the subject is asked to describe the quality of his private sensations', and not merely to report or react to 'the identity or non-identity of the sensations evoked by different stimuli'. Class B observations cannot be replicated on animals.

The above-mentioned methods show how sensory ordering is the basis for sensory classification. A sensory class, it might be said, is a collection of objects that are to be treated in the same way for certain purposes. As we have been saying, this is a simplification. In the case of a determinable sensory class, there is a degree of variation among its members, illustrated by the above relations of confusability and association. Thus, it is appropriate to think of a sensory class as a collection of objects united by some degree of similarity. Fuzzy logic is the appropriate logic for such sets, since their membership is not determinate (cf. Kay and McDaniel 1997/1978). However, we shall ignore this complication in this book: here, sense-features are treated as discrete entities with determinate boundaries, and talk of sensory ordering is generally assimilated to the simpler logic of sensory classification.

At any rate, from the above and other observations concerning sensory variation and comparison, psychophysicists arrive at a set of quantitative *distance* measures between stimuli taken pairwise. Intuitively speaking, the distance between two stimuli corresponds to the dissimilarity between them, and this will depend on the extent of variation along the relations of sensory intensification described in the previous section. A feature A that is a *lot* redder than another one B is more dissimilar to B than C which is only

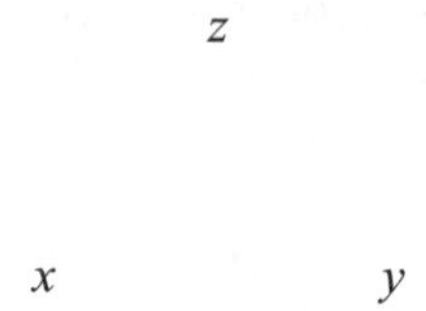

z

x   *y*

If the distance *xy* is equal to *yz*, and *xy* is equal to *xz*, then *x*, *y*, and *z* cannot be placed on a line; they must be placed on a plane. A fourth point equidistant from all three will have to lie outside the plane of the paper.

FIG. 3. Representing Equal Similarity.

a little redder than *B*; this comparison can be captured by a distance measure: *A* is further away from *B* than from *C*. This comparison can also be displayed graphically: on a line that represents a progressive intensification of *red*, *C* will lie in between *A* and *B*. Such distance measures are somewhat variable from human observer to human observer, but retain a statistical correlation across humans.

As suggested above, dissimilarity measures behave mathematically like spatial distances. They enable mathematicians to arrange sense-features graphically in a spatial structure, known as a *similarity space*—'quality space' and 'resemblance ordering' are other terms that have been used for the same structure. Using the methods of *multidimensional scaling*—see Clark 1993, Chapter 4 and Appendix, for an excellent description—these pair-wise distance measures are integrated into a single multidimensional graphic representation, in which the distances between all pairs is preserved. An important geometrical principle at work here is that if you have *n* points pair-wise equidistant from one another, you will need an $n - 1$ dimensional space in order to arrange these points to display these relations. Take three points *x*, *y*, and *z*. If these points are equidistant from one another, i.e. if $xy = yz = xz$, then *x*, *y*, and *z* cannot be accommodated on a straight line (a one-dimensional space), but can be placed on a plane (which has two dimensions). Add a fourth point equidistant from all three, and you need a three-dimensional solid (see Fig. 3). The aim of multidimensional scaling is to generate a model of the pair-wise distances between stimuli in as small a number of dimensions as possible.

A nice example of multidimensional scaling is drawn from musical pitch. Nelson Goodman (1972/1970) sets the stage with a question:

Surely, pitches are the more alike as they differ by fewer vibrations per second. But are they? Or is middle *C* more like high *C* than like middle *D*? The question is argument enough. Similarity of so-called simple qualities can be measured by nearness of their position in an ordering, but they may be ordered, with good reason, in many different ways. (ibid., 445)

When Goodman says that these notes can be ordered 'with good reason, in many different ways,' he presumably means that if we were merely thinking about the physical stimuli, there would be no observer-independent reason to prefer one ordering over another. For instance, there is no reason to think that middle *C* is like high *C* independently of human auditors. For as Roger Shepard (1982, 306) rightly says, 'The cognitive psychological approach looks for structural relations within a set of perceived pitches independently of the correspondence that these structural relations may bear to physical variables.' Thus, Goodman's point can be stated thus: when we consider *perceived* similarities in pitch, it makes no sense to ask about orderings 'with good reasons'. That we perceive two things as similar has nothing to do with rationality.

This leads us to a puzzle concerning Goodman's argument. Suppose that middle *C* is perceived as similar both to middle *D* and to high *C*. Why does Goodman suggest that we have to *choose* between these two perceived similarities—similarity by adjacency (middle *C* similar to middle *D*)[5] and an ordering by octaves (middle *C* similar to high *C*)—or posit separate orderings for them?

There is simply no conflict between these two relations: the methods outlined above allow us to eat this particular cake and have it too. It is true that closeness in frequency does influence perceived similarity—traditionally, closeness was thought to be proportionate to the difference in the logarithm of frequency, though this is modified by other effects (see footnote 5). It is *also* true that octaves are perceived as similar. We accommodate both these truths by representing the sequence of ascending notes in a three-dimensional similarity space. Thus, as Fred Lerdahl (2001, 43) tells us, 'M. W. Drobisch suggested [in 1855] that pitch height be represented on a helix, with octave recurrences placed proximally on the vertical axis of the turning axis.' If the slope of this helix is shallow, high *C* would actually be closer to middle *C* than middle *D*, but in a different direction—high *C* would lie on the turn of the helix above middle *C*, but middle *D* would lie along the helical twist. One would expect from this that tone and height would be perceived as distinct components of pitch, the former being arrayed on the circumference of the circular projection of the helix, and the latter along its axis.

As it turns out, Drobisch's helix is too simple: it fails to account for the special status of the fifth and of the enhanced similarity of notes adjacent in the *chromatic* scale (as opposed to the sharps, which are off this scale, but in between with respect to frequency), at least in those acculturated to this scale. Roger Shepard (1982) shows how the representation of these relations

---

[5] Worrying about adjacency seems to be a mistake in any case, for notes separated by a significant interval such as a fifth or an octave sound more alike than those separated by a smaller but less significant interval (Shepard 1982, 307).

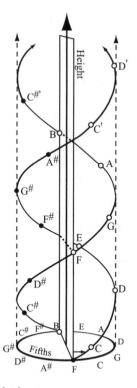

Fig. 4. Shepard's 'Melodic Map'.

Source: Shepard (1982) with author's permission.

demands a double helix (Fig. 4). Note that even in this rather simple example, sensory similarity cannot be equated to the physical similarity responsible for the effect that a stimulus has on the sensory receptors.

In such representations, each sense-feature takes its place in an *n*-dimensional
similarity space which consists of all the features in its exclusion range. This
similarity space preserves the distance measures derived from similarity
judgements. Figure 5 is a representation of the similarity space of colour
which preserves the just-noticeable-difference distances as equal.

Discounting a variety of complicating factors, such as reduced input sensitivity at the extremes of the spectrum, the underlying representational space
of colour is usually schematized as in Figure 6. The exact status of such simplified schemata is contested—it is not clear how well they correspond with
perceptually based representations (see Mollon and Jordan 1997)—but this
need not concern us here. Johnson's thesis prefigures the idea that our perceptual grasp of colour leans on our grasp of the relations of intensification
along the axes of such diagrams.

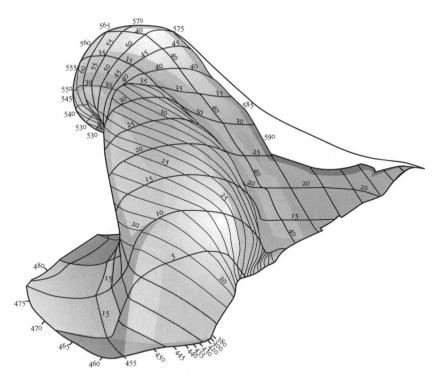

FIG. 5. Colour measured by Just-Noticeable Difference.

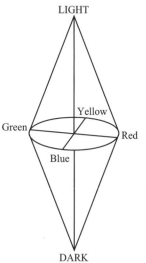

A perceptually based colour space, in which the vertical axis represents lightness or brightness, the angle around a circular cross-section at any level represents hue, and the distance along any radius represents saturation. All colours that lie along the central vertical axis, thus, are achromatic, and all colours that lie along any vertical line have the same hue.

FIG. 6. HBS Colour Space.

This kind of representation of sense-features, i.e. in terms of position in a space, is known as *vector coding*. The Feature Exclusion Principle stated in section I.4 is a necessary accompaniment of vector coding: every exclusion range consists of features arrayed in an unified similarity space; every determinate feature in the exclusion range has a unique vector representation; every feature different from it has a different vector coding; no place in sensory colour space can be assigned two codes at the same time.

III. Representational Invariance in Graphical Representations

1. *Conventional Aspects of Mathematical Representation*

That the characteristics of a certain domain of phenomena can be mapped into a space-like structure does not mean that the domain *literally* displays all the spatial relations that one can extract from this structure. Not all aspects of the spatial map are dictated or constrained by the data. How should one go about determining which aspects of a map reveal some aspect of objective reality and which do not? Which aspects of the above mapping of colours reveal some aspect of external reality and which do not?

One way of proceeding is to consider alternative representations of the same data. Here is a simple example. Suppose that in physical space, a point *a* is displaced by 3 cm from another point *b* in one direction, the *x*-axis, and 4 cm away from it in an orthogonal direction, the *y*-axis. By Pythagoras' theorem, the straight-line distance between the two points is 5 cm (assuming that the space is Euclidean). Now, these numerical measures of distance can be changed. In another system of representation—for example, where the above distances are expressed in inches (instead of centimetres), the displacement along the first direction will be (roughly) 1.2, along the orthogonal direction 1.6, yielding a straight-line distance of 2. The numerical values are different in the two representations, but the relationship given by Pythagoras' theorem, i.e. $z = \sqrt{(x^2 + y^2)}$, is invariant. This is because the Pythagorean relationship reflects something real about the underlying quantities, while the numerical values given these quantities in a particular representation are merely conventional measures. If in a representation of certain data, we find invariances that were not explicitly built into the representation, we may infer that these invariances must result from something other than the method of representation. Representational invariance that does not result from explicit constraints on the representational scheme must have *some* other source. They call out for explanation.

The converse inference is not correct. That is, not every fact that receives alternative representations is conventional. Here is a simple illustration. On the Fahrenheit scale, the numerical measure of temperature on a spring day, 60°, is twice that on a cold winter day, 30°. But it is clearly a mistake to say that the *temperature* in spring is twice that in winter—on the Celsius scale, the numerical ratio is roughly −15. One might think that this shows that since temperature ratios vary with the representational scheme, there is no right or wrong about the way in which one scheme represents these ratios, that by contrast with lengths, where ratios have a clear meaning, the differences between the Fahrenheit and Celsius scales show that temperatures ratios are conventional. One might trace the differences between the two temperature scales to the conventionality of the zero point in these scales for measuring temperature, and one might hastily conclude that by contrast with the zero point for length, zero points are generally conventional for measures of temperature.

As it turns out, this would be a mistake. It is an important empirical fact that there is a non-conventional way of fixing the zero for temperature. In statistical mechanics, temperature is identified with the mean kinetic energy of the underlying molecules. Thus, one can fix the zero in an objectively valid way as the temperature that corresponds to an absence of molecular motion. The Kelvin scale takes this into account: the absolute zero in the Kelvin scale corresponds to a total absence of kinetic energy in the underlying molecules. In the Kelvin scale and other absolute systems of measurement, temperature ratios do have meaning; these ratios are representational invariants in absolute scales of measurement.

This shows that not all representational variability is a consequence of the conventionality of representation. In certain cases, variability results from a poor choice of representational schemes. The realization that the zero point of the temperature scale is not arbitrary makes it appropriate to introduce some constraints on the system of representation. Such constraints are needed if we are to capture certain relations that we have discovered to obtain in the domain of phenomena being represented. In properly constrained systems of representation, all invariants require explanation from outside the representational scheme.

2. *Spatial Representations*

The methodology of similarity spaces considered in the previous section has application in a number of fields other than psychophysics. Consider the diagrams that biological taxonomists use to illustrate the distinctness of species. Various species of finch, for example, can be measured in terms of such parameters as beak-size and curvature, body-weight, body-length, etc. We can plot biological specimens in the n-dimensional space defined by these parameters: this is the structure that taxonomists call 'morphospace'(see Figure 7).

Now here is an important fact revealed by this form of representation. Members of single species cluster together in morphospace, with unoccupied regions in morphospace. This is a graphic illustration of the fact that despite Darwinian variability within species, members of a single species are generally

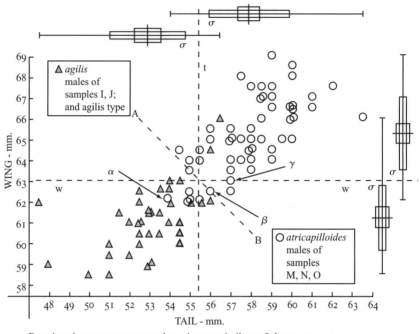

Does it make more sense to say that α is more similar to β than to γ in the two dimensions combined?

FIG. 7. Representation of Biological Specimens in Morphospace (Drawn by William A. Lunk).

more similar to one another than to members of other species. This clustering of specimens is a representational invariant: it does not depend on the scaling of the graph. Clustering is an objectively valid phenomenon, and demands explanation by evolutionary theory. Thus, there is no question but that the representation of organisms as occupying points in morphospace does capture some important facts about them.

Though the graphic representation does reveal clustering, one cannot assume that it licenses certain further inferences concerning the domain of finches. For instance, it is not clear what it might mean to say that the *integrated* or *overall* similarity of one specimen to another—the total similarity that results from differences in all of the separate parameters combined—is measured by the linear distance between the points they occupy; indeed, it is not clear what might be meant by talking about overall similarity of one specimen to another.

Consider once again a space that represents just two characteristics, wing-length and tail-length. In Figure 7, you will find one specimen, α, that has wing-length just under 62 mm and tail-length 54 mm, while for another, β, the corresponding measurements are 62.25 mm and 56 mm. The difference in terms of each of these characteristics is well defined, but what would it mean to talk about *the* overall similarity with respect to these two parameters taken together? The straight-line distance between these specimens in the graphic representation shown in Figure 7 happens to be about 17 mm. However, this distance is not a representational invariant. If we distorted the graph by changing the scale of one of its axes, this distance would change. Nor is there some fact about the relationship between wing-length and tail-length that constrains us from distorting the graph in this way. Thus, though the ratios of wing-length and tail-length that we can take from the figure correspond to reality, there is nothing in objective reality that corresponds to oblique straight-line distances in the graph. It follows that the clustering of specimens of the different subspecies in the figure is really a clustering in each independent dimension: there is no composite property that clusters.

One cannot even use the distance between α and β as a *comparative* measure of similarity. On the face of it, α is more similar to β, being only 17 mm away from it, than to a specimen γ from which it is 20 mm away. But this comparative measure can again be changed by rescaling the graph. If we were to shrink the scale of the dimension in which γ is more dissimilar to α and magnify the dimension in which β is more similar, γ could get placed closer to α than β. Nothing would be misrepresented by such rescaling—there is, after all, no quantity to which the straight-line distance corresponds. Rescaling the axes of morphospace would not be like rescaling a map of Vancouver by shrinking the north-south dimension. There is something that gets misrepresented by so transforming the map of Vancouver—actual straight-line distances in the vicinity—but there is nothing in biological species that gets misrepresented in this way. Again, consider the *directions* of various lines in a space-like representation of morphological characteristics. In Figure 7, the subspecies *agilis* lies 45° 'southwest' of *atricapilloides*. What does this tell us about these subspecies? Nothing beyond the information about the individual parameters encoded in the diagram itself—namely that the difference in wing-length is roughly the same in absolute terms as the tail-length.

In the graph, wing-length and tail-length are equally scaled. This might reflect the taxonomist's opinion that the variance in these parameters is roughly the same. But the criterion is not absolute. There could well be contexts in which one would be inclined to give more weight to one of these parameters than to the other. Rescaling changes the orientation of lines. Since distance and direction in a particular representation have no further significance, the geometrical properties of the representation are simply artefacts of the display. Morphospace is 'space-like' in that distances and directions are there to be measured; it is not literally a space because not all of the measurable quantities correspond to real characteristics of the things being represented. Oblique straight-line measures and directions have no significance independently of contingent features of the graphic representations. The x and y axes of the diagram capture all the information that the domain provides; other geometrical magnitudes measured in the plane defined by these axes lack representational significance.

Of course, it could turn out that there *is* some physical or biometrical law or generalization in which the supposed combined distance measure serves as a parameter. If so, then we would need to privilege those representational schemes which preserve the comparative distances that this law demands. The situation would be the same here as in the case of absolute measures of temperature: recall that absolute scales are privileged because they preserve relationships that are significant in statistical mechanics. Here too there is a mutual interaction between representational invariance and underlying laws. When we discover a representational invariant such as clustering, we are inclined to look for explanations of the phenomenon. When we discover an underlying law that *should* lead to representational invariants, we privilege the class of representations within which the invariance is preserved.

In general, we need to distinguish between the geometrical features that are artefacts of the representational scheme we use to display similarity relations in a domain, and those that are forced on us by something other than the way we represent these relations. It is reasonable to think that representational invariances arise out of the latter. Hermann Boltzman[6] once distinguished between 'diagrams of illustration, which merely suggest certain relations to the mind of the spectator' and 'diagrams drawn to scale, from which measurements are intended to be made'. More particularly with respect to the present discussion, one should distinguish between those parameters which are drawn to scale in a given diagram, and those quantitative measurements that may be made in the diagram, but which give us no information about the things represented therein, even though they might be suggestive of certain relations. Representations of biological morphospace are suggestive in that they demonstrate that specimens cluster in many dimensions: if these dimensions were separately represented, this convergence would not be as easily grasped. On the other hand, the *joint* representation of these dimensions, the representation of them as axes of a space, engenders certain quantitative characteristics that have no counterpart in the domain being represented—for instance, the straight-line distance between specimens. The straight-line distance 'suggests to the mind of the spectator' a measure of overall similarity, but since the relations among the dimensions cannot be 'drawn to scale', this

---

[6] Boltzmann's article on diagrams, cited by Goodman (1976, 171), is in the eleventh edition of the *Encyclopedia Britannica*, which is currently available (in an uncorrected optically scanned version) at http://www.1911encyclopedia.org/.

is misleading. There is nothing in the specimen pool against which to check whether the equal scaling of wing-length and tail-length is right, as opposed to some other. It simply makes no difference.

IV. Representational Invariances in Sensory Similarity Spaces

We saw in section II that similarity relations among sense-features can be encoded as similarity spaces. Keeping the relativity of scaling in morphospace in mind as a basis for comparison, we may now ask what features of a sensory-similarity space are invariant. What is 'drawn to scale' by these diagrams? Answering this question will help us to appreciate which facts concerning sensory similarity spaces stand in need of explanation, and which can be written off as artefacts of the representational system.

We come now to a *crucial*, but largely unremarked upon, characteristic of the component structure of sense-features. We have seen that sense-features are experienced as possessing intensifiable components—each experienced colour has a *red-green*, a *blue-yellow*, and a *dark-light* component; each musical sound has pitch, loudness, and timbre; and so on. The crucial fact to which we must now attend is this: these components are not sensed as *separate* elements; rather, each sense-feature is associated with a *unitary* experience within which the components can be discerned.

Here are some examples. When you mix sugar into your coffee, it acquires a new taste in which sweetness is more pronounced than before: the sweetened coffee does not present you with two taste-sensations side by side, one remaining the same, and the other added or intensified. Another example: Emma Kirkby's voice is purer than Maria Callas's, in the sense that in Kirkby's voice, the overtones are weaker. But when Kirkby and Callas sing the same note, say middle *C*, their voices sound holistically different; the fundamental frequency is not heard separately from the overtones—rather, the greater strength of Callas's overtones expresses itself as a middle *C* that has a different sensory quality, specifically a different timbre. Again, when you add green to blue, you get *turquoise*. This new colour is not *two* colours, an added green sensed separately from the initial blue, but rather a new and distinct single colour, recognizably greener than the original shade. All of these sense-features are experienced as composite yet unified and distinct; the components can vary independently of one another, modifying the single complex experience, as they do so, making it sweeter, or richer, or greener.

The phenomena just described confirm Johnson's contention that our grasp of sense-features has a relational aspect. What do we mean when we say that turquoise is greenish? We do *not* mean that *green* itself—*green* unmixed with any other colour, 'unique green' as this unmixed green is called—is a component of the colour. No, for when we look at a turquoise surface, we simply do not see unique green sitting there, in the same place but distinct from, a unique blue of roughly the same brightness. Rather, we mean that if certain aspects of our experience of turquoise were to be intensified, and others made weaker and ultimately annulled, *then* our experience would become the same as that of unique green. In other words, when we describe turquoise as greenish, we are describing it in terms of its relation to a particular colour pole. The same goes for the other mixtures mentioned above. It is noteworthy that these descriptions are very closely related to the way that we experience sense-features. For as noted in Chapter 3, section VII, subjects can easily be taught the vocabulary that enables them to provide such descriptions with a reasonable degree of consistency. *These are the relationships of intensification on which Johnson relies to generate fully determinate features top-down.* They are the relations by means of which we are able to describe the entire similarity space of colour.

In this way, the relationship between pitch and timbre within the auditory experience of Emma Kirkby's voice, or the relationship between *red* and *yellow* within the visual experience of orange, is quite different from, say, the relationship of sizes, shapes, and colours in the visual experience of a painting by Mark Rothko. In the Rothko, we find certain shapes—squares, stripes, blobs, etc.—each of a certain size and a certain colour. If one were to place a coloured transparency over a square or a blob, thereby changing its colour, one would not thereby change one's experience of its shape—the square remains a square of the same size, the blob a blob of the same size and shape, though each takes on a different colour. In the case of the intensification of sense-features, by contrast, the addition of sweetness, richness, or greenness modifies the sense-quality itself. It makes no sense to say that you can hear Kirkby's middle C *in* Callas's *with the addition of some overtones*: rather the *quality* of Callas's middle C is distinguished from Kirkby's by the addition of overtones. This is how sense-features are experienced as possessing components that are subject to intensive variation.

The non-separability of the components of sense-features gives reality to a multiplicity of *paths* in similarity space, which in turn gives representational significance to *direction* in similarity space. Consider a lamp in which there are three differently coloured light sources: red, blue, yellow, for example. Three rotary knobs allow you to control the strength of these light sources, thus changing the colour emanating from the lamp. This test lamp is changed by small increments and then compared against a fixed reference light. Now imagine the following experiments.

> A. Both lights start at the same colour F and the test light is augmented by n just-noticeable-difference steps of red. The result is a new colour G which we may describe as $F + nR$. Now, G is augmented by m steps of blue, yielding a third colour, H which is $F + nR + mB$.

This procedure establishes one 'path' in similarity space from the original colour F to the final colour H; this path passes through G. Path A is only one of those available between the two hues. We can generate another by reversing the order in which we add blue and red. Thus:

B. Both lights start at the same colour F and the test light is augmented by m just-noticeable-difference steps of blue. The result is a new colour J which we may describe as $F + mB$. Now, J is augmented by n steps of red, yielding a third colour, $F + mB + nR$. This destination colour is the same as colour H in example A: the additions of blue and red 'commute'. (This assumes that the *red* dimension is not stretched or distorted in this different region of similarity space.) However, the intermediate colour, J, is distinct from G.

Here is a third.

C. n small increments of red and m of blue are alternated; this yields a step-wise 'diagonal' path between F and H. This path does not pass through G or J.

Paths A, B, and C all lie in different directions in colour space, and because of how component variables combine to yield new features, the paths are *phenomenally* different also—that is, they pass through phenomenally different shades as intermediate points.

Now, the distance from F to H, measured in just-noticeable-difference steps along the diagonal path C is generally different from (most often less) than the distance along the path through G or the path through H. (The deformed surface shown in section II is a map of these distances.) Consider the following schema:

The distance along one side of a triangle is less than the sum of the distances along the other two sides.

This schema, generally entitled the *triangle inequality* is *usually* (though not invariably) a feature of sensory spaces. (Notice that in the diagram of colour similarity space, some areas bulge, allowing for the possibility that a curved path between two points could be shorter than a 'straight' one.)

In morphospace, on the other hand, the triangle inequality is neither true nor false: distances in different directions are not properly defined. This is an important difference between the diagram of perceived similarity relations incorporated in a similarity space and the diagram of organisms arrayed in biological morphospace. As we observed earlier, diagonal distance depends on the relative scale of the axes on which independent parameters are plotted. This relative scaling marks a merely conventional decision in morphospace diagrams (where the parameters being plotted vary independently of one another), but is constrained in the case of similarity space. Rescaling similarity space so as to disturb the interrelationships of distance between paths will distort sensory experience: it will make it appear that one path comprises more just-noticeable-difference steps than another, when in fact it does not.

Similarity Involving more than One Exclusion Range

Now, to mark the contrast, let's revisit similarity judgements involving the simultaneous comparison of sensory qualities drawn from more than one exclusion range. (The comparison of the colour-altered Rothko shapes is an example.) Here is what happens when observers try to grade the similarity of objects that differ from one another with respect to features from *two or more* exclusion ranges, for example, objects different from one another in both colour and shape:

> We saw that *within* an exclusion range, two items that are dissimilar to any degree are always holistically different from one another. Composite items that vary with respect to features in different domains are not component-integrated in this manner. But when you make a red spot *larger*, your experience of the red does not thereby change. The original shade of red is (disregarding contrast phenomena and the like) a *separate* and *unchanged* part of the altered experience. Thus, even if it makes sense to say that colour and size are two components of one's experience of a red expanse, or that tail-length and wing-length are different components of one's experience of a particular kind of bird, they are components in a quite different way than *red* and *black* are components of *brown*—they are separate components.
>
> Because there is no 'new' feature to be placed in the space—there is no single experience that constitutes sensing a red spot of a given size—the larger red spot cannot be compared to the smaller green one in a single act of comparison. Rather we perform a two-step comparison compounded out of the two separate components—comparison of colour and comparison of size. This two-step comparison displays the same kind of indeterminacy as biological morphospace. In the finch diagram, the direct distance between two points is a quantity that corresponds to no real relation among specimens. Similarly here. How much does the difference of colour count for, as against the difference is size? What, in other words, is the right relative scaling of these two parameters? Since we rate these parameters differently in different contexts of judgement, there is no *right* answer. In within-exclusion-range comparisons, within colours, for example, the scaling of components is delivered by sub-personal systems in the form of composite experience. Here, scaling is left open. Thus, the direct distance between a large red spot and a small green spot does not mark a measure that is valid across persons, contexts, and criteria of comparison.
>
> Judgements about scaling will also be context-dependent. 'Stroop tests' illustrate this: when confronted with the word 'red' written in blue, observers get confused, and take a longer time to read the word or

identify the colour. This suggests that such an inscription is in some sense more like the word 'blue' than the word 'red' written in red, or perhaps in normal black.

A subject will take a significantly longer time to make the judgement when there is variation in two such parameters than when the variation is confined just to one.

Since the only representationally invariant measures are the component distances, some philosophers say that the difference is a sum of these component distances, each appropriately scaled (Gärdenfors, 2000, 24–6)—something along the following lines:

> Integrated distance = C * distance in colour + D * distance in shape (where 'C' and 'D' are scaling constants that depend on the observer, the context, etc.).

The resulting distance measure is known as the 'city-block metric': to get the overall dissimilarity between two items with respect to both shape and colour, an observer must first traverse the dissimilarity in colour, and then the dissimilarity in shape, just as a city-walker has to traverse the streets and the avenues separately in order to get from one place to another—no diagonal shortcuts.

What can we learn from these differences between comparisons involving several different sensory exclusion ranges and comparisons *within* the exclusion ranges? The comparisons involving more than one exclusion range are made by our epistemic faculties and are subject to the explicit control of contexts of comparison. The comparisons within exclusion ranges, on the other hand—comparisons between different colours, different musical sounds, different tastes, etc.—are automated, delivered by sub-personal system over which we have little or no control. A proper explanation of sensory phenomenology has to include an account of these space-like characteristics of the sensory array; it is necessary to account for the interaction between the components producing new features.

The predictability of sensory comparisons, underwritten by the existence of single qualia at each point of a sensory similarity space, is crucial to the identification of sense qualities by components. As we saw in Chapter 3, section VI, subjects are able to describe sense-qualities by means of quantitative comparisons of their components. After a little practice, they are able, for instance, to imagine a shade of brown that has twice the ratio of *red* to *yellow* as a given target shade. (Byrne 2003 makes the interesting point that though ratios of the basic colour components make sense in this way, absolute quantities do not. There is no such thing as two *browns* which differ from one another in absolute quantities of *black, yellow*, and *red*, as opposed to ratios of these components.)

In similarity spaces that represent two separate exclusion ranges, such comparisons make no sense. It makes no sense, for example, to ask that a coloured spot be so modified as to increase its *red* to *round* ratio by 30 per cent.

What accounts for our ability to identify sense-features by their component structure? This is the topic under investigation in Chapter 5.

5

The Sources of Sensory Similarity

The Göttingen psychologist, Georg Elias Müller attempted to explain sensory similarity by means of four 'axioms' he formulated in 1896. These axioms link sensations with underlying neurophysiological events and processes. Here are some excerpts:

> 1. Every state of consciousness is based upon a material event, a so-called psychophysical process . . .
> 2. An equivalence, similarity, or difference in the character of the sensations corresponds to an equivalence, similarity, or difference in the character of the psychophysical process, and vice versa . . .
> 3. [C]hanges or differences having the same direction in psychophysical processes always correspond to changes or differences of the same direction in sensations. If then a sensation can be changed in direction x, the psychophysical process upon which it is based must also be susceptible to change in that direction, and vice versa. (reprinted in Herrnstein and Boring 1965, 257–8)

Clearly, Müller's axioms are not true a priori. It is not even clear at this stage what they mean. We saw in Chapter 2, section I, that (as Berkeley argued) it makes no sense to say that a sensation resembles its object. It is similarly vacuous to compare a neural process to a sensory experience without further explanation. In Chapter 4, section II, for example, we saw that the similarity space of musical tones is a double helix. Increasing pitch corresponds to upward progression along one of the strands of this figure. What would it mean to say that the underlying neurophysiological process is also a double helix, or that increasing pitch was progress along a helix in this process? What would it mean to say that the process underlying colour perception is variable in three dimensions?

Commenting on Müller's third axiom, Davida Teller remarks

The proposition that similar sensations arise from similar physiological states is involved in discussions of the Benham top phenomenon, when we propose any explanation that assumes that the neural signals produced by the Benham top stimuli must be similar to the signals produced by the chromatic stimuli they resemble. These assumptions are not logical necessities; yet, if one did not make these assumptions, it is not clear how one would go about searching for an explanation for the Benham top phenomenon, or recognize an explanation when one had found it. (2002/1984, 299)

At first glance, it appears that Teller is better off than Müller in that she is at least comparing things in the same category—neural signals to neural signals. On closer examination, however, we find traces of the same obscurity. Her claim is first that Benham's top—a black and white pattern that appears coloured when spun—produces *sensations* similar to those elicited by coloured objects, and second that this can only be explained by showing that Benham's top produces *signals* similar to those produced by 'the chromatic stimuli they resemble'. There are *two* relations of similarity alluded to here, one on the domain of experiences and the other on the domain of neural signals. If two stimuli produce similar sensations, Teller says, then they must produce similar neural signals. Assuming that it is introspectively evident what kind of similarity of sensations is involved here, the question still remains: What kind of similarity of neural signals will suffice to explain the similarity of experiences? These are examples of the questions we will attempt to illuminate, if not definitively answer, below.

Müller's axioms are plausible, as we shall see by the end of section III below, but we will need to clarify them before we can embrace them.

I. Explaining Sensory Similarity

In the traditional paradigm, sensation is regarded as the more or less exact counterpart in consciousness of the energy patterns that affect our outer sensory receptors. In other words, the tradition regards the following principle paramount:

*Similarity of Effect

x and y will appear similar only to the degree that they have physically similar effects on sensory receptors (thus causing these receptors to have physically similar outputs).

Similarity of Effect is at the heart of the Cartesian paradigm; it is the source of the idea that sensation is raw and unprocessed, the output of an analogue measuring device. In an analogue weighing-machine, weight affects an electrically conducting wire monotonically—150 lbs stretches this wire more than 140 lbs and less than 160 lbs; as a direct consequence, the 150 mark on the dial is between 140 and 160. The traditional paradigm supposes that the effect of coloured light or pitch on outer receptors is similarly monotonic, and that this is the source of the sensory ordering we experience. The relationship of tones that we experience as a slide when a vibrating string is lengthened, the relationship of colours across a rainbow: these are supposed to be analogue phenomena, phenomena that result directly from the monotonic effect of ambient energy or our external sensory receptors, phenomena that precede classification. In Chapter 3, section I, we quoted Nelson Goodman saying: 'Where the task is gauging or measuring, the analog instrument is likely to play its chief role in the exploratory stages, before units of measurement have been fixed.' The traditional paradigm goes a bit further: not only does it maintain, in effect, that sensory receptors are 'analog instruments', but holds also that *sensation* is the output of these instruments, the read-out on their faces.

Notwithstanding the strength of such intuitions, Similarity of Effect is false. Here is a counter-example drawn from colour vision. Long-wavelength light signals affect the colour-sensitive cones quite differently from a short-wavelength signal: the former excites the long-wavelength receptors but not the shortwave receptors, while the latter does just the opposite. Yet, these signals have a certain commonality: both appear reddish. Because of this, signals from the opposite ends of the spectrum are perceptually more similar to one another than either to a signal in the middle, which might appear greenish or yellowish—see Figure 8, which shows how the spectrum is aligned in HBS space. For another simple example of the failure of Similarity of Effect, see the discussion of similarities of musical tones towards the end of Chapter 3, section II: two tones an octave apart may sound more similar to one another than two separated by a fifth, even though the latter pair are closer in frequency. Similarly—an example discussed in Chapter 9—the sounds that we hear as constituting a single phone like /d/ in the words 'dig' and 'dog' are acoustically quite disparate.

The divergence between Similarity of Effect and sensed similarity should not be surprising at this stage of the argument. In Chapter 1 we encountered the idea that sensory classification need not reflect any pre-existing mind-independent similarity—for example, an aspect of similarity important for physical prediction. Hayek's sorting machine (Chapter 1, section I.2) placed an apparently heterogeneous collection of balls into the same receptacle: 'the machine will always place the balls with a diameter of 16, 18, 28, 31, 32, and 40 mm in a receptacle marked A, the balls with a diameter of 17, 22, 30, and 35 in a receptacle marked B, and so forth.' We can imagine that this machine sorts balls by diameter, and then uses some routing mechanism to send balls of predetermined diameters into particular receptacles. It is this final destination that constitutes sensory classification: it is not necessarily relevant how the balls enter the machine.

Suppose that sensory *similarity* corresponds to the *proximity* of the receptacles in Hayek's machine: suppose that the balls in the receptacle marked A are experienced as more similar to those in B than they are to those in C, and so on. Then, the similarity relationships among the balls would have little to

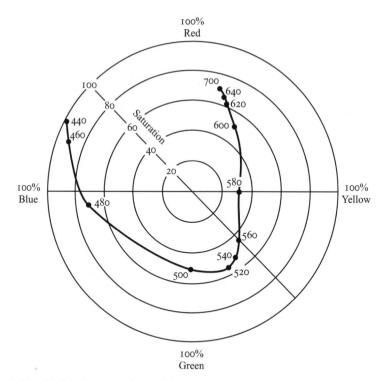

FIG. 8 The Visible Spectrum in HBS Space.

Source: Hurwich (1981, 84) with author's permission.

do with the relationships among their diameters, or with how these diameters interact with the machine's receptors. Hayek says: 'The fact that a ball is placed by the machine into a particular receptacle thus forms the sole criterion for assigning it into a particular class.' One might hold in an extension of this conclusion, that the sole reason why two things appear similar is that the sensory system assigns them to classes that it places close to one another. The objection to this extreme conclusion is the same as that which was advanced against Hayek's Extreme Nominalism in Chapter 1, section I.4. An organism's sensory system is constrained by various environmental and functional considerations, and cannot simply impose on the domain of representation any arbitrary similarity structure. Though similarity is created by the system, it is constrained. This is an outline of the framework within which we will try to explain observed failures of Similarity of Effect.

In the case of colour vision, it so happens that the system is interested (among other things) in whether the signal reaching the eye contains more energy at the ends of the visible spectrum or in the middle. To determine this, it subtracts the energy received at the two ends from the energy received in the middle of the spectrum. Let us call the resultant quantity *R*. It is defined roughly as follows:

R
A* (energy in long waveband + energy in short waveband) − B*energy in middle waveband (A and B are scaling constants).

If the result of this differencing operation is positive, then there is more energy at the ends of the visible spectrum than in the middle. ('More' is an inexact but serviceable way of speaking, since the scaling constant B is different from A.) If the result of the differencing is negative, there is more energy in the middle of the visible spectrum than at the ends. (Why is the system interested in the value of this particular variable? Perhaps for no better reason than that it is a convenient way of maximizing the information extracted from the outputs of overlapping colour receptors.)

R is an example of a numerical data-extraction process referred to in Chapter 3, section IV. The results of this process are made available to the perceiver by means of different experiential qualia. Positive values of *R* are signalled by a reddish look, the greater the positive value, the more reddish the look. Correspondingly, negative values of *R* are signalled by a greenish look, the greater the negative value, the more greenish something looks. (This is oversimplified. The correspondence between opponent processing and colour experience is much more complicated than this: see Mollon and Jordan 1997.)

Similarity of Effect is falsified by the use of measurements like *R*. Stimuli that are similar with respect to looking reddish may not have similar effects on the outer receptors: stimuli that stimulate the long-wave but not the short-wave receptors, and those that stimulate the short-wave but not the long-wave receptors both yield positive values of *R*, and as a consequence, they both look reddish. Thus, violet at one end of the spectrum and red at the other are more similar to one another than either is to green in the middle (since green is component-incompatible with red). *R* is an odd classificatory instrument, no doubt, but since sensory systems construct categories that are useful to the organism, whether or not these categories correspond to the categories of physics, this should be something we can take in our stride. Later, we'll question the relevance of asking whether such categories correspond to those of physics, but for now let us just try to assimilate the consequences of accepting that *physical* similarity—similarity defined in terms of some physical variable—is not mirrored in experienced similarity.

In the light of operations such as *R*, it has been suggested that Similarity of Effect should be replaced by the following principle:

Similarity of Process
Two stimuli appear to be similar because the sensory process they occasion results in physically similar output.

Müller advanced just such an idea. His second psychophysical axiom reads in part: 'An equivalence, similarity, or difference in the character of the sensations corresponds to an equivalence, similarity, or difference in the character of the psychophysical process, and vice versa.' Given the kind of phenomenon we have been discussing, we cannot simply assume that stimuli that send similar signals to the sensory receptors will be treated as similar. So one might think that it is the *output* of sensory systems that determines similarity, not the input. Note, however, that Similarity of Process explicitly juxtaposes similarity relations defined on incommensurable domains. Thus, it is too weak. As we shall see in section II below, there are far too many relations of physical similarity for this principle to have any bite: two output states might be similar in brain-location, in strength, in the shape of the cells in which they occur, and so on. Similarity of Process makes a claim about physical similarity explaining similarity of appearance, but we still have no idea what relation of physical similarity is intended. Let us try and tolerate this vagueness for a time.

It is worth noting that, even if replaced by Similarity of Process, Similarity of Effect does not completely lose its grip. After all, sensory systems pass information from their outer receptors down through several layers of data-processing. As we have been saying, this data-processing will often involve treating highly similar inputs differently, or highly disparate inputs similarly. However, even in the presence of such manipulations, similarities in receptoral activity are often passed on passively; to treat adjacent signals differently takes, as it were, a deliberate decision, and such 'decisions' are relatively few and far between.

This is evident in cases like the following. My office wall is off-white illuminated from the windows on one side. There are subtle differences of shading, but overall any one part of the wall looks similar in colour to any other. Why? Because the different parts of the wall are sending similar signals to the eye. One could put the point like this: the more similar are the effects of two stimuli on sensory receptors, the higher is the *prior probability* that they will be similar to one another. If two stimuli send virtually the same message to the eye, it is very likely (other things being equal) that they will look similar to one another. Thus, note that in Figure 8, neighbouring wavelengths are perceived as similar, though the ends of the visible spectrum curve around.

To summarize then: Similarity of receptor response may often propagate through the system. For this reason, one can expect *some*, often substantial, correlation between the effect that stimuli have on sensory receptors and their appearance, though, as response condition *R* illustrates, this correlation will often break down: small (often purposeful) distortions of the neurophysiological signal can accumulate over the range of signals received by the system. While Similarity of Process is the overriding principle, Similarity of Effect often constitutes a partial explanation why two stimuli happen to be processed similarly.

We have made some progress. Similarity of Effect takes ambient energy to be the sole locus of sensed similarity; Similarity of Process recognizes the signal-processing contributions of the system, and is thus a better principle. However, Similarity of Process is ultimately unsatisfying. It does not *explain* the output of sensory systems, but merely asserts that it arises from the sensory process—Similarity of Process is deficient in exactly the same way as Hayek's principle that the system's activity determines classification. It makes sense to ask *why* things evoke the same process, i.e. *why* they are co-classified, why they look similar to one another. The inquiry that such a question occasions will lead to more fundamental principles. (Müller himself was merely correlating sensory experience with neural phenomena. This was the point of the axiom just stated: he was not concerned, in this context anyway, with explaining similarity of process.) Similarity of Process should be regarded as an explanandum rather than as an explanation. It is an explanandum in exactly the way that the Sensory Classification Thesis is: given that a sensory system creates certain classes, we may ask why it does so.

II. Similarity and Its Woes

Sensory similarity must be explained in the context of certain puzzling features of the logic of similarity relations in general. Important studies of similarity by Nelson Goodman (1972/1970), and Amos Tversky (1977) show that the similarity judgements that people make are sensitive to the perspective and interests of the person who is evaluating similarity—we shall be presenting these studies in the present section. Now, we saw in the previous chapter (section IV) that certain experienced similarities are robust; they do not vary with subjective attitudes taken up by the perceiver. However, there does not seem to be good reason for thinking that sensory similarity is exempt from the vagaries that Goodman and Tversky find in the logic of similarity in general. The robustness of sensory similarity must, therefore, be explained in a way that accommodates the interest-sensitivity of similarity in general.

Let's review the reasons for saying that similarity judgements are sensitive to perspective. Intuitively, we expect similarity to behave like a measure of overlap. Start with an individual **a**. The criterion of this individual being more similar to another individual **b** than to **c** in a certain respect is that there are more behaviours, responses, and effects that **a** shares with **b** than with **c**. Consider similarity with respect to weight. Two things that are closely similar in weight will share the following sorts of responses and effects: there will be more people who can lift one easily if they can lift the other; there will be more surfaces that are deformed by the one resting on them than are deformed by the other. And so on. Of course, similarity in this particular respect does not imply similarity in any other. Two things may be similar in weight, but not be similar in colour. The behaviours, responses, and effects that count towards similarity in colour are different from those that make up similarity in weight.

Since similarity is based on this sort of overlap, and since overlap is symmetric—C is the overlap of A and B if and only if it is the overlap of B and A—one might expect that similarity would be symmetric. In other words, if **a** shares a certain set of responses with **b**, then **b** must share them with **a**. So whatever the degree of similarity (in this respect) **a** bears to **b**, the same degree of similarity must hold between **b** and **a**. One would also expect similarity to be objective and invariant from situation to situation, since the behaviours that constitute the domain for overlap seem themselves to be objective and invariant.

Now, it turns out that if you ask people simply to make similarity judgements where more than one sensory exclusion range, or *type* of sense-feature, is involved—ask them flat out whether one thing is more similar to another than a third, or ask them to group things by similarity, without mentioning the respect of similarity—the logical expectations based on overlap are not met.

> It turns out, for example, that many psychologically relevant sorts of similarity are not symmetrical. To adapt an example from Tversky (1977), Canada reminds most foreigners of the US, but the US does not always remind them of Canada. If you were asked which one of the following was the closest match with Canada—the US, China, Russia—the chances are that you would pick the US. But if you were asked to match one of the following with the US—Canada, China, Russia—the chances are much lower that you would pick Canada (particularly if you are not Canadian). This is because (to non-Canadians especially) the US has a large number of salient features, only a small portion of which belong to Canada, while Canada has a relatively few salient features, many of which it shares with the US. It follows that in response to the simple question, 'Which is the most similar to the US?', you will answer 'Canada' only if the features that first come to your mind are those that the US shares with Canada—and since there are many features that you could pick in the case of the US, the chances are higher that you will pick something that is not shared by Canada. This shows that the kind of similarity that underlies psychological association is 'path-dependent'—i.e. dependent on the starting point of the associative process—and hence not symmetric.

> Assessments of similarity also depend on point of view. For there is such a plethora of comparisons to be made amongst things, that, as Goodman tells us, anything can be *overall* as similar to another thing as it is to any third thing—for any respect in which the first is more similar to the second, one can adduce a different measure of similarity that makes the first more

similar to the third. Normally, you might be inclined to adjudge two twins, A and B, more similar to one another than either is to an unrelated third person C. But suppose that (only) one of the twins A belongs to the same college, club, or regiment as both you and the third person, C. It might well be that in such a case, the rules, traditions, shared history, and dress of this collegial body might (from your point of view) trump A's physical similarity to the outsider B. In this case, you might think—at least in some contexts—that A is more similar to C than to B. Any judgement of similarity that distinguishes one pair from another is in this way dependent on bias—on a selection of respects of similarity relevant to the comparison task being undertaken and the person undertaking it. Classifications based on similarity are not absolute.

As we saw in section IV of the previous chapter, there is no unique measure of integrated sensory similarity. Similarity in respect of colour, of shape, of size, etc. cannot be non-arbitrarily combined into a single measure of overall similarity. Conversely, similarity in a given respect— for example, similarity with respect to colour or shape—cannot unambiguously be distilled from overall similarity, and this is a task hardly worth performing, in any case, since the latter notion shifts with context.

Why do people make similarity judgements that so depart from the logic of overlap? Most likely not because the logic of overlap is inapplicable to similarity, but because the questions these people were asked do not properly specify parameters of evaluation. When you are asked which is most similar to Canada, the US, Russia, or China, you are left to decide similarity with respect to what. And you will make a decision based on your frame of mind at that particular instant. When you make the converse judgement, you may well choose a different parameter, and thus arrive at a different answer. If you were asked to evaluate similarity relative to some precisely specified parameter— size, wealth, governmental system, or geographical location—your answer would be much more predictable.

This is why judgements of overall similarity—similarity judgements in which more than one parameter of comparison is involved—are so disorderly. On some occasions, the component parameters of overall similarity might be clear, but how they are to be combined ill-specified. When asked to compare things which differ in both colour and shape, people will weigh differences in colour against differences in shape differently in different contexts. Hence, they will arrive at different results. On other occasions, the parameters themselves may not be well specified. Here is an example of a *well*-specified parameter. If you are asked to judge similarity with respect to weight, you will do certain predictable things—you will try to lift things, or (if they are similar in size and shape) observe the indentations they make on similar surfaces—and though there are well-known errors in this regard (for example, people tend to overestimate the weight of large things), outcomes are reasonably orderly. For contrast, here is an example of an ill-specified parameter. If you are asked to compare people with respect to intelligence or beauty, all sorts of incoherence will result, since what counts as intelligence in one context may not correlate with what counts in another; again, some of a person's features may make for beauty, others may not.

Now, we have seen that to a great extent, sensory similarity *within* an exclusion range like colour, shape, or pitch, is exempt from situational or perspectival fluctuations.[1] Judgements of similarity with respect to colour, like judgements of similarity with respect to weight, are broadly consistent from one person to another, and from one context to another. This means that sensory similarity is well-specified, as is similarity with respect to a physical quantity, by contrast with similarity with respect to intelligence or beauty: that is, one can use sensory experience to make similarity judgements in this domain in a reasonably consistent and orderly way. Should one conclude that similarity is absolute here, and that perspectival influences can be disregarded?

This, in effect, is the suggestion made by Alex Byrne (2003, 641): he claims that the sensed similarity of *blue* to *purple* is 'genuine', while any judged similarity of *blue* to *yellow* is 'gerrymandered'. This is a wrong move. The moral that we should take from Goodman and Tversky is not merely that similarity is perspectival when it fluctuates, but that there is no such thing as similarity *tout court*. Byrne speaks, for example, of aspects of similarity that 'will be evident at the level of the canonical physical description' (642, n. 5). Why should such aspects of similarity be privileged? 'Similar' is not a term that appears in the canonical terminology of physics. *Physical* similarity can be defined in many ways, and it is not clear why some ways of defining it should be thought preferable to others. Why, for example, should we regard similarity with respect to mass (closeness in numerical value of mass) more 'genuine' than similarity in weight (closeness in numerical value of force exerted on a body in a particular gravitational field)? It is true that 'mass' is more fundamental in physics than weight; nevertheless, similarity in weight can be defined as unambiguously as similarity in mass. Isn't a clear and unambiguous definition enough for an aspect of similarity to be 'genuine'? Why not? What grounds could we have for preferring one well-specified respect of similarity to another?

Two things that are similar in one respect may be dissimilar in another. And the consequence is that we need to specify what exactly we mean. *Blue* is more similar to *purple* than to *yellow* in that they are so experienced; *blue* is more similar to *yellow* than to *purple* in that the first two, but not the third,

---

[1] Dustin Stokes (unpublished) urges that feedback mechanisms involving motivation and desire may change how we see things—he calls this 'orectic perception'. This, and attentional changes in perception, are important phenomena, but their effects on perception are relatively small compared to their effect on conscious and deliberate assessments of similarity.

occur in the Swedish flag. Byrne would perhaps attempt to accommodate this flip-flop by calling the first relation of similarity 'genuine', and the latter 'gerrymandered'. But this is a dubious move, since both relations are well-specified. Neither similarity is more 'genuine' than the other. The right way to accommodate the variance is by explicitly introducing the parameter of evaluation. *Blue* is more similar to *purple* than to *yellow* with respect to sense experience; it is more similar to *yellow* than to *purple* from the point of view of Swedish heraldry.

Sensory similarity is not ontologically privileged; it is no more genuine than any other kind. Why then is it stable? (Robert Nozick [2001, ch. 2] shines a bright light on questions of this sort.) It was suggested earlier that the illogic of people's similarity-judgements might stem from their taking up different respects of similarity, and weighting these differently, in different situations. By contrast, our sensory systems always respond to situations in the same way: they process incoming data in ways that are inflexible and broadly consistent across organisms of the same species. The 'perspective' that these systems adopt hardly ever changes, and so with very few qualifications, they deliver pretty much the same similarity relations. This is why sensory classification is stable; this is why it can serve as a basis for conditioning, learning, induction, and so on. Suppose you assessed 'beauty' by the rigid application of certain quantitative criteria. Your assessments would then be consistent from occasion to occasion. But this would not mean that your conception of *beauty* was objectively any more 'genuine' or more well-founded than a more subjective approach. The consistency of your judgements simply reflects the rigidity of your assessments.

The consistency of sensory similarity judgements thus does not show by itself that they are 'genuine' or objectively valid. But we still have no good reason to adopt the opposed position, namely that sensory similarity is purely 'subjective', solely the creation of sensory systems. Sensory systems may be biased processors of information; they may fasten on aspects of the situation that are of particular interest to the organism they serve. However, the fact that a report is biased does not necessarily imply that it is fabricated. Bias implies that some things are given importance for reasons peculiar to the subject and other things are downplayed. It is plausible to think that evolution makes sensory systems biased in this sense. This does not imply that what they report is flat out false. So there is room for realism in the idea that sensory systems are biased. We'll return to this theme in section IV below and again in Chapter 8.

III. The Internal Origins of Sensory Similarity

What exactly do sensory systems contribute to sensory similarities? Do they simply create similarities? Or do they record similarities that exist independently of themselves? We'll explore these questions further by examining the origins of sensory similarity spaces such as those described in the previous chapter.

One interesting answer to the above questions can be taken from the work of C. R. Gallistel (1990, ch. 14). His argument can be summarized in three propositions:

(1) There is a limitation on the precision with which neurons represent conditions in their receptive fields.

(2) In ancient times, evolution solved one problem posed by this limitation—the problem of how to locate a stimulus in space—by adopting a certain form of spatial mapping.

(3) Later, evolution extended and adapted this method to other non-spatial sensory representations. This is why the system represents the inter-relations of sensory features in ways appropriate to space.

Let us examine these three propositions more closely.

1. *Limited Representational Precision*
The representational system used for spatial mappings is forced by a certain limitation on the precision with which neurons represent information. We'll illustrate this by means of a contrast. Think first of a measuring instrument that displays its reading on an array of light-emitting diodes (LEDs). Suppose it is a speedometer on a bicycle. The LEDs are arranged next to numerals in an increasing sequence:

$$0 \quad 5 \quad 10 \quad 15 \quad 20 \quad 25 \quad 30 \quad 35 \quad 40$$
$$\circ \quad \circ \quad \bullet \quad \circ \quad \circ \quad \circ \quad \circ \quad \circ \quad \circ$$

When the bicycle is running at 10 km per hour, the LED next to the figure 10 glows (•), and all the rest are off (o), as represented above. If the bicycle had been running at 15 k.p.h., the LED next to 15 would have glowed, and the rest would have been off. Somewhere between 10 and 15 the first light would be extinguished, and the second light would come on.

Call this *narrow-band tuning*. This kind of display has two key characteristics. The first is that one and only one LED lights up at a time, namely the one corresponding to the speed-range that the instrument has detected. The second is a consequence of this. The range of the 10 light has to extend from where the 5 light goes off to where the 15 comes on. Thus the 10 light encompasses a wide range of speeds. This form of representation is quite imprecise.

Now, suppose that because of some intrinsic property of the LEDs or of the speed-detecting system, *many* LEDs light up for any given speed of the bicycle, but with different strengths—weak (.), medium (ø), strong (•)—while some stay off (o). So we might get a display like this:

0	5	10	15	20	25	30	35	40
o	o	◉	●	◉	◉	o	o	o

One might suppose that each light indicates a probability that the bicycle is going at the corresponding speed: in the above display, the 15 light expresses the strong probability that the bicycle is running at 15 k.p.h., the 10, 20, and 25 lights express medium probability for their values, and so on. Taken as a whole, this pattern is biased below the median value, 20, by the highly confident 15, and above its strongest value, 15, by the preponderance of readings at the high end, though these are not as strongly confident. Further, the display would have been symmetric around 17.5 if 20 had lit up strongly, and so the speed here must be lower. We might guess that this display corresponds to 17 k.p.h. or so.

This illustrates *broadband tuning*: each LED is tuned to many values; each responds to some values at maximum strength, but to many others at less than maximum strength. Conversely, many LEDs light up with different strengths at each speed. We estimate the speed of the bicycle by calculating the weighted average of displayed values. Notice that this way of estimating the speed of the bicycle leads to a value intermediate between the discrete values inscribed on the display. Thus, the *whole* display is capable of indicating values in between those that its components indicate. Even if the individual LEDs are imprecise with respect to what speed they indicate, the entire display is relatively fine-tuned. To revert to terminology used in Chapter 2, section III, broadband tuning is more closely packed than its inputs are. They are, in this sense, more nearly analogue. Further, given certain assumptions about how well behaved these LEDs are with regard to the strength of their responses, it may well be that taken as a whole this display is a more accurate indicator of speed than the one that is narrow-band tuned. Broadband tuning can be regarded, therefore, as a way of overcoming the representational limitations of individual LEDs. The only drawback is that it takes some computation to figure out what the display as a whole indicates: look at the reasoning that took us to the conclusion that the broadband speedometer display above indicates 17 k.p.h. Such reasoning is, in effect, a form of analogue conversion, as defined in Chapter 3, section IV.

Now, neurons in the brain are broadband tuned. That is, they respond to a number of different values, but with different strengths representing different 'confidence levels'. This is a limitation in their individual expressive precision. The superior colliculus (SC) is a mid-brain structure concerned with the location of stimuli for the purpose of diverting our visual gaze and attention to places where some sudden movement is occurring. An individual neuron in SC responds most strongly when there is motion in its receptive field. Let's consider a particular neuron in SC, the receptive field of which

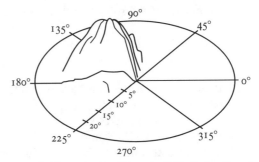

Neurons respond with varying 'confidence levels' to the location of a
stimulus. Response depends on the vector sum, not on the strongest response.

FIG. 9 Broadband Tuning.

Source: Adapted from Gallistel (1990, 483) with author's permission.

happens to be in the 'north-west' portion of the visual field. Call this neuron
NW. If *NW* were narrow-band tuned, it would not respond under any other
condition. But this is not how neurons work in fact. Generally speaking, *NW*
will also respond to motions in other locations, but less strongly—for
instance, it might fire when motion is present in the 'west north-west' or
'north north-west' portions of the visual field, but in these circumstances it
will respond less strongly than when motion is detected at its preferred location. The response range of the neuron overlaps—a number of different neurons will fire when the north-west motion is present, but all with strengths
weaker than that of *NW* (see Figure 9).

Thus, sensory processing does not result in just one neuron being activated,
but in a pattern of activation of several neurons, all firing with different
strengths. Gallistel states the principle of broadband tuning in this way: 'The
activity of an individual unit is an "assertion," given with a "confidence" specified by the firing rate' (1990, 491)—as we noted in Chapter 2, section III,
neurons assign a 'Bayesian' or subjective probability value to the propositions
that constitute their response conditions. *NW* can be interpreted as 'asserting'
that motion is detected in its receptive field, with a confidence level proportionate to its firing rate. Other neurons will fire at the same time, each 'voting'
for their own locations, but with different levels of confidence.

2. *Spatial Representation*
How is a system supposed to respond to a broadband display? How is it supposed to discern what value the whole display indicates? Gallistel supposes that
some sort of additive or averaging operation is used in determining the cumulative effect of such a display. Here is an example of an additive operation. Let
us suppose that each unit commands the system to react in a certain way.

Let us suppose further that when *two* units are active, their joint effect on the system is as if the two had been acting at the same time. For instance, suppose that the broadband speedometer display discussed above is connected to a accelerator-brake cruise-control system which attempts to keep a vehicle moving along at precisely 20 k.p.h. This result might be achieved if each LED below 20 commanded the system to accelerate at a rate proportionate to the difference between its value and 20, and each LED above 20 similarly commanded the system to brake. All of the accelerate/brake impulses act on the system simultaneously. By adjusting how strongly each unit contributes to these effects in proportion to its activation level, we might get a reasonably effective resolution of the display. Then the output of the entire display would be a function of the speed of the vehicle. Cumulatively, these operations would be roughly equivalent to an averaging estimate, such as the one provided earlier. The interactions among the neurons would amount to a kind of analogue computer which calculates the value indicated by the whole display. Enabling this kind of computation is another reason for the (near) analogue character of the medium of representation noted in Chapter 3, section IV.

Now what about multidimensional variables? There are parts of the brain devoted to localizing stimuli in space. The superior colliculus directs the eye to new stimuli as they suddenly pop up in the field of view. SC simply maps the retina. Any sudden change on the retina induces units in the corresponding locations in SC to fire. But the SC map is broadband tuned, as are all feature-maps in the brain. Each neuron codes a stimulus-position, *and, proportionate to its strength, influences the eye to move to that position.* The position coding is two-dimensional, since it is a mapping of the retina. The impulse sent to the muscles of the eye will also be two dimensional; it will contain a message about the *direction* in which the muscle is to move, as well as the displacement from north. The cumulative effect of the broadband display will be the summation of all the messages with regard to these two directions. In one dimension, simple addition suffices. Here, we need two directions represented separately, added separately, and to send out two separate directional messages to the effectors, one for movement in the up-down dimension, and one for movement in the left-right direction. In short, we need something like (suitably scaled) vector addition. Just as the entire broadband speedometer display denotes a single value for speed, so the entire SC map displays a single value for the position of the changing stimulus. The process of vector-addition that stands behind the action reflects this single result—the movement of the eye in the direction of the new stimulus.

3. *Extending Spatial Representation*
Colour experience is a composite of information carried by separate channels in precortical stages of visual processing. Why does this information need to be integrated? Why is there a unified experience corresponding to each

ordered set of values for red-green, blue-yellow, and black-white dimensions of colour, instead of three different features belonging to separate exclusion ranges? Given that these values are carried in separate channels in the initial stages of colour processing, colour information *could* have been presented as three separate sense features, instead of one. Why was all this information combined? Presumably the answer has to do with how we use colour information; the use of this information is enhanced—made more reliable, made more sensitive—by collating the information carried by all of the channels. For example, as Barlow (1972) suggests, colour experience is not merely a sum of information available in each channel: it is more strongly determined by the channel that is most sensitive to the colour-range of a given stimulus. It may be useful to know that an object satisfies the condition R discussed above, but it is presumably more useful for various purposes to assess this information against the background of how it fares with respect to the other colour channels as well. Primates use colour information for contrast in fine patterns, for the identification and reidentification of objects, and for signalling. Presumably, natural selection found that these tasks are better performed when colour information is integrated. It is not a necessary truth that this should be so; we can only infer that evolutionary trial and error discovered that it was so.

Now, given that colour information is going (for whatever reason) to be combined into a single composite, the question arises how this is to be done. Given broadband tuning for the read-out of each of the three channels, how is the system to deliver a single value for the integrated feature? Gallistel makes an intriguing, though conjectural, suggestion regarding the coding of such features as colour: that it derives from the way that the brain represents *space*, actual space. In the case of location-coding discussed above, the brain uses a system that allows the eye-muscles automatically to resolve the broadband display and to move correctly to the location of the stimulus. The mapping from retina to SC preserves spatial detail, and the translation to muscular action has spatial correctness conditions. In the case of colour-vision, there is no corresponding problem of resolving a broadband display for the purpose of muscular control. But Gallistel speculates that the human brain simply adapts the locational coding used in evolutionarily old areas like the superior colliculus to the resolution of broadband displays generally:

The facts about color vision suggest how deeply the nervous system may be committed to representing stimuli as points in descriptive spaces of modest dimensionality. It does this even for spectral composition, which does not lend itself to such a representation. (1990, 518).

The claim is that the different dimensions of colour-experience are arranged in a space-like map in the brain, as illustrated in Figure 10, and that the vector addition operation process used in the SC-map is simply readapted to resolving broadband tuning in the colour maps. In other words, vector

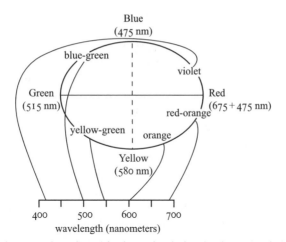

Gallistel suggests that colour vision is copying the locational systems when it creates a map of colours.

FIG.10 Colour-tuned Cells within the 'Blobs' of the Primary Visual Cortex.

Source: Gallistel (1990, 516) with the author's permission.

addition in colour vision is just a retooling of vector addition in motion-guiding parts of vision which have to deal, quite literally, with a space. *Note that in implementing the colour map, the system automatically scales the different components of sensory colour.* The option of discretionary flexibility of scaling is lost once evolution was committed to this form of combining the components. If the information from the three channels had been kept segregated, the colour information in different channels would have constituted three different exclusion ranges, and then colour-perceiving organisms would have been stuck with the disadvantages and advantages of discretionary scaling with its city-block metric (see Chapter 3, section IV). This freedom was lost, long before humans came onto the scene, when the system was designed to combine the components automatically.

In the spatial map, the result of resolving broadband tuning was a single motor command to move the eye in a certain direction. In colour maps, the result is analogously a single *experience* corresponding to location in the colour map. The similarity-space of colour derives its structural characteristics, then, from the actual space to which eye-movements and the like are adapted, not from any characteristics that colour possesses in itself:

The brain's representation of color may indicate its general approach to the problem of representation because this way of representing reflectance spectra is in no way dictated by the formal properties of those spectra or by constraints on the behavioral outputs. (*ibid.*, 519–20).

The use of space-like representational form is not dictated by external constraints on spatial coding—as it was in the case of locational coding in SC—but simply as a means of resolving broadband tuning. A point in the space-like arrangement of colour is an ordered triple of values corresponding to the dimensions of colour experience. These values have no intrinsic connection to one another: in this respect, they are just like the axes of biological morphospace discussed in Chapter 4, section III, and unlike physical space. However, in order to resolve broadband tuning and enable analogue computation, the system introduces operations that compute complex functions of the dimensions. This gives meaning to oblique directions and distance measures in the space of colour. With physical space, direct distances and directions exist first, and are simply reflected by vector notation. Here the choice of representational form dictates the fixity of these measures.

As emphasized earlier, Gallistel's suggestion is conjectural. Whether it turns out to be correct or not, however, the idea that space-like coding is useful for the purpose of resolving broadband tuning is illustrative of a hypothesis that traces the resemblance ordering of sense-features to the integration of information carried by distinct colour channels in a single feature-map. It is reasonably well-accepted that these distinct colour channels *are* recombined into a single map *somewhere* in the visual pathway in between the lateral geniculate nucleus and V4 (see Chatterjee and Callaway 2003, who cite DeValois et al. 2000). Gallistel's idea has the attraction that it diagnoses the need for such information-integration to characteristics and functioning of the sensory system, rather than to characteristics of the stimulus domain— attractive because (as he rightly says) the stimulus domain seems not to 'lend itself to such a representation', at least not independently of the characteristics of the processing system.

There is a single experience corresponding to each combination of values for the dark-light, blue-yellow, red-green channels because this makes it possible to conduct vector-summation operations on such combinations. Vector representation is not necessary for the representation of colour, but given that it is implemented in this case, the invariance of direct distances is a necessary consequence. The existence of integrated colour comparisons is not an *absolute* representational invariant, but invariant only given the kind of system natural selection has thrown up.

We now have a clarification of Müller's psychophysical axioms, quoted at the beginning of this chapter. These axioms turn out to have an unexpectedly literal interpretation. When psychophysical measurements of the sort described in Chapter 4, section II yield a similarity space in n dimensions, it is likely that this space is isomorphic to an n-dimensional map of the sort just described. This map is the locus of the 'analogue conversion' of digitized or numerically calculated sensory information that was described in Chapter 2, section III. It need not literally be a spatial array, in the way that Gallistel imagines the colour map to be, but it will represent the shape of experienced similarity in some functional way. It is possible that certain additional elements of variation will express themselves in non-spatial dimensions of variation in the underlying neurophysiological map. For instance, the loudness of musical notes is not represented in Shepard's double helix, and may correspond to the level of activity of units in the tonal map (cf. Müller: '[W]ith a raising or lowering of the intensity of a sensation, the psychophysical process increases or lessens, and vice versa'). But we may hypothesize that each exclusion range is represented by a map, and that directions within this map correspond to some important dimensions of variation within the exclusion range.

IV. Sensory Similarity and Correspondence Realism

Looking ahead to Part III, let us briefly preview the issue of realism. We can put one question aside here. As we have seen (Chapter 1, section I. 7), there is a traditional divide between those who think that colour is a property of sensations, and those who think that it is a property of distal stimuli: the former are anti-realists in one important sense; the latter are realists. In the next section, and more fully in Part V, we come down firmly in the latter camp: sensory classes are classes of stimuli; sensations label them. So one form of irrealism is dismissed immediately: contrary to phenomenalists like Carnap (1928) and Goodman (1977/1951), *blue* is not a class of sensations (see McGilvray (1994), however, for a recent defence of the phenomenalist position).

Here, however, is another pair of questions concerning realism—a positive answer to either question constitutes what we may call *Correspondence Realism*.

> Does the classificatory basis for sensory classes reflect some system-independent property of distal stimuli?
> Does the experienced similarity of stimuli correspond to some similarity relation that can be specified in a system-independent way?

It might seem that Gallistel's hypothesis would imply that the answer to the second question is negative. For Gallistel maintains that the similarity ordering of sensory classes is a device that the sensory system uses to solve certain internal problems, and while it is useful in affording us a grasp of sense features relative to one another, it may not reflect the similarity metric that a physicist (for instance) would choose. And this would suggest that sensory classes also fail to correspond to system-independent properties.

This is how many philosophers (most influentially, C. L. Hardin 1984) argue. They claim that the non-correspondence of colour similarity space to physical similarities of wavelength, reflectance, etc. shows that *colours* (as well as colour similarity relations) are 'in the head'. Such irrealist arguments are discussed in greater detail in Chapter 8, section II. For the moment, I want simply to show that irrealist conclusions do not follow from positions like Gallistel's. Even if stimuli are grouped together for system-related reasons, there may still be some correspondence between system-generated categories and those that exist outside.

Begin by recalling this numerical variable R calculated by neurons involved in the processing of colour information:

> R
>
> A*(energy in long waveband + energy in short waveband) − B*energy in middle waveband (A and B are scaling constants)

Clearly, R is an idiosyncratically chosen quantity: it is not forced on the system by external realities. Does this mean that it marks a similarity relation with no external significance?

We need to distinguish three claims about the external significance of a quantity like R.

> A. The reason for selecting resemblances based on R is 'subjective' in the sense that it depends on the evolutionary history of the organism and its kind, rather than any property of the stimulus domain existing independently of evolution.
>
> B. The classifications that arise out of R have no place in physics.
>
> C. There is no way of stating R in the language of physics. That is, R corresponds to no physically specifiable quantity.

We have already conceded that A is true, and A gives B credence: most biological categories are outside the scope of physics. So let us concede B as well. Even so, B does not imply C. In fact, C is clearly false: R *is* physically specified—just look at the definition above. But there is another point to be considered. Though a sensory class is created by the activity of a sensory system—this is the content of the Sensory Ordering Thesis and the principle of Similarity of Process, above—this might not be the end of the story. Two things may not be similar *only* because they are treated similarly by the sensory process. There might be something external that explains and justifies the sensory process.

Here is one example of a principle that attempts to explain Similarity of Process.

Similarity of Functional Relevance
If x and y are similar from the point of view of an organism's way of life, then the organism *may* gain an evolutionary advantage if its sensory systems treat them as similar to one another.

Similarity of Functional Relevance is, obviously, neither an absolute principle nor a complete one. It offers no guarantee that the co-classification of functionally similar stimuli will lead to an advantage, and in any case it is neither necessary, nor in many cases even possible, that all such evolutionary advantages will be realized. Nevertheless, Similarity of Functional Relevance clearly does have a role in explaining a number of sensory phenomena.

For example:

> Primate cone-cells are 'tuned' to enhance the similarity among fruit in a certain class, and to exaggerate their difference from foliage. This makes the fruit stand out against a background of foliage. The resulting ease of spotting edible fruit even at a distance serves foraging monkeys well. (This example is discussed further in Chapter 7, section II.)

> The human speech perception module is designed to categorize phonemes according to the muscular 'gestures' that speakers use to produce them, even though the sounds that encode a single phoneme may be acoustically quite diverse (see Chapter 9, section I).

> Certain characteristic phenomena serve as danger signals for animals that are prey. For instance a large shadow cast by an overhead object leads small mammals to freeze or run for cover. Obviously, these shadows may be a diverse lot in terms of darkness, size, shape, and so on. The 'looming' characteristic that serves as a danger signal is an example of what J. J. Gibson calls a 'higher-order invariant', and has to be extracted from receptor activity patterns by active data-processing.

> Two surfaces of very different brightness will appear to have the same colour when contextual clues make it likely that the difference of brightness is explained by differences of illumination rather than of reflectance. When, on the other hand, contextual clues suggest that the difference of signal is due to the reflectance of the surface, the same surfaces look as if they are differently illuminated. This is related to the phenomenon of colour constancy (see Chapter 6).[2]

Similarity of Functional Relevance qualifies Similarity of Effect, for not everything that affects the sensory receptors similarly will play similar roles in an organism's way of life, and not everything that is similar in functional

---

[2] It used to be thought that this phenomenon is wholly explainable in terms of certain properties of cells reacting to the *boundaries* of the colour contrast—see Clark (1993, 21)—and the adaptation of a cell to temporally extended stimulation. Psychologists held in effect that there is no functional explanation for Similarity of Process. However, Surajit Nundy and Dale Purves (2002) and Purves and R. Beau Lotto (2003, ch. 3) show convincingly that something like Similarity of Functional Relevance is involved: the system is trying to emphasize reflectance and discount illumination.

relevance will affect the receptors in similar ways. The subjectivist overtones of Hayek's principle, and of irrealism based on failures of correspondence, are subverted by Similarity of Functional Relevance. Hayek and Hardin suggest that criteria of co-classification and of similarity are dictated by the system, not by the nature of the distal stimulus. Similarity of Functional Relevance has the useful corrective effect of drawing our attention to the fact that the system might converge on functional similarities, or even natural similarities—though admittedly these similarities (e.g. the similarity among ripe fruit as distinct from leaves) lack interest from a purely physics point of view.

Now consider Gallistel's conjecture. The idea is that the similarity relations among colours arise from an arrangement which enables the output of colour neurons to be vector-added. This arrangement demands an array of colours along certain qualitative dimensions; it is the substrate for the experienced similarity space of colour. The same point can be made here as was made with regard to R—it is a convenience for the sensory system, not an attempt faithfully to reflect a similarity relation relevant to the laws of physics. Does this indicate an irrealist position?

No, for two reasons. The first is that Gallistel's conjecture is compatible with the existence of a purely physical description of the similarity space of colour—the account of opponent processing in Chapter 6, section I is an outline of such an description. This purely physical description is a kind of key or code-book which enables the psychophysical theorist to extract the message embedded in colour similarity relations: the reddishness of a stimulus indicates that it is emitting light that satisfies R.

The second reason for not giving up on realism is that Gallistel's conjecture does not imply that the arrangement of colours in similarity space is completely arbitrary. Sensory systems are constrained in the ways they can arrange data; they are not free to impose just any relations on the stimulus domain. As we saw in section I above, Similarity of Effect is still a boundary condition on sensory processing, since physically similar signals will propagate through the system, and are preserved in the output unless active data-processing intervenes. Thus, while the ordering of electromagnetic signals by frequency is disrupted by sensory processing, it is not completely scrambled.

Moreover, the incongruity of colour-similarity space with the physical spectrum is compatible with Similarity of Functional Relevance playing a role in the construction of colour similarity space. That is, while it may not correlate with an objectively measurable similarity relation that figures in physical laws concerning ambient energy, it may still incorporate some relation that gives us a handle on distal objects. Roger Shepard (1997/1992) has suggested that

[T]he principal criterion of success of the visual system's chromatic analysis is not that it represents the full complexity of the spectral reflectance function for each surface but that it ensures that the (possibly reduced) representation of each such function is constant under natural variations of illumination. (328)

In accordance with this delineation of the function of colour vision, Shepard suggests that the most important variations of colour in naturally illuminated scenes are such that colour constancy is best achieved in a similarity space constructed as ours is—even though the discriminations that this similarity space affords us are relatively crude.

These considerations show that there are a number of external constraints on the shape of similarity space. As far as Gallistel's account is concerned, it comes in the end to this. Suppose that similarity space is constructed so that it is possible to get a single response to sensory stimulation despite the blurring effect of broadband tuning. Suppose further that several different orderings will resolve broadband tuning. It is still possible to choose between these orderings, for some will result in unambiguous but inappropriate responses to sensory stimulation, while others will result in appropriate responses. To the extent that there is selective pressure to avoid inappropriate responses, there is not only an external constraint on the shape of similarity space, but—plausibly—a right or wrong concerning the choice of similarity orderings. (This demands further argument, which will be attempted later.) This is a kind of realism. We will return to the consideration of this and other forms of realism in Chapter 8.

Part II: Afterword

The Stages of the Sensory Process

It will be helpful at this stage to clarify the logic of sensory classification and sensory ordering as it has been presented up to this point. It was proposed in Chapter I that sensory systems are classificatory instruments which assign stimuli to various classes. There we distinguished items that belong to three different stages of the sensory process:

A. Stimuli: distal stimuli (things out there), and proximal stimuli (the packets of energy that distal stimuli send to our sensory receptors).

B. Sensory classes: the groups that the system makes of the stimuli, and sense-features, the properties that stimuli in a given sensory class share.

C. Sensations: events in sensory consciousness with a particular subjective 'feel'. These events are like labels that the system attaches to stimuli in order that we may know that they have been assigned to a particular class.

In Part II, we argued further that sensory systems order sense-features in a similarity space. This similarity space is the basis of our treating things the same or differently: when stimuli are assigned to classes that are close together in the ordering, they are likely to be treated similarly; when they are assigned to classes that are far apart, they are likely to be treated differently. For instance, if we are conditioned to react in a certain way to things that have feature F, then the probability that we will treat something with feature G the same way depends on the closeness of F and G in their shared similarity space. The similarity space within which features are arrayed also affords us a way of identifying features and comparing them with others.

Now, when we talk about sensory classification and sensory ordering, it is important to keep the above stages of the sensory process separate, and to be clear about their primary application. For instance, certain stimuli appear blue—things like pieces of cloth, ink-marks, the sky, water, and so on. What is the significance of this appearance? The broad categories listed above help us get a clearer idea of this.

The most natural and straightforward view of the matter is that *blue* is a sense feature: the feature shared by things assigned by vision to a certain class, i.e. the class of blue things. Stimuli *look* blue because they are assigned to this class. The sensation as of a blue thing is the *label* by which we are able to identify a thing as having been assigned to this class (rightly or mistakenly). The reader might ask: 'In what sense are they "labels" ?—Obviously, they are not *literally* so.' Answer: No they are not, but the idea of sensory labelling is, as we shall see in Part IV, more than merely a metaphor: it is more like a structural analogy. For the moment, let us just use the term without worrying too much about how we will back it up. Our grasp of the relationship between such labels and the sense-features with which they are associated is intuitive and innate: we don't have to *learn* that the sensation of something's looking blue means that it has been assigned to *blue* rather than to *orange*. This connection is innate, not empirically discovered.

Taking this idea seriously—the idea that a sensation is a label for a sense-feature—we propose that the relationship between a sensation, a sense-feature, and a stimulus is analogous to that between a descriptive word, the attribute it designates, and the individuals that possess this attribute.

> (a) Biologists co-classify cats, and label the class or attribute so created *'felis'*.
> (b) We call a particular individual, Leo, a *felis*—we use this word to describe him—because we believe that he possesses the attribute designated by the word *'felis'*.
> (c) He *is* a *felis* if we are right in so believing.

The relationship between the sensation and a stimulus is similar.

> (a') The visual system co-classifies blue things and labels the class so created with the look of blue.
> (b') The Cross of St Andrew **looks** *blue*—figuratively, the visual system 'calls it blue'—because it has been assigned to the class so labelled.
> (c') It *is* blue if this assignment is correct. (More about the logic of this in Chapter 11.)

The vector coding spaces that we encountered in the previous section are orderings imposed on sensory classes by Similarity of Process. The sensory system makes this ordering evident to us by graded sensations of similarity. Some philosophers are fond of saying things like this: Colours are points (or regions) in Hue-Brightness-Saturation (HBS) space (or whatever their preferred similarity space for colours is). This is wrong: colours are sense-features; HBS space is a descriptive structure that colour vision uses to identify and compare these features. The *location* of a colour C in HBS space is an essential characteristic of C: this is why we can use its location to identify C. However, there is an emphatic difference between saying that colours are located in HBS space, or even that they are essentially located in this space, and saying that they *are* regions of HBS space. Colours are features shared by classes of stimuli which are encoded by location in HBS space.

This account of the matter enables us to avoid certain confusions that traditionally surround the relationship between sensations and stimuli. Descartes and Berkeley, for instance, think that when we call something 'blue', we are improperly 'projecting' a sensation onto distal material objects. *Blue* is primarily a characteristic of sensations, they say, and when we characterize a stimulus as blue, we are improperly characterizing it in terms of an attribute that properly belongs only to mental events, i.e. to sensations. We can now see that this criticism of everyday practice is not justified. (The criticism is, moreover, methodologically suspect, as we shall see in Chapter 8, section II.) There is an intermediate entity here—the sensory class—that Descartes and Berkeley fail to notice; the relationship between sensations and sensory classes allows us to clear up their mistake.

What is correct in Descartes's and Berkeley's account is that sensations do indeed play a role in our coming to know that something appears a certain way. How do we know that the sky looks blue, rather than orange?—By the character of the visual state that the sky occasions in us. The *mistake* in their account is to think that *blue* is the attribute of sensations that allows us to do this. When we say that the Scottish flag is blue, we are *not* assigning it to a class of sensations (see a'): rather, we are assigning it to a class identified by the sensation (see b'). Compare: when we call Leo a *felis* we are not assigning him to a class of word-utterances (a): rather, we are assigning him to a class designated by the term '*felis*' (b). So, a sensation as of a blue thing identifies the class to which it assigns a stimulus. This *sensation* is not itself a member of the class of blue things, nor are the blue things members of the class of sensations of that sort.

To summarize:

> *Descartes's Theory*: *Blue* is a class of sensations; when we say that the Scottish flag is blue, we are assigning it to that class, and saying in effect that the cross is a sensation (which is necessarily false).

> *Sensory Classification Perspective*: *Blue* is a class of stimuli labelled by a particular kind of sensation; when we say that the Scottish flag is blue, we are saying that it belongs to the class so labelled (which happens to be true).

There is no metaphysical error in our everyday practice. The Sensory Classification Perspective shows why.

In a similar vein, there are traditional confusions about sensory similarity relations. Some think that when we say that blue things are more similar (with respect to colour) to turquoise things than to red things, we are projecting onto distal objects a similarity relation that properly belongs to the realm of sensations. Once again, this overlooks sensory classes. The thread of Part II has been to show how sensory similarity relations order sensory *classes*, or sense-*features*, giving us thereby a descriptive relation (similarity) among stimuli. What would it mean to say that *sensations* are similar to one another in ways that are captured by the corresponding similarity space? What would it mean, for instance, to say that the sensation as of blue is more similar to the sensation as of turquoise than to the sensation as of red? We saw that when we say that x and y are similar, we mean that they are likely to be confused with one another, that a conditioned response to one transfers to the other, that an inductive inference drawn from the occurrence of x will also be drawn from an occurrence of y, and so on. Notice that it is the *stimuli* that we are talking about here. After all, we are not concerned here about *sensations* getting confused with one another or *sensations* becoming associated with one another by conditioning or learning—we are interacting with *stimuli* in confusability judgements and in inductive inference, not sensations. Stimuli are treated similarly because the classes to which they have been assigned are relatively close to one another in the sensory similarity ordering.

Again, the analogy with language is helpful. Consider this: 'lion' and 'tiger' represent things that are similar to one another, but it does not follow that the *words* are similar, orthographically or phonetically considered. The words are similar only in a semantic sense, i.e. in that they designate things that are biologically similar. In just this way, the *sensations* as of blue and as of turquoise are not similar to one another with respect to their own properties: they represent distal objects as being similar to one another. It is only because we tend to associate stimuli from neighbouring sensory classes that we can say that these classes are close together in the sensory ordering—not (primarily) because we tend to associate the sensations themselves.

That sensory similarity orders features (primarily) and stimuli (derivatively), not sensations, suggests that Descartes's Theory got the matter exactly backwards. It supposes that we (mistakenly) project properties and relations that properly belong in the realm of sensations on to distal objects. I am claiming that some philosophers and psychologists tend (equally mistakenly) to project similarity relations that properly belong in the domain of stimuli and sense-features back on to sensations. They mistakenly think that the sensation as of *blue* is similar to the sensation as of *turquoise* on the grounds that *blue* is similar to *turquoise*. That is the real 'Error Theory'.

Summary of the Argument

Philosophers have long held, on grounds of introspection, that the sensory image is pictorial in character, and that it does not come labelled, either with classificatory tags, or with internal links of similarity. It has sometimes been assumed that this pictorial image is a projection into consciousness of energy patterns incident on the outer sensory receptors. Parts I and II have argued that this wrong. The senses are essentially classificatory systems. They assign stimuli to classes, order these classes in similarity relations, and provide sensory consciousness with awareness of the results of this activity. Thus, sensory consciousness is articulated in terms of class membership, in the subsumption of individual stimuli under classes, and similarity relations.

In Chapter 5, we saw that sensory similarity is not a simple projection of energy patterns in the external world. It is an artefact of a representational system used to solve certain problems. We suggested, however, that this did *not* imply an anti-realist position with regard either to sensory classes or sensory similarity. It can still make sense to claim that the system is right or wrong in its construction of classes and their similarity metric. In Part III, we will investigate the role of the organism's own purposes in constructing sensory classes and similarity, and articulate a kind of realism appropriate to sensory systems.

PART THREE

Specialization

6

Perceptual Specialization and the Definition of Colour

In Parts I and II, we discussed the nature of sensory classification. Parts III and IV are an inquiry into the ecological and functional significance of sensory classes. In Part III,[1] we begin with an investigation of colour? What is it? What do we get to know about the real world when we see it classified by the colour vision system? If two things look the same with regard to colour, what property do they seem thereby to share? Or, to put this question in a slightly different form: On what basis, in virtue of what purported similarity, does colour vision co-classify stimuli?

In defining colour—in answering the questions just posed—philosophers standardly appeal to one of two things: the nature of colour experience, or the nature of the real properties that are supposedly detected by colour experience. Their approach, more often than not, is anthropocentric: the properties standardly cited in such definitions are those detected by the *human* system, the experiences cited those that humans have. Traditionally, this form of anthropocentrism is adopted because philosophers do not think that the restriction makes a difference. What humans perceive is what there is to be perceived, it is assumed, and therefore just what the members of any other species would perceive unless they lack the appropriate receptors.[2]

---

[1] Part III derives, with many additions, deletions, and revisions from a paper entitled 'The Disunity of Color' (Matthen 1999), which first appeared in the *Philosophical Review* 108 (copyright, 1999 Cornell University), and was reprinted in *Philosophers' Annual* 22 (2000). Such overlaps as there are appear by permission of the publisher. I thank Jonathan Cohen, Larry Hardin, Alex Rueger, Evan Thompson, and the editors of the *Philosophical Review* for helpful comments on various drafts of that paper.
[2] Some of the philosophers criticized below for their commitment to anthropocentrism— C. L. Hardin and David Hilbert, for example—do not subscribe to this thesis that members of other species perceive the same things. On the contrary, they adopt anthropocentric positions because their awareness of species differences moves them deliberately to exclude certain kinds of system from the class of colour-vision system. It will be argued below that such exclusion is undesirable: one should not be in the position of denying that honey bees have colour vision

Such perception is manifested in terms of characteristic kind of experience, these philosophers say. It has been thought to follow that colour is defined by the human experience of it: if other animals lack the same experiences, they lack colour vision.

We shall see in this chapter that the narrowness of scope that anthropocentrism brings is an obstacle to an adequately general understanding of colour vision. We shall argue for the following

> *The Disunity of Colour Thesis*
> I. There is no *ecologically characterized* class of properties such that colour vision *must* consist (in whatsoever kind of organism it may occur) in the capture of some or all of the members of this class.
> II. There is no *subjectively characterized* class of experiences such that colour vision *must* consist (in whatsoever kind of organism it may occur) in having some or all of these experiences.

Colour vision is variable across species: the principles of classification vary; the colour experiences vary too. Even if we did manage to gather together all colour classification schemes in all existing kinds of animals, there is no reason why another kind of organism could not have existed with a different colour classification scheme. This variety confirms a point emphasized in Part I: the ecology of organisms, and the activity of their sensory systems, are factors that influence the sensory classifications they perform. The conclusions reached in this chapter are mainly negative; Chapters 7 to 9 present a framework for understanding this variability.

I. Colour Appearance: Some Preliminaries

Before we begin to evaluate anthropocentric views of colour, we will need to review some features of human colour experience.

1. *Opponent Processing and Colour Experience*
Cone Cells. Humans possess three types of cone cell, or 'visual pigment'. When light of a given frequency falls on a cone cell, the cell emits a neural signal of strength equal to the strength of the signal multiplied by the *sensitivity* of the cell to light of that frequency. Each such cell is selective in its sensitivity: it is sensitive to light only in a particular waveband, and differentially sensitive to different wavelengths within its band. Conventionally, the cone cells are named after the wavebands of sensitivity with which they are associated: long (L), middle (M), and short (S). This characterization is

---

simply because of differences between their visual system and ours, or because they probably have no conscious experience of colours. Such a denial flies in the face of their ability to discriminate between surfaces on the basis of their colour.

somewhat inaccurate, since the so-called long-wavelength cone (L) is actually also sensitive to light of short wavelength: an important detail as we shall see in a moment.

Opponent Processing. The output of the cone cells gives us redundant and overlapping information. The waveband of each type of cell overlaps with that of the others. Suppose that both an L-cell and an M-cell is responding to a particular light signal. Nothing much can be gathered from this fact about the spectral distribution of the signal, i.e. about how its energy is distributed across the visible spectrum. The fact that both L and M are responding tells us only that the signal has energy either in each of the non-overlapping parts of the two wavebands *or* somewhere in the overlap of the two wavebands. Both distributions will activate both cells.

The system reduces this ambiguity by subtracting the overlap of the two cells. If the difference is non-zero, then the signal contains more energy in one waveband. If the difference is zero, then it contains the same amount of energy in both. This process is called 'opponent processing'. There are two such processes. The first subtracts the output of the medium cone from that of the long cone. Since, as noted a moment ago, the 'long' cone is also sensitive to light at the short-wavelength end of the spectrum, this operation in effect tells us how strong a signal is at the *ends* of the visual spectrum (long and short) as compared to the middle. The second opponent process subtracts the output of the S cone from the sum of the other two: thus, it computes the function $(L + M) - S$. This tells us how much of the signal's strength is in the middle and long wavebands relative to the short.

Colour Experience. If the $(L - M)$ opponent process yields a positive value, then the signal is cumulatively stronger at the ends of the spectrum. In this case, the signal will look *reddish*. If it is stronger in the middle of the spectrum than at the ends, the value of the function will be negative, and it will look *greenish*.

If the $((L + M) - S)$ process yields a positive value, the signal is stronger in the long and middle part of the visible spectrum than in the short-wavelength part. In this case, the stimulus looks *yellowish*; if it is stronger in the short waves, it looks *bluish*.[3]

The values of these two functions constitute two axes of colour similarity space; the experience of a colour as reddish or greenish, and as yellowish or bluish are the internally available 'labels' that enable us to place stimuli in this similarity space. Together, these two computed values constitute *hue*.

The third component of colour is 'lightness' (or 'brightness' in the case of luminous objects)—how bright or dark a surface looks relative to others in the scene.

---

[3] It should be noted that there is presently no robust consensus among colour scientists on the exact mathematical function computed by the opponent-processing channels, or the exact relation between these channels and the Hering primaries of red-green, blue-yellow—see Mollon and Jordan (1997).

TABLE 1 Colour Appearance and Opponent Processing

CATEGORY (SENSORY LABEL) ⟹ ⇓	More energy at the ends than in the middle (REDDISH)	More energy in the middle than at the ends (GREENISH)
More energy in long-wavelength half than at the short-wavelength end (YELLOWISH)	**I** COMBINATIONS OF RED AND YELLOW	**II** COMBINATIONS OF GREEN AND YELLOW
More energy at short-wavelength end than in long-wavelength half (BLUISH)	**III** COMBINATIONS OF RED AND BLUE	**IV** COMBINATIONS OF GREEN AND BLUE

We need to make a distinction here between the basis for co-classifying stimuli, and the experiences that reveal the various classes to us. For instance, stimuli are placed in the middle column of Table 1 because they send a signal to the eye that contains more energy at the ends of the visible spectrum than in the middle. That a signal contains more energy at the ends of the spectrum is the *basis* for placing it in one of the cells in the middle column of Table 1. That certain stimuli fall into one of these cells is conveyed to us by the fact that our experiences of them have a reddish component. So in accordance with the Posteriority of Appearance thesis articulated in Chapter 1, section II, things are not co-classified because they look red; rather they look red because the sensory system has co-classified them.

Now, the classification that defines the columns is initially kept separate from that which defines the rows—that is, the red/green channel is initially separate from the yellow/blue one. As we saw in Chapter 5, the channels are combined into a unified vector representation in the primary visual cortex. In this brain area, we have hue represented as a composite. Notice that in Table 1 the most dissimilar pairs of hues—the most dissimilar in terms of experience because they share no components—are the ones that are diagonally opposed to one another—**I** and **IV**, and **II** and **III**.

From Table 1, we can derive the sequence of hues found in the rainbow. Consider a linear ordering of monochromatic lights, ranging from the short-wave at the left to long-wave at the right. It is arranged like this as in Table 2. The most experientially opposed kinds of hues—those in cells **I** as compared to **IV** of Table 1, and **II** as compared to **III**—are not maximally far apart in the spectrum. That is **III** and **I** are experienced as more similar to one another (they share a red component) than **III** and **II**, though the latter pair are closer together in the spectrum. This is why the visible spectrum takes a horseshoe shape in the similarity space of colour (see Figure 8 in Chapter 5, section I).

TABLE 2 Opponent Processing and the Visible Spectrum

SPECTRAL SECTOR (wavelength increases towards right) ⇒	SHORT WAVE-LENGTHS	SHORT TO MEDIUM WAVE-LENGTHS	MEDIUM TO LONG WAVE-LENGTHS	LONG WAVE-LENGTHS
SIGNAL DOMINATED BY LIGHT AT ⇒	SHORT & ENDS	SHORT & MIDDLE	LONG & MIDDLE	LONG & ENDS
RESULTING EXPERIENCE ⇒	RED + BLUE (**III**) (red diminishes towards right)	BLUE + GREEN (**IV**) (blue diminishes towards right)	GREEN + YELLOW (**II**) (green diminishes towards right)	YELLOW + RED (**I**) (yellow diminishes towards right)

The transformations of the data rendered by the opponent-processing stream are, in the sense outlined in Chapter 2, section II, classificatory in nature: they sort the activation patterns of the cone cells into different classes according to whether they satisfy the conditions that define the cells of Table 1. Notice that by dividing activation patterns into these four types, colour vision throws away a lot of information. The reddishness of a particular stimulus indicates that how much stronger the light it sends to the eye is at the ends of the spectrum than in the middle—many different energy profiles will be the same in this respect and thus be classified the same way. The differences between these profiles is lost in the classification process. This is the phenomenon known as *metamerism*.

Some philosophers take metamerism to be a problem for realism, since opponent processing results in the co-classification of signals of widely differing spectral distribution. This is a mistake: there is no reason why every realistic classification scheme should respect similarity in spectral distribution. Hayek's ball-sorting machine (Chapter 1, section I.3) gathered balls of widely different diameters in the same cell of its classification scheme. This does not imply (though Hayek thought it did) that the classification scheme does not correspond to reality. Here is an analogy that helps bring the point home: suppose we calculated the *gender inequality* of a couple by subtracting the income of the wife from that of the husband and dividing the result by the larger income. (Gender inequality would be negative by this measure if the wife earned more.) This calculation would result in a lot of 'metamers': for instance, a couple whose incomes were $40,000 and $30,000 would have the same calculated gender inequality value as one whose incomes were $80,000 and \$60,000. This does not mean that this measure of 'gender inequality' corresponds to nothing real. The case of colour metamerism is precisely analogous.

2. *Colour Contrast and Colour Constancy*

Opponent processing dictates the nature of the similarity space within which colour classes are arrayed, but it is not the whole of the process by which an individual stimulus is assigned to a colour class. For it has very long been a fundamental truth of colour psychophysics that two stimuli may send the same signal to the eye, but still look different, or send different signals to the eye, and still look the same.

A distal stimulus takes on very different appearances depending on the colours with which it is surrounded. A light patch will look darker in a light surround, lighter in a dark surround. Consequently, an orange will look brown if surrounded by objects much lighter than itself; it looks orange only in 'normal' contrast situations, i.e. when it is not by far the darkest object in the scene. Why? Because lightness of its surround adds black to the reddish-orange of its normal appearance, thus creating a brown. The principle extends to the component brightnesses of a given colour appearance. A reddish object will look less red when surrounded by intensely red things: its appearance is pulled towards the green, and this admixture makes its appearance less saturated. These are phenomena of *simultaneous* colour contrast. There is also an effect of colour adaptation that takes place over time: the cone cells can become fatigued by constant exposure to light in their waveband of sensitivity, and as a consequence, respond less strongly. (This is responsible for a variety of after-images, etc.) These phenomena arise from the nature of the cells and how they respond to light; however, they seem also to play a role in the system's strategy of 'discounting the illuminant' (a phrase used by von Helmholtz), while determining surface colour.

Because of how the system uses colour contrast, objects are less variable in colour appearance than one would expect given variations in the signal they reflect in different conditions. The signal that arrives at the eye from a given object varies quite a bit with the illumination in which it stands. For instance, a white cloth bathed in the red light of a fireplace emits a signal quite a bit richer in red light than the same cloth lit by the cold bluish light of a snowy field. However, we find that colour experiences are stabilized somehow—though the white cloth looks different in front of the fireplace than it does in the snow, there is something in the two experiences that enables us to identify its colour, as well as something about how it is lit. In other words, the colour-vision system is able, in a wide range of viewing conditions, to separate out the surface property (i.e. the reflectance) of an object from the illumination in which it is being viewed. A white object will look white in many different conditions of illumination, though it may not look exactly the same in all these conditions. This is the phenomenon known as *colour constancy*.

It is important not to exaggerate how much the colour image is stabilized in this way. Bradley and Tye (2001), and Byrne and Hilbert (2003), take colour constancy to indicate that colour vision detects an illumination-independent property of objects. This is something of a stretch, given how much our colour experiences of objects actually varies with circumstance. (I was guilty of the same stretch in Matthen 1988.) This is why the definition of colour constancy offered in the previous paragraph relies on the fact that in a certain range of circumstances, colour vision separates out two different distal causes of the proximal visual stimulus; within this range of circumstances, it reports (not always with perfect accuracy) on *both* a property of distal objects, and the state of the illumination in which they are placed. As emphasized earlier, one does not want to say that a white shirt looks the *same* in reddish and in bluish light; colours are not constant in *this* way. In red light, the shirt looks like a white object in red light (and different from a red object in white light); in blue light, it looks like a white object in blue light (and different from a blue object in white light).

In certain circumstances, the colour vision system may fail correctly to separate out these components. For instance, in the yellow sodium light of a parking lot, a green car simply looks black. In this unnatural circumstance, the colour vision system may give us all kinds of misleading information about colour and illumination. It may tell us (falsely) that the car is black and the illumination normal; it may tell us (also falsely) that the car is black and the illumination yellow. It may also convey the false message that the car is black, with no determinate message about illumination. All of these sorts of failure are known to occur across the range of situations faced by perceptual systems. Consider perception of size. If you are looking at a row of same-size cubes receding into the distance, they will (in normal circumstances) all look the same size though at different distances away. If, however, you are looking down at a highway from an airplane, the scene looks like a picture or map at an indeterminate distance, with the cars and houses seen as little specks or models. In the latter case, the visual system fails to extract information about distance, the customary cues being absent, and consequently arrives at a wrong estimate of size.

The idea that constancy is separation of independent variables is supported by recent work by Surajit Nundy and Dale Purves (2002) and Purves and Beau Lotto (2003). Consider the familiar contrast phenomenon of a grey patch looking darker against a light background than against a dark one. This phenomenon is, as we saw earlier, a component of colour perception: colours appear as if they contain more black when they are surrounded by lighter objects; an orange will appear brown, a green more olive, and so on. As it turns out, this effect is enhanced when the scene contains cues which indicate that the darker background *is caused by a shadow*. Significantly this can happen in two ways. First, the object supposedly casting a shadow can explicitly be included in the display. Second, the dark background can be made to look more like a shadow by the addition of a fuzzy penumbra. In both cases, the effect is enhanced: in both, the light patch looks even lighter because it is diagnosed as standing within a shadow than it does against a similar background of indeterminate origin.

Notice that two components of the scene have been separated in these presentations: when the dark patch is diagnosed as a shadow, the lighter patch is diagnosed as darkened by the shadow. Since the lightness of the latter is attributed to illumination rather than intrinsic reflectance, it is co-classified with other more reflective surfaces and presented as lighter. In more ambiguous presentations—i.e. where the origin of the dark background is unclear, the system apportions responsibility for the contrast more equally to illumination and reflectance. So the lighter patch does not look quite as pale against the dark background (Purves and Lotto 2003, 49–55). Nundy, Purves, and Lotto conclude, quite plausibly, that the appearance of brightness is a probabilisticaly weighted estimate of its reflectance given information concerning illumination. Two surfaces transmit the same signal to the eye: when it appears from contextual cues that one of the two is in shadow, it appears lighter than the signal would indicate on its own; when it is unclear whether or not it is in shadow, it appears less so.

As we saw, some philosophers argue that colour constancy shows that colour experience corresponds to properties of external objects, not of light. This conclusion seems too strong. A better conclusion to draw from constancy is that colour vision is functionally adapted to separating out the sources of appearance of external objects.

II. Narrow Anthropocentrism

With these details about the nature of colour vision in the background, we turn now to evaluating some standard philosophical theories of colour.

1. *Anthropocentric Conceptions of Colour.* Descartes defined the colour of an external object in terms of the character of the human colour experience it produces: a thing is called 'orange' if (in normal circumstances) it produces orange sensations in us. Let us say that a concept is narrowly *anthropocentrically defined* if it is defined relative to human response (cf. Averill 1985): Descartes's definition is anthropocentric in this sense.

Such anthropocentric definitions of colour are odd for several reasons. First, as we have noted (in Chapter 1, section II and in the Afterword to Part II) the experience that a stimulus produces in us is an internal 'label' by which we come to know that it has been assigned to a certain sensory class. To define a class by its label is to get things the wrong way around: it is like defining *cat* as the class of things called 'cat', a mistake since the label is only contingently attached to the class. Secondly, the fact that a class of things evokes similar reactions from humans is no guarantee of its scientific or physical unity—while it is often true that physically similar causes produce physically similar effects, it is not always true that similar effects are caused by similar causes. Indeed, we know that very different kinds of physical property are the cause of colour experiences (Nassau 1980). According to Scott Atran (1990), pre-scientific 'folk' schemas and other early botanical taxonomies grouped plants together according to their medicinal properties. He records a complaint of systematists in the early modern period that 'the more [such human centred taxonomies] enriched medicine, the more they threw botany into confusion' (18–19). Is it clear that anthropocentric conceptions of colour—definitions in terms of human sensation—do any better? What guarantee do we have that classifications based on similarity of human colour experience are not the source of similar 'confusion'?

2. *David Lewis's Definition of Colour.* Let's look at a typical anthropocentric definition. David Lewis (1997, 327) proposed the following as a schema for defining colour terms.

D1. Red is the surface property which typically causes experience of red in people who have such things before the eyes.

D2. Experience of red is the inner state of people which is the typical effect of having red things before the eyes.

Lewis claims that the truth of the above pair of statements is preserved when any other colour term, for example 'green', is substituted throughout *D1* and *D2* in place of 'red'. He concludes that:

A *colour* is any first component of a corresponding pair. A *colour experience* is any second component (ibid, 335).

This is not quite right. Other terms, such as 'square', 'smooth textured', 'speckled', 'six feet away', and 'looming' (when they are properties of surfaces), would also satisfy *D1* and *D2* when substituted for 'red'—and of course they are not colours. But this over-inclusiveness presents no great difficulty, at least not given Lewis's general approach to these matters. Lewis avers that colours are *reflectance* properties of surfaces. He also allows that other properties such as luminance are colours. Let's call these other properties *associated* surface features in virtue of the fact that they create in us the same experience as reflectances. Then, to get a general conception of colour out of his definitions, we need to amend *D1* accordingly: '*Red* is the *surface spectral reflectance* or associated property which typically causes . . . etc.' The idea is that we identify the experience of red by reference to a surface spectral reflectance in the first instance, but then other properties come along for the ride.

Consider, then, the following amended formulae:

> $S1$ x is the class of surface spectral reflectances and associated properties which typically cause *experience of* x in people who have such things before the eyes.
> $S2$ *Experience of* x is the inner state of people which is the typical effect of having a thing with a surface spectral reflectance or associated property in the class x before the eyes.

Lewis's theory, slightly amended, is that colours are the 'first components' of pairs that satisfy these formulae, and colour experiences are second components—colours are, in other words, the things that can truly be sub-stituted for 'x' in $S1$, while colour experiences are those that can simultan-eously be substituted for '*experience of* x' in $S2$, keeping the x constant. This is not the whole of Lewis's theory (as we shall see in Chapter 8, section III). The theory fragment given so far is 'narrowly anthropocentric' but, as we shall see, Lewis's full theory is not.

3. *Novel Colours and the Inadequacy of Narrow Anthropocentrism.* The narrowly anthropocentric definition of colour contained in the schemas $S1$ and $S2$ and the accompanying stipulation that colours are the 'first com-ponents' of pairs that satisfy these schemas immediately bump up against the problem of 'novel colours'.[4]

Imagine an organism, O, very much like humans as described in section I above, but with its short-wave receptor shifted towards the ultraviolet. (O could be an atypical human for the purposes of this discussion.) O will be capable of seeing ultraviolet reflectances. If nothing else was changed from the neurocomputational process described above, O would experience ultra-violet in much the same way as we see violets (that is, as occupying cell I of Table 2 and thus appearing bluish-red). Ultraviolet cannot be substituted for x in $S1$: spectral reflectances in this range do not 'typically' cause 'people' to have any sort of experience at all, even when they are 'before the eyes'. However, $S2$ admits O's experience of ultraviolet; it is the very same 'inner state' which, in people, is the typical effect of having *violet* things before the eyes (not ultraviolet since there is no such inner state in humans). Lewis is thus obliged to say that although O experiences ultraviolet as a colour, specifically as violet, ultraviolet is not a colour. In other words, O has colour experiences that issue from something *like* a colour, but correspond, never-theless, to no colour. This odd result, which is incongruent with the general idea of pairing colours with colour experiences, shows how Lewis's definition turns on contingent features of *human* colour experience. It does not allow

---

[4] The following discussion of novel colours owes much to Thompson (1992). For informa-tion about the pigeon discussed below, see J. F. Nuboer (1986), and Francisco J. Varela, Adrian G. Palacios, and Timothy H. Goldsmith (1993).

us to focus on the idiosyncratic character of human colour vision and its classifications—it prevents us from recognizing that humans have just one type of colour-vision system. Such a definition is obstructive when we wish to consider colour and colour vision in a general setting.

The problem becomes acute when we consider colour-similarity spaces different from our own. The pigeon has eyes with photoreceptors similar to our own, and retinal cells that treat the output of these receptors by a more complicated version of opponent processing, the neurocomputational scheme described above. However, the pigeon has four visual pigments. We are trichromats in the sense that we are able to duplicate a light of any hue by varying the strength of three different colours in a light mixture; in virtue of their extra pigment, pigeons are tetrachromats in the sense that for them it takes four different lights. A pigeon's chromatic experience is richer and more complex than ours—this is why it takes more different lights in a mixture to duplicate a given colour experience. The pigeon's fourth pigment is sensitive to ultraviolet, and it is thus capable of seeing reflectances in the ultraviolet range of the spectrum. Further, it computes three difference values concerning information drawn from four wavebands, not just two such difference values drawn from three wavebands, as in Table 1. Consequently, pigeon colours vary in *three* hue-dimensions (plus *black-white*); the colours they experience are not completely describable, as ours are, in terms of *two* such components—*red-green* and *blue-yellow* in our case. When pigeons look at the feathers of other pigeons (which tend to have a high short-wave reflectance), they not only see reflectances there that we cannot see, they also experience them in ways we cannot imagine by means of projection from our own colour experience. We have already seen that narrow anthropocentrism fails to accommodate ultraviolet 'colours'. In addition it excludes the pigeon's colour experiences because they do not correspond to any inner state of people, and thus fall outside the scope of *S2*. This is arbitrary.

Lewis was perhaps of the view that 'red', 'blue', etc. are *our* terms, human terms, and that the colours that a pigeon experiences should not be named by these terms. This seems unobjectionable. It is perfectly reasonable to say that, to a pigeon, the feathers of another pigeon are not blue or bluish, but some other colour that we cannot name or even adequately describe in the conceptual scheme for colours backed by our own colour-processing system. (This proposition is actually validated by the Thesis of Pluralistic Realism of Chapter 8, section IV.) Thus, we might allow that Lewis's anthropocentric definitions of 'red', 'blue', etc. are appropriate for these human colours—we'll need parallel columbicentric definitions to define pigeon colours. However, it is not so reasonable to define *colour*—colour in general—anthropocentrically. *Colour* is not 'our' term: we can make it so only at the exorbitant cost of abandoning the comparative (i.e. cross-species) study of colour vision. A general conception of *colour* and *colour experience* should allow us to treat the human and the pigeon colours, and their systems, as instances of a general kind. Failing that, we need a principled reason for excluding the pigeon from the domain of colour perceivers, or for counting the matter as indeterminate.

Conclusion 1: Anthropocentric accounts that restrict colours to those detected by humans, or colour experiences to those that occur in humans, cannot account for colour vision as it occurs in other species.

III. Flexible Anthropocentrism and Colour Experience

Some philosophers suggest that the way to handle the pigeon's experiences is to include them, provided they sufficiently resemble the human case. This is a flexible procedure in broad agreement with that recommended by C. L. Hardin (1988, 147): 'We can begin with the human case, in which we know there to be genuine colour vision, and extend the concept of a colour per-ceiver outward to other species.'

To someone new to this area, this 'family resemblance' approach must seem rather timid. Why not eliminate the reference to human experience altogether, and eliminate the oddity that we noticed at the beginning of the previous section? This is what many colour scientists in fact do. They define colour vision *functionally*, like this:

> *F* (Functional Definition of Colour, first pass)*
> Colour vision is the perceptual discrimination capacity underlying differential responses to light differing in wavelength only.

On this account, the colours would be properties that are discriminated by distinguishing light differing in wavelength only. (We'll refine this later.)

One problem with *F**, emphasized by Hardin (1988, 148) and David R. Hilbert (1992), is that it requires very little by way of an internal repres-entation of colour. Hilbert presents us with the following sort of case: some invertebrates have wavelength-sensitive behaviour that can be modelled on a system consisting of one receptor sensitive to long wavelengths connected to a motor that makes them move towards the light source, and another receptor sensitive to short wavelengths that makes it move away. Such a visual system responds differently to red and blue, but it is doubtful that it has colour vision, Hilbert says, because it has no integrated representation of colour. Hilbert concludes that 'the empirical literature is not going to provide us with an independent characterization of colour vision that will be helpful' (ibid, 359).

Hilbert's criticism is a little obscure at first sight. Why *can't* one say that this organism has colour vision, albeit of a primitive sort? Perhaps the point is a little like the one we made in connection with Descartes's claim that animal sensory systems do not classify (see Chapter 2, section II). Some reactions of organisms can be attributed directly to the causal effect of qualities of things in the environment, without the need to posit that the organism forms representations of these qualities. A strong wind will knock you over without your needing to represent it as strong, or for your sensory systems so to classify it. And some organisms may have evolved ways of taking advantage of such direct effects of environmental causes. For example, maples evolved seeds with a boomerang-shape that enables them to take advantage of winds for the purpose of dispersion. It would be far-fetched to suppose that these seeds represent the presence of the wind as they are swept along. They just respond to the wind without the need to represent it: they are 'designed' so that they can do this. This point is not obviously changed when such evolutionary design is linked to behavioural response to colour. Certain plants have an elaborate biochemical system that 'measures' the long hours of daytime blue light in summer, and initiates the more profuse flowering appropriate to that season (Imaizumi et al. 2003). Is this a reason to say that these plants are *representing* colour? What would motivate such a view? Words and pictures are paradigms of representational entities. Can one reasonably maintain that the plant's internal state relates to summer as words to their meaning?

This much acknowledged, it is puzzling why Hilbert should say that 'the empirical literature is not going to provide us with an independent characterization of colour vision'. (Perhaps he meant no more than that the empirical literature does not take up the question explicitly, and not that the question has no empirical implications.) As a matter of fact, there *is* a widely used empirical test of whether an animal *represents* colour, or merely *responds* to it. The test is whether an animal can be conditioned to respond differentially to different colours. Suppose that an animal is rewarded when it responds to a stimulus x, which possesses sense-feature F, with behaviour B. This, let us say, leads it to respond to stimulus y, which possesses the same sense-feature F, with behaviour B. This response is causally dependent on a past occurrence, i.e. on x's being F having led to B being rewarded. In some implicit way, the animal has to be *comparing* the two stimuli x and y with respect to the sense-feature F. But the past stimulus y is not, or at least need not be, present to affect the organism. Thus, x's past possession of F has to be recorded somewhere inside the organism, as a memory or in some other form.

Conditioning, learning, and other such capacities involve, in this way, not just an organism's capacity to respond to a sense-feature F, but its capacity to modify its own state in response to F (perhaps by 'storing' occurrences of F in memory) and thus to modify its future response to F. (In this way, perception leaves a *trace* in the system.) This capacity is not specific to the feature F: if the organism had been rewarded when it responded to another feature G (in the same exclusion range) with behaviour B', then it would have so modified itself that when another G thing came along it would respond with behaviour B'. Thus, conditioning is a capacity that conforms to something like the following:

Meta-response (Trace) Schema
For some class of features R and some class of behaviours S, if organism O is rewarded when it responds to a stimulus that has feature **r**, which is a member of R, with behaviour **b**, which is in S, then the probability that O will respond to a future **r**-thing with **b** rises.

The claim is that this capacity is more complex than that of merely responding differentially to features in R; it involves creating a record of these features. It is a 'meta-response' capacity, in the sense that it is a capacity to acquire a response-pattern to any feature (in a range) if that feature is presented in a context of 'reward'. It is perhaps still not exactly transparent why the animal should be said to *represent* the past state of affairs, or why its achievement should count as vision. But the existence of a meta-response schema at least distinguishes it from Hilbert's organism, and gives the representational idea some initial plausibility. We'll return to the issue of representation in Chapter 8 and attempt to motivate a more demanding, and more foundational, account.

These observations indicate that if you want to know whether a creature classifies or represents things as red—as opposed to merely responding to the presence of red—then you must at least attempt to find out whether it can be trained to press a bar or push a lever when a red light is presented, and not to press it when a blue or green light of equal brightness is presented. This, rather than simply finding out whether it responds differentially to different outputs of receptors, is the appropriate test. This suggests the following definition of colour vision, slightly modified from F^* above:

Functional Definition of Colour Vision
Colour vision is the visual discrimination capacity that relies on wavelength-discriminating sensors to ground differential *learned* (or conditioned) responses to light differing in wavelength only.[5]

---

[5] The *Functional Definition* has been modified in two ways since it first appeared in Matthen (1999) under the name *F*. First, in a poster presented at the Society for Philosophy and Psychology in 2002, Peter Bradley (unpublished) argued that the infra-red skin sensors of the pit viper would count as colour vision by the original version. To accommodate this point, I have specified that colour vision is a *visual* capacity, as presumably that of the pit vipers is not. I take it that vision is defined in historical-evolutionary terms by reference to the use of lenses to create an image on the retina, and the retinal rod and cone cells that transduce this image—I am assuming, in other words, that all visual systems trace back to an ancestor that possessed some rudimentary version of these devices. Secondly, I have insisted that the system must rely on wavelength-discriminating sensors in order to accommodate the fact that rod monochromats are in fact able to respond differentially to stimuli differing in colour, but not on the basis of information from such sensors—see below.

Correspondingly, *colour* can be defined as follows:

Functional Definition of Colour
A colour classification is one that is generated from the processing of differences of wavelength reaching the eye, and available to normal colour perceivers only by such processing.

These *Functional Definitions* correspond quite closely to empirical practice in comparative studies of vision.

Hilbert might balk at this too; certainly Hardin displays unease with the idea that honey bees (which possess colour vision by the Functional Definition, but probably do not see colour or anything else *consciously*) should be brought into the fold. The reason why many philosophers are reluctant to accept definitions like the above Functional Definitions is that they omit reference to the *conscious* phenomenology of colour. In this context, they tend to quote or paraphrase P. F. Strawson (1979, 56): 'Colours are visibilia, or they are nothing'—this is taken to imply that colours must conform to human visual phenomenology, since they are phenomenologically defined by humans. So colour should be defined in terms of colour *experience* — human experience, that is. This seems to be why Hilbert, whose guiding intuition is a paraphrase of Strawson—'Colours that cannot be seen . . . are not plausibly colours at all' (1992, 359)—insists that, although 'colour vision plays rather diverse roles in different organisms', an adequate conception of colour must focus on, or at least start from, human phenomenology. The idea is that colour vision is a perceptual system that produces something like human colour phenomenology.

There are several ways that resemblances to human phenomenology have been invoked in the recent philosophical literature; and I shall come back to Hilbert's own way in the next section. (A principal aim of the present chapter is to undermine all resemblance accounts, including those that appeal to 'family resemblance'.) First, let us consider the views of Evan Thompson (1995), who was among the first to point out the philosophical relevance of colour vision in other animals. Thompson thinks that in deciding whether other animals possess colour vision, we should stay close to the structure of colour as humans experience it.

I agree with Hilbert that we can have an independent phenomenological route to colour vision. What this route reveals [however] . . . is that colour vision, whatever else it might be, is the ability to see visual qualities belonging to the phenomenal hue categories, red, green, yellow, blue. (9)

Hardin (1988, 14) takes a similar position: he says that opponent processing accounts for 'some of the deepest features of the internal relations of colors'.
Thompson's words suggest a

*Strong Phenomenological Constraint on Colour
If an organism does not experience red, green, yellow, and blue, it does not experience colour at all.

But in fact Thompson (personal communication) intends something weaker. He is interested in the computational and physiological basis of human colour phenomenology and recommending that colour vision be defined in terms of resemblances to the mechanisms that produce the 'phenomenal hue categories' in humans. Thus he is advocating a

Weak Phenomenological Constraint on Colour
If an organism does not possess colour experiences that result from multiple pigments and opponent processing, it does not experience colour at all.

To illustrate some of the difficulties this kind of proposal brings, let us first test the Strong Phenomenological Constraint by reference to a phylogenetic scenario described by J. D. Mollon (1991, 311): 'Our colour vision seems to depend on two, relatively independent, subsystems—a phylogenetically recent subsystem overlaid on a much more ancient subsystem.' The ancient subsystem, he says, detects a very simple characteristic of the wavelength distribution of a spectral signal, roughly whether it is stronger in the short- or the long-wavelength end of the visual spectrum. (This corresponds to the second opponent process described in section I.1 above.) The ancestral organisms that possessed only this subsystem would have been dichromats. Subjectively, it is the primordial subsystem that divides our own colour sensations into warm, cool, and neutral. Our dichromatic ancestors would have had colours that correspond to this classificatory system in ourselves.

Here is the question. Consider a species that possesses the 'ancient' subsystem, but does not know Thompson's 'hue categories, red, green, yellow, blue'—does it have colour vision? On grounds of phenomenology, and in isolation, one might well be inclined to say 'No': in our colour phenomenology, warm and cool seem to be characterizations that sit on top, as it were, of the colours, and there is a strong tradition of ascribing colour vision only to trichromats. But when we remember that warmth/coolness is pretty much the same as the long/short-wavelength determination that forms the basis of our blue-yellow categories, we should hesitate. Clearly the primordial subsystem has access to one of the two dimensions of our richer experience of hue. To deny that it represents the world in colour seems as invidious as for a tetrachromatic pigeon to sniff at us. Not only that. We noted earlier that since the pigeon has more complex colour experiences: it likely does not experience red and green either, or experiences them only in a quite different way. So it too might, for all we know, be excluded by the Strong Phenomenological Constraint. Moreover, there are humans who can respond to colour differences even though they have, because of brain damage, lost the ability to experience colour—a condition known as colour blindsight. These people too would be excluded by both varieties of Phenomenological Constraint outlined above, and by Strawson's approach generally.

The Weak Phenomenological Constraint does not license the extreme conclusion rehearsed above: the ancient subsystem does not know the hue categories Thompson fastens on—*warm-cool* becomes *blue-yellow* only when the additional hue category is in place—but it does have opponent processing, the neurocomputational basis of these categories. So let us now turn to the weaker (and much more plausible) hypothesis that opponent processing is a defining condition of colour vision. (Keep in mind that the Functional Definition only constrains the front end, the receptors, and therefore admits systems that use processing systems other than opponent processing to extract information concerning wavelength-dependent features from the incoming signal.) In order to test this Weak Constraint, imagine a primate that during the course of evolution came to live in caves. In the dim light available there, its opponent-processing system is of little use, because the colour-sensitive cone cells put out small values in poor illumination, and the differences between these outputs are smaller still. However, the *addition* of signals from the three cone cells—what corresponds to the *achromatic* channel in human daytime vision—is still useful. Let us imagine that the primate retains the achromatic channel, but loses the differenced chromatic channels with the passage of evolutionary time.

Now, though the achromatic channel delivers our daytime perception of black and white and grey, it is most sensitive to light in the waveband of greatest overlap between the three cones, i.e. in roughly the middle of the visual spectrum. This is why yellows and greens seem bright to us—two kinds of cone cell contribute amplitude to our perception of these colours at close to their peak sensitivity, thereby nearly doubling their brightness—while the reds and violets at opposite ends of our spectrum, which activate only one cone, seem relatively dark. So, in effect, our primate distinguishes (what we call) yellow from blue and red (just as our own daytime achromatic vision does). But it will do this without experiencing *hue*; it merely experiences yellow things as bright. And in the dim but uniform lighting of the cave, it might well be able to use this phenomenal difference between yellow things and blue things to discriminate between different kinds of things. Does it have colour vision? Does it 'remember' an aspect of colour much as the ancient subsystem anticipates it?

Compare the primate's vision with that of a rod monochromat, the latter resulting from a congenital absence of colour-discriminating cone cells. Rod monochromats rely for vision entirely on the rod cells that most of us use for night vision only. There is a resemblance between what such monochromats see and what we experience as black, white, and grey: one such individual, Knut Nordby (quoted by Sacks 1998, 14), says that *phenomenologically* his vision 'has some resemblance to that of an orthochromatic black-and-white film'. However, there is a difference: what such an individual (and the rest of us at night) perceives as 'bright' is not the same as the brightness we have just been talking about, that is, that of yellow and the other 'bright' colours. The rod monochromat's vision is based on the output of one type of cell only. This cell will be more sensitive to light of certain wavelengths and less so to light of other wavelengths. But it will respond equally to a less bright object in its peak sensitivity range and brighter object outside this range. Since the difference between peak sensitivity and minimum sensitivity of a single cell-type is much smaller than the range available to the primate in virtue of its summative channel, it is unlikely that a rod monochromat could use this cue to distinguish colours. Thus, our imaginary primate's vision is closer to the trichromat's in one crucial respect that is relevant to our perception of colour— even though its experience is phenomenologically similar to that of a rod monochromat.

Taking only phenomenological resemblance into account, there may be very little to distinguish the primate from the rod monochromat. The range of qualia available to both is pretty much the same—as our own night vision reveals, rod-based vision is in black and white and grey. Nevertheless, the correspondence that does exist between the primate's vision and that of a colour perceiver is significant with respect to how it is classified. It is not merely the extent of the similarities and differences amongst these three systems that makes the difference regarding which are, in some sense, perceivers of colour, but how the comparative phenomena are explained. Considering the evolutionary connection it has with other primate colour perceivers, it makes sense to insist that, as in the case of the dichromatic system that experiences warm and cool colours, this animal's perception of certain surfaces as bright and others as dark is a manifestation of one aspect or dimension of colour vision.

It is also relevant here to note that rod monochromats can also discriminate colours, and display a surprisingly good ability to use standard colour vocabulary. How do they achieve this? Justin Broakes (conference paper, 2002) suggests that they may be using cues like the following. A red object will darken less than a blue one at dusk since the light is reddish at dusk, and the red object will reflect more of the available light. Equally, those parts of a red object that are in shadow at dusk will show more contrast with directly illuminated parts than in the case of a blue object. However, these rod monochromats are not using wavelength-discriminating sensors to make colour discriminations. So by the Functional Definition they lack colour vision. This definition has the somewhat surprising consequence, then, that it is possible perceptually to discriminate colours without possessing colour vision. (The definition could be modified to admit rod monochromats, but on the whole it is preferable to say that they do *not* possess colour vision.)

The cases we have just discussed show that we cannot define colour vision by phenomenology or by the cognitive mechanisms that produce a particular phenomenology. Of course, we already knew this from our consideration of narrow anthropocentrism. But there is a further point that we can take from our discussion so far. When we are dealing with human colour vision, we have a more or less fixed object of investigation. There is no urgent need to decide what is essential and what is accidental about this system; we can take it as we find it, subject to such variation as exists amongst individuals of this and closely related species. When we investigate colour vision *in general*, the point of taking the human case as a paradigm becomes less clear. In the first place, it is unclear why we should assume that the human system is the norm rather than some kind of oddity or specialized adaptation. In fact, primate colour vision *is* a singularity, having evolved, independently of other such systems, from the dichromatic vision of nocturnal mammals. It can be expected, for this reason, to possess some of the peculiarities of its evolutionary antecedents, and to be different in some respects from other independently evolved trichromatic systems. Secondly, treating *human* colour vision as if it gave us an unambiguous paradigm is, in any case, somewhat dangerous. There are many differences among individual humans with respect to colour vision, and the methodology of establishing a norm even among humans has never been adequately discussed (see Cohen 2003*b*; Hardin 2003).

This is why flexible anthropocentrism is not a principled approach. It does not offer us an understanding of deeper issues. The complaint is not that it fails to offer us precision—perhaps no approach can do that. The problem is that some kinds of resemblance are more relevant than others. Arranging things by similarity to the human case may well be a useful preliminary to sorting these out, but it is the *explanation* of similarity and difference that must in the end form the basis for the classification of visual systems.

Conclusion 2: Defining *colour vision* by its family resemblance to the human case falls short of articulating *explanatory* principles that govern the classification of colour-like experiences in other species.

IV. Anthropocentric Realism

It might be thought that the difficulties of flexible anthropocentrism can be traced to its failure to deal with *real* colour—the properties of stimuli that account for them being co-classified by colour vision. So far, we have been looking at colour experiences without considering the other half of Lewis's dual schemata, the environmental qualities that occasion colour experiences. Is it not possible that all colour-vision systems detect and discriminate among certain independently existing qualities, while differing from one another in how they represent these qualities? If so, the differences that have preoccupied us above are unimportant. They simply reflect differences in the form of representation, rather than in what is represented. In the remainder of this chapter, we consider successively less demanding versions of this idea, arguing that each is unable to deal satisfactorily with the facts of comparative colour vision, because it is impossible in principle to set bounds on the qualities that colour vision is able to detect.

Hilbert (1992) responds to the shortcomings of the rigid and exclusionary anthropocentrism considered in section II by formulating an approach he calls 'anthropocentric realism'. He starts with the idea that

(1) It is possible to identify our own colour experiences introspectively as 'an aspect of our visual experience that is clearly different from figure, texture, depth'.

He then suggests that

(2) The human colour experiences so identified have the biological function of detecting surface spectral reflectances.

This, he thinks, makes it plausible that

(3) Colours are surface spectral reflectances.[6]

In short, Hilbert agrees with Thompson in identifying human colour experience by means of its phenomenology, but instead of taking the essence of colour vision to reside in the perceptual mechanisms that produce this phenomenology, he concentrates on its environmental significance. He proposes that, regardless of what species it occurs in (and disregarding phenomenology in species other than humans) a visual system should be identified as colour vision if, as in the human case, it detects spectral reflectances via colour-like experience.

So long as it is applied in a disciplined way, this form of anthropocentrism is harmless, Hilbert claims.

The claim is not that human beings have the best colour vision or that human characteristics are more central than that of other organisms. They may possess visual abilities that humans lack and as long as we are careful to classify organisms as having colour vision only on functional grounds we will only impose similarity on organisms that really are similar in relevant ways. (1992, 364)

Hilbert's reliance on environmental qualities allows him to extend the scope of a conception like Lewis's to colours not visible to humans. The pigeon's detection of the ultraviolet in bird feathers is a colour-vision state because it is a colour-like experience that detects reflectance. Presumably, this makes

---

[6] In making (2) part of the ground for (3), Hilbert relies on an argument made in some detail by myself in Matthen (1988). However, I noted that a more encompassing definition was required in order to accommodate luminous and transmitted colours. Later, in Matthen (1992) I abandoned (3) in response to Thompson et al. (1992). I shall argue below that (2) should also be rejected. In Part IV, I offer a different account of the function of sense-perception in general.

ultraviolet a colour, and pigeon's system a colour-vision system. Further, if we allow Hilbert the assumption that both the rod monochromat and the imaginary primate discussed above have colour-like experiences, a contentious but not indefensible claim, he might well arrive at the same conclusions as we did with regard to them, since primates makes wavelength-based distinctions among spectral reflectances, using wavelength-discriminating sensors, while rod monochromats do not. These are good results. By stressing the reflectance-detection function of colour vision, Hilbert is able to include a wide range of experiences of other species. And by introducing a criterion based on function, he goes beyond vague and non-explanatory considerations of overall resemblance to human phenomenology.

Hilbert's conception is not all good, unfortunately. Let's look again at the pigeon's ultraviolet vision. The atmosphere scatters ultraviolet light more than light of longer wavelengths; consequently, light coming from a direction perpendicular to the sun tends to have a high concentration of ultraviolet, while light from the direction of the sun tends to be unbiased as to frequency, that is, white. J. F. Nuboer (1986) speculates that with its ultraviolet vision, the pigeon is able to navigate in an aerial environment which not only lacks 'landmarks' but extends deep into three dimensions (by contrast with our own environment which does not normally extend far below our feet or above our eyes). Even in its trackless space, the bird can determine direction in heliocentric coordinates. But both the narrow anthropocentrist of section I and Hilbert are committed to saying that it is not doing so by detecting *colour*. The narrow anthropocentrist is forced to say this for the uninteresting reason that since humans do not see in the ultraviolet, ultraviolet is not a colour. Hilbert is forced to agree with this blinkered conclusion, but his more interesting reason is that he identifies colours by what *human* colour-vision detects, which (according to him) is surface reflectance. The pigeon detects a property of direction, and direction is not a surface.

This is not so good a result. We discriminate and locate surfaces by the colour experiences induced in us by light differentially reflected from them. This is at least part of our justification for saying that colour is a property of surfaces. The bird discriminates *directions* by the colour-like experiences induced in it by light differentially scattered from different directions. This should incline us to say that to the bird, directions look coloured: the direction of the sun looks white, and directions at right angles to the sun look ultraviolet. In short, for the bird, colour is a property of directions as well as of surfaces. For it surfaces are comparable to directions with respect to colour: for instance, directions perpendicular to the sun are the same colour as ultraviolet plumage. All of this makes pigeon-colour a different property than the one we see. And this suggests that colour cannot be defined as a specific environmental property.

Hilbert, however, refuses to truck with the permissiveness of the previous paragraph:

The only way an objectivist can meet the challenge posed by the apparent fact that colour vision functions to detect different properties in different kinds of organisms is to deny that this really [is] the case (1992, 365).

Accordingly, he *denies* that the bird's experiences of direction are experiences in colour. Colours are what *human* colour experience detects. We *could* have called directions coloured, but given how we have fixed the reference of colour terms, it turns out that we do not. This conclusion seems infelicitous— it seems, on the face of it, that anthropocentrism should be incompatible with objectivism, so if objectivism *implies* anthropocentrism, objectivism is inconsistent. But let us eschew this kind of argument: a lot of our intuitions count for little in the unfamiliar territory of interspecies comparisons. It would not be wise to exclude Hilbert's thesis on the flimsy ground that it conflicts with intutions concerning anthropocentrism.

Still it is fair to ask: why is it so important to Hilbert that only reflectances be included among the colours? This is what he says:

Colour objectivism requires that there be some mind-independent property that is colour. If . . . there is no single property that all organisms with colour vision are capable of visually detecting, the objectivist . . . must either deny that possession of colour vision entails that the organism has the ability to visually determine the colour of a surface or give up his claim that colour is an objective property. (1992, 358)

This, again, is obscure; it is far from clear why the objectivist must insist on there being a *single* mind-independent property that is colour. Why not allow that a plurality of mind-independent properties might fall under the genus, colour?

Hilbert's intuition is based on a realist interpretation of the dimensional structure and separateness of sensory exclusion ranges. As we saw in Part II, we make judgements of comparative similarity within sensory exclusion ranges; these reflect the multidimensional vector coding of the features that constitute an exclusion range. The realist (or 'objectivist', to use Hilbert's term) seeks to ground this similarity order in an *objective* ordering of the qualities that colour vision detects. He seeks a field of qualities that (a) exists independently of our perception of them, and (b) displays the same resemblance ordering (relative to some physical quantity) as experienced colour.[7] This seems to be what Hilbert is trying to do.

Spectral reflectances are real, and they can be arranged in a numerically measured similarity space (in the sense of Chapter 4). Hilbert (1987) claims that they provide him with the similarity-ordering that he is looking for.

---

[7] Byrne (2003) sees the problem pretty much in these terms, though he defuses it by denying that colours stand in similarity relations—only stimuli do, he says (see the Afterword to Part II for a discussion of Byrne's position).

If we think of triples of integrated reflectances as coordinates in a three-dimensional space, then similar colours will occupy adjacent regions of that space . . . . Every reflectance will have a location in this space.

Colour space is [thus] specified completely objectively, so the various colour relations have an objective basis. Colour space is also structured in the same way as our perceptual colour judgements so that there can be no conflict between true perceptual judgements and the objective facts. The reference of colour terms and the relations and properties they instantiate are objective although anthropocentric. (1987, 117–18; cf. Edwin Land 1977, 108–28)

The properties of directions and the like would not be a part of reflectance space—that is, they are not representable as 'triples of integrated reflectances'. This is why Hilbert would like to exclude them from the field of colours.

There is a decisive empirical refutation of this approach. As Leo Hurvich and Dorothea Jameson established in the 1950s, the similarity space of human colour is essentially determined by the opponent processing of outputs from retinal cone cells (see section I above). The similarity relations that opponent processing spawns do not correspond to similarities defined on reflectances, and cannot be explained by them. They are generated by sensory systems, as we saw in Chapter 5. Opponent process theory had unfortunately not entered the general philosophical consciousness when Hilbert wrote his doctoral thesis (1987). (I made the same error in Matthen (1988), as did Paul Churchland (1988, 148–9)—Churchland revised his argument in the second edition of his book. See, however, Keith Campbell (1969) for an early exception to this.) Hilbert himself was aware of opponent processing when he wrote, though he thought it irrelevant: in view of the attention it has garnered in the philosophical literature since then, he probably regrets not tackling the issue head-on. As far as this goes, flexible anthropocentrism, which is based on the phenomenal structure of human colour vision, does a great deal better, though, as we saw in the previous section, it is untenable for other reasons.

Putting this shared embarrassment aside, there is another problem with the idea that colour vision is directed to a 'single property'. The proposal leans too heavily on the claim that reflectance is the one and only thing that human colour vision functions to detect. What we have learned from the case of the pigeon is that the mechanisms of colour vision can be used, and *are* used, to detect other things. So even if the distal colours detected by humans did happen to be unified by physically defined similarity relations among reflectances, it is by sheer luck. Let the pigeon try a 'columbicentric' definition in the style of Hilbert's anthropocentric realism—let it define *p-colour* as whatever its own kind of experience properly detects—and it would pull in a heterogeneous collection of properties, not only properties of surfaces but properties of directions as well. In the case of the pigeon, then, the introspected unity of colour experience fails to guarantee that the external properties that correspond to its experiences constitute a single resemblance ordering in the strong sense Hilbert demands. So, the objectivist would be ill-advised to demand, in general, that the unity of colour experience be replicated in the real world. If it is so in the human case, it is because of the fortuitous fact— if it is a fact—that our colour experiences detect one thing only. If *our* experience had pulled in a heterogeneous collection of environmental features, as the pigeon's does, the resemblance ordering of reflectance would not have provided so neat a way of adjudicating dodgy colours.

Once this point has been made, it is hard not to notice that in the human case too, colour experience *does* seem to gather in a heterogeneous collection of spectral emission properties—reflectances, to be sure, but luminances and transmittances as well, for lights and stained-glass windows seem not only to be seen in colour, but to be experienced in ways that are comparable, in exactly the above sense, to how surfaces are experienced. (The red of a stained-glass window is the same as that in its creator's cartoon. It might be judged more similar to the orange of a traffic light than to the green of a leaf.) Indeed we are more like the pigeon than Hilbert is ready to acknowledge. Not all of our colours are reflectances, not all are properties of surface. Not every colour of which we are aware is even *located* in a surface—the blue of the sky has a direction (like the pigeon's ultraviolet?) but no obvious surface. Is it not wishful thinking to suppose that all the colours we perceive can be accommodated in reflectance space? And if human experience detects all of these different kinds of property, is there any good reason for insisting that directions—which the pigeon detects by ultraviolet scattering, and other organisms, such as the honeybee, may detect by polarization—are not coloured?[8]

Conclusion 3: Anthropocentric definitions of *colour* in terms of the alleged real unity of colours as detected by humans cannot accommodate the diversity of properties detected by colour-vision systems.

---

[8] In Matthen (1988), I mentioned the need for a generalized definition of colour, which would include surface reflectances as a special case, but generalize to radiant and transmitted colour. Similarly, Byrne and Hilbert (1997c) say that 'the extension of our account to light sources and transparent volumes is a matter for another time' (265). Cf. Lewis (1997), 'My restriction of the topic [to surface colours] leaves unfinished business' (330). Byrne and Hilbert (2003) attempt to make good on their 1997 promise with their notion of a 'productance', but their definition is problematic when it comes to luminance—it implies that a light is less 'productive' in bright light than in the dark, which is counter-intuitive since it has the same luminance—and in any case, they haven't yet incorporated pigeon direction-colours and the like.

7

The Disunity of Colour

In this chapter, we explore the specialization of colour vision in an evolutionary setting. We discuss how specialization evolves, and show how a proper conception has important consequences for how we should understand colour experience. We shall find that perceptual specialization is best accommodated by the Sensory Classification Thesis.

I. The Multiple Emergence of Colour Vision

It is a remarkable fact about good colour vision (trichromatism) that (a) only a few types of animal possess it (aside from birds, among which it is relatively common), and that (b) these are phylogenetically widely separated. Among mammals, only some primates have trichromatic colour vision. But good colour vision occurs in nearly every broad group of animals: insects, reptiles, birds, fish, mammals. The wide phylogenetic separation of colour perceivers suggests that colour vision is latent in almost all phylogenetic groups, a genetic possibility that can emerge with relative ease when the circumstances are right. For if you pick two colour-seeing species from distinct phyla—pigeons and humans, for instance—you will find that there is no direct line of descent that links these two species to a common colour-seeing ancestor. In other words, good colour vision arose independently in these two organisms.

It seems, then, that trichromatism emerged *de novo* in each phylogenetic group in which it occurs. Some evolutionary theorists assume that this is a case of convergence, that is, a case where exactly the same function evolves independently in more than one species. This is implied also by most philosophical views, for they do not admit the possibility that colour vision could have different functions in different phyla. After all, the function of colour vision is to detect colour, is it not? How could such a function be differentiated in its multiple occurrences? In this section, we argue that these tendencies are off the mark. Through a consideration of how biological speciation occurs, we will argue that the history of colour vision consists of the emergence of *different* functional specializations, albeit on the same biochemical substrate.

Normally, the independent emergence of any one trait in different phylogenetic groups is regarded an improbable conjunction of events. How then can colour vision have emerged independently so many times? In order to answer this question, we must first look at what all biological colour-vision systems share. The chemicals in cone cells that are sensitive to different wavebands are based on protein molecules known as 'opsins'. Opsins evolved about a billion years ago in bacteria, where they were and are still used for photosynthesis. They were then co-opted for differential colour response relatively early in their history (Allman 1999, ch. 1). In *Halobacterium salinarium*, a unicellular organism which lives in salt marshes, a light-sensitive pigment closely related to rhodopsin, which is used for colour vision in vertebrates, is used to guide the organism towards sunlight. In another unicellular organism, *Chlamydomonas*, another pigment closely related to vertebrate rhodopsin is used to guide the bacterium towards its energy source. Significantly, *Chlamydomonas*'s use of colour information requires short-term memory, since it demands the comparison of light intensities over short periods of time. (Thus, it has some claim to satisfying the Functional Definition of Colour Vision stated in Chapter 6, section III.) This shows that the *material basis* for colour vision— i.e. the opsins—is very ancient, and can likely be traced to a common origin, or at least to a few independent events that occurred very long ago in bacteria. In time, these opsins came to be localized in structures specialized for differential wavelength sensitivity, the cone cells. Cone cells incorporate stacks of photosensitive membranes incorporating the opsins; they can be activated by the capture of just a single photon. Notably, these cone-cell membranes are descended from bacterial cilia. This progression from ancient opsins to highly sensitive cone cells marks a classic case of evolutionary optimization.

Now, possessing a single opsin is not enough for colour vision. Good colour vision requires three different visual pigments, as we saw in the previous chapter (section I.1). What is required, then, is the emergence in an organism of several opsins, each sensitive to a different waveband in the visible spectrum. Now, the opsins of the short-wavelength cone differ from those of the long by the substitution of one amino acid for another. Opsins proliferate by just such small substitutions. There is, however, a limit to the number of such substitutions, and thus a limit to how many classes of cone cells are available to natural selection. On the other hand, all visual organisms possess *some* opsins, and thus the proliferation of photoreceptor types within the above-mentioned limits is frequently available to natural selection. For judging from the considerable variety in cone-cell sensitivities over the human population, mutations that modify opsins occur regularly, and these mutations will be selected and persist if they bring an advantage. This explains the latency of colour vision in all phyla. On the other hand, new and different colour-sensitive receptors have never evolved. The front-end of colour vision, the receptors that are differentially sensitive to light of different wavelengths, is (a) of ancient origin, (b) more or less fixed in structure, and (c) readily available.

Now, given that colour vision is latent in all phyla and readily available to all classes of organism, why don't *all* organisms possess it? Would it not be an advantage for all organisms? There has been, as we saw a moment ago, steady improvement in photoreceptor sensitivity and structure. Why has there not been a similar steady and universal improvement in colour vision? The answer is to be found in a principle enunciated by Darwin. Darwin realized that speciation occurs when a sub-population of a species specializes. This sub-population distances itself from the ancestral population by developing the ability to exploit environmental resources in novel ways. By doing this it benefits from reduced competition. Thus, if a species is able to modify a pre-existing facility to help forge a new way of life, it is enabled to exploit resources that are not available to other species, and it frees itself (and the ancestral species) from competitive pressure. This is called the Principle of Divergence. (Gould 2002, 234–50, is an informative discussion.) It suggests a reason why natural selection takes up the opportunity for trichromatism so sporadically. The reason is *not*, as many have found obvious, that it is an advantage for all; rather, it is a specialization which enables some organisms to occupy a niche that their predecessors did not occupy. I remarked two paragraphs ago that the optimization of photosensitive receptors was a steady progression. My present point is that the history of colour vision is not similarly a story of progress across all branches of the tree of life: colour vision emerges by divergence.

When colour vision emerges, it is because it enables a particular species to distinguish itself from the ancestral population by exploiting a resource that this ancestral population could not use. *Ex hyposthesi*, the ancestral species lacks colour vision, and continues on without it. Among mammals, colour vision emerged among old-world monkeys. The ancestors of this group, the new-world monkeys, lack good colour vision for the most part. These two branches of the phylogenetic tree exist simultaneously: there are still monkeys that lack colour vision. This implies that the non-colour-seeing monkeys are able to exploit their distinctive niches without using colour vision. Thus, one should not assume that colour vision is advantageous for all forms of life. We should look for its value in the difference between populations that possess it and ancestral populations that do not. If most vertebrates lack colour vision, it is not because evolution could not have provided it: it is rather that in most vertebrates this facility has utility only relative to a specialized and differentiating style of life.

Colour vision is widely assumed to have the *same* function wherever it occurs. The Principle of Divergence shows that this is unlikely (at least if the function is fully specified). The pressures that made colour discrimination valuable for a honey bee in competition with its ancestors are unlikely to have been exactly the same as those that made it valuable for old-world monkeys in a quite different situation. Thus, we should expect that old-world monkeys use colour vision in a different way from honey bees. This argument generalizes: since colour vision supports divergent modes of life in the widely divergent species in which it occurs, it is to be expected that colour-vision systems in divergent groups will possess different characteristics. However, as we saw earlier, the front-end of colour vision—the receptors that discriminate wavelength differences in incoming light—is more or less fixed. Consequently, the differences needed by the Principle of Divergence are achieved by specializations downstream of the receptors: (a) the addition of filters, polarization detectors, and other such gadgets, and (b) new forms of colour-processing. It is here that the causes of specialization is to be found.

These considerations suggest that each different type of trichromatic colour-vision system will focus on different colour-detectable environmental characteristics. It is not the detection of colour as such that provides each colour-seeing organism with an advantage, but the use of colour differentiation for other purposes. The idiosyncrasies noted in the previous chapter are signs of the specialized nature of the niche that various colour-seeing organisms occupy. Since each species performs a different set of tasks, each must measure the environment in its own way. Each colour classification scheme must adapt to different external realities.

II. Specialization in Primate Colour Vision

Now, what is the differentiating advantage that human, or more accurately, primate colour vision provides? J. D. Mollon and co-workers (Regan et al. 2001) have advanced the hypothesis that it co-evolved with the colours of small fruits and berries.

(i) Most primates eat fruit, and many eat it in large quantities . . .
(ii) At the same time, the plants whose fruits the primates eat are competing for seed dispersal. Effective dispersal of seeds is critical to reproductive success in plants . . .
(iii) The set of traits shared by fruits dispersed by a particular class of consumer can be interpreted as adaptation to that dispersal agent, and is known as a dispersal syndrome. Characteristics of the primate seed-dispersal syndrome are a yellow, orange or red colour, which makes the fruits conspicuous (at least, to a trichromatic consumer) . . . (234).

It seems that certain plants evolved fruit that are nutritious to primates, and visible to them, while primates evolved the kind of vision that makes it easy to find these fruit from a distance against a leafy background, and under leaf colour. This relationship is a specialization for both parties: it turns out, for example, that fruits less conspicuous to primates are specialized for consumption by nocturnal animals, while the conspicuous fruit are particularly well suited for dispersion through the digestive tracts of primates with colour vision. This whole system of mutual dependence starts with colour. The fruit-colour evolves in such a way as to be conspicuous to primates with emerging trichromatic colour vision; primate colour vision in turn evolved and took hold because it offered its possessors the opportunity to focus on these particular kinds of fruit. (A competing hypothesis holds that primate colour vision evolved to aid in foraging for young leaves, which are often red in colour—see Dominy and Lucas (2001) and Surridge et al. (2003). No attempt is made here to adjudicate this dispute; we stick with the fruit hypothesis for no other reason than convenience.)

Now, what exactly is the specialization that colour-seeing primates possess? In order to answer this question, we must compare these primates with their dichromatic cousins. It will be recalled (Chapter 6, section II) that the ancestral mammalian colour-vision system simply divides the visible spectrum into long-wavelength and short-wavelength halves, measuring which is dominant. This corresponds to the 'warm' and 'cool' colour sensations. It turns out that this ancestral system is ill-adapted to searching for fruits among foliage, 'because it has poor spatial resolution, and the fruits eaten by primates, when seen at a distance, are usually too small to be resolved by this subsystem' (Regan et al., 2001, 241). The ideal colour-vision system for the task would make the fruit 'pop out' against the background; that is, it would minimize the search time for such fruit, and make it relatively invariant relative to the number of green leafy distractors. This enables a monkey surveying the arboreal scene from afar quickly to detect where its chosen fruit are, rather than having to inspect each tree close up.

Now, it is likely that fruit colour evolved just so as to be conspicuous in this way to colour-vision systems with the peculiar characteristics of primate colour vision. For what is needed is that the chromatic difference between these fruit and the leaves be maximized, while the difference among the leaves themselves should be minimized. As Regan et al. say, 'We therefore consider the optimal photopigments to be those that maximize signal-to-noise ratio for detecting fruit targets against the visual noise of the leaf distractors, rather than the number of fruits that lie one or more JNDs (just-noticeable-difference steps) from the leaves' (2000, 240). In other words, it is *not* sufficient that these kinds of fruit should simply be distinct from the leaves, for instance that they should cluster in one half of a straight line in colour space while the fruit cluster in the other half. Instead of this kind of difference in degree, there needs to be some sort of sharp qualitative difference which enables them to pop out. It turns out that the peak sensitivities of primate colour receptive cones are well spaced with regard to differentiating *red* and *orange* from *green*.

There are, then, two contributions that primate colour-vision systems make to carving out an evolutionary niche that includes the consumption of a particular set of fruit. The added colour information provided by this system is (a) fine-grained enough that it can detect relatively small fruit from a distance, and (b) it makes the fruit pop out against a background of leaves. Notice that the niche-creating advantages provided by colour vision do *not* include the discrimination of colour close up in good light. The special advantage that primate colour systems possess is not that they can process relevant information about these fruit from close up.

Keeping these specialized functions in mind, a comment made by Gerald Jacobs, an eminent student of comparative colour vision, becomes highly relevant. According to Jacobs (1981):

In testing large numbers of subjects from various mammalian species, some of which have 'good' color vision, I have frequently observed that given a luminance difference as cue, the animal frequently uses that as a basis for discrimination even if a color difference known to be discriminable is also available. (169)

In other words, if information about a particular surface-feature is available in luminance differences, the organism will appeal to the latter. Thus, 'given a luminance difference as cue, [an] animal frequently uses that as a basis for discrimination even if a color difference known to be discriminable is also available' (ibid., 159). Thus, in 'a multi-hued world in which objects appear to merge and contrast by virtue of their differences in color', people often mistake luminance-contrast for colour contrast. We may think that we are using colour discrimination whenever we open our eyes: in fact, we often use black and white information in its place.

Jacob's comments make sense of an observation of Robert Boyle reported by John Mollon (1991). Boyle had occasion to observe a young woman who had lost her colour vision after a high fever. He reported that she was nonetheless able to perform most tasks that depend on colour discrimination reasonably well. However, she lamented that she was unable to pick small flowers in meadow, 'tho',' as Boyle writes, 'she kneel'd in the place where they grew.' Along similar lines, Mollon (2001) quotes a report on colour blindness delivered to the Royal Society of London by J. Huddart in 1777. Speaking of a shoemaker named Harris, Huddart says:

He observed also that, when young, other children could discern cherries on a tree by some pretended difference of colour, though he'd only distinguish them from the leaves by their difference of size and shape. He observed also, that by means of this difference of colour they could see the cherries at a greater distance than he could, though he could see other objects at as great a distance as they; that is, where the sight was not assisted by the colour. Large objects he could see as well as other persons; and even the smaller ones if they were not enveloped in other things, as in the case of cherries among the leaves. (Mollon 2001, 10)

Diagnosing this particular pattern of failure, Mollon says: 'We need color vision when the target is embedded in a background that is varying randomly in lightness and in form', a 'dappled and brindled' background, as he says elsewhere. Mollon is suggesting that we do not need to use colour vision to discriminate large targets against invariant backgrounds of contrasting colour. True, but we can go further. With respect to such large targets, colour-blind people are not just able to discern them against the background, but can often make accurate estimates of what colour they are—and this applies, as we saw in the previous chapter, section IV, not only to dichromats, but also rod monochromats. This is why Ishihara plates are used in the diagnosis of colour-vision deficits: these plates consist of a field of equiluminous dots, with a letter or numeral picked out in one colour against a background of dots in another colour.

To summarize again: colour-blind people are somewhat hampered, but not completely disabled, in colour-naming and colour-discrimination tasks where the contrasting colour blocks are large, especially where the light is good. They are completely disabled only when it comes to performing colour-discrimination tasks in fine spatial detail. It is the latter sort of task that seems to have been involved in differentiating colour-seeing primates from their dichromatic ancestors.

III. Questioning the Colourist Intuition

The facts recounted in the previous section threaten what we may call the *Colourist Intuition*, a persistent fallacy in philosophical approaches to colour. Imagine a scene that contains a variety of richly coloured things: the interior of a grand cathedral, say, with intensely coloured lights, stained glass, gilt, jewels, polished wood, coloured stone, diffraction fringes from the glass, and so on. Now take a high resolution, natural contrast, black-and-white photograph of the coloured scene. What is missing? Intuitively, the answer seems obvious: *colour*. Colour seems to be something discrete: something taken from a palette and added to a monochromatic scene, much in the manner of a colourist jazzing up an old black-and-white movie for uncouth contemporary audiences. Intuition tells us that when we change from black and white to colour, we substitute certain experiences for others—reds, greens, etc. in places where previously there was only black and white and grey. In traditional sense-datum theory, as captured in what David Lewis (1999/1966) calls 'colour mosaic' theory, there is actually *nothing* shared between a colour photograph and one in black and white (unless there happens to be a monochrome object depicted in the former). Each and every pixel in the one has been replaced by a different pixel in the other.

The Colourist Intuition encourages a particular form of Universalism about colour. We could introduce it by means of an analogy. Though there are many different kinds of coloured things in it—lights, transparent panes of glass, prisms, reflective surfaces—a coloured painting or photograph reduces all the diverse colour-making properties into surface reflectances: the surface red of a painting that depicts a translucent red pane of glass is recognizably the same colour as the pane. Similarly, a television image renders all of the kinds of colours in terms of luminance colours; a colour transparency or slide photograph renders them all in terms of colour transmittances. Thus, it seems possible for just one kind of thing—wavelength-differentiating illumination in the case of the television image, reflectance in the case of the colour photograph, transmittance in the case of the transparency—to capture all of the kinds of colours present in the heterogeneous scene.

The Colourist holds that in something like the same way, colour *experience* renders all of the different kinds of colour—reflectance, transmission, illumination—into a single medium and takes the measure of them all. Generalizing this across species, he argues that there must be a common measure of all the properties available to any colour perceiver. A bird discriminates heliocentric directions in colour, but what does this mean? Surely, the Colourist insists, that it has experiences similar to those that we have when we view the cathedral, and that it is instinctively able to use these to identify directions. We may see a variety of things in colour, and when we take other species into account, the variety expands even further. But all of these things are seen in colour: the way of seeing them all is the same. There is a palette of pre-existing experiences characteristic of colour vision, however diverse might be the properties that are delivered to us in colour. This is the Colourist Intuition. (Anybody who holds a dispositional theory of colour—the theory that colours are dispositions in external objects to evoke colour-qualia in perceivers who view them— is committed to this intuition. So too are the recent 'relativists', who also define colour in terms of colour experience: Jackson and Pargetter (1987), Jonathan Cohen (2000, 2003*b*), and Brian McLaughlin (2003*a* and *b*).

The Colourist Intuition sits uncomfortably with the kinds of data that we considered in Chapter 6 and the observations recorded in the previous section. Why is it reasonable to think that a pigeon has exactly the same set of experiences that we do, given (a) that its colour vision is tetrachromatic, and (b) that its colour awareness is holistically tied to experiences of other properties? Why should we cling to the belief that our own experiences of colour are separate in the way that the Colourist proposes when it is possible to make a lot of the same colour discriminations using information only about luminance? Is it really tenable to think that colour is something of which we find out solely through the operation of the colour-vision system? Despite these perplexities, the Intuition is extremely persistent and difficult to overcome. It is not enough to question or reject the Colourist perspective; we need to replace it with a new approach.

Consider four species: humans and a closely related dichromat species, H', honey bees and a closely related dichromat insect species, B'. Humans and honey bees have advanced colour vision; H' and B' do not. There are two ways of making groups out of these species.

Functional groups

A. The species with good colour vision: humans and honey bees.
B. The dichromats: H' and B'.

Phylogenetic groups

C. The primates: humans and H'.
D. The insects: honey bees and B'.

It might seem obvious that since we are investigating colour-vision, it is the functional groups that are important. Clearly, they *are* important to the comparative study of colour-vision. The species in group *A* can make complex discriminations of colour, which, in the case of actual biological organisms, means three or more visual pigments and opponent processing. The species in group *B* lack these endowments, or possess them only in an etiolated form. Nevertheless, it is a mistake to conclude right off, as the Colourist does, that there must be a characteristic kind of datum that is shared by the organisms in the functional group *A*, or that there is some one thing about which they possess information, in contrast with the organisms in group *B*. Because humans and honey bees have no common ancestor with colour vision, there is no reason to think that the two colour-vision mechanisms developed as a response to comparable environmental challenges. Humans have single-lens eyes, their colour processing extends beyond the retina into cortical areas of the brain, and they use colour concepts in language-like representations of objects. On all counts, bees are different. On the other hand, bees are tetrachromats and use polarization as an integral part of their visual representations, including colour, and use colour vision directionally. Humans lack these refinements. Why then should we suppose that human colour discrimination is *phenomenally* or in terms of information comparable to that of bees?

This account of specialization in visual systems leads us into a different way of thinking about the effects of adding of colour dimensions to an ancestral fewer-dimensional system. The Colourist Intuition is influenced by the idea that sensation corresponds to the retinal image. In this Cartesian paradigm, it is natural to think that colour is discrete—it is retrofitted to the ancestral system, replacing much of what in that system was represented in black and white (or warm and cool). Generalizing to other modalities: there is an ambient store of discrete features awaiting capture by the sense modalities. Evolution picks items from this store, and adds them one-by-one to an animal's repertoire as needed.

The Sensory Classification Thesis of Part I offers a completely different perspective. Sensation corresponds to the answers to certain questions posed by sensory-feature detectors: it is a record of specific conditions, of whether or not they obtain. Taking this approach, we see that the questions asked by a specialized sensory system will generally add to, modify, or complement those asked by its ancestor. From this perspective, it is much more comprehensible why the phylogenetic groups listed above would share more in the way of sensation than the functional groups, even though the members of the former differ with regard to colour. The phenomenology of added sensory specialization is strongly influenced by what was there before. Evolution is not like a Colourist, painting colours into a scene already delineated. It is much more like a technician tweaking the performance characteristics of a system—changing the sensors, adding filters, rerouting data, fiddling with 'gain'—to create new discriminations within an older format. This is why colour experience is very likely closely tied to phylogeny. And it is why the phylogenetic groups given above are at least as important in the characterization of colour vision as the functional groups.

Colour is a disunity, then. There is neither a single phenomenology of colour vision nor a set of shared concepts that defines colour wherever it may occur. There is a commonality in the informational material from which colour concepts are constructed; this is inherited from the opsins that constitute the basis for any colour-vision system. Consequently, there is a functional commonality in the mechanisms that are needed to gather this information, but, as the Disunity of Colour Thesis stated at the start of Chapter 6 implies, no one mind-independent property that all colour perceivers track or detect, no one ecological problem they all try to solve. Considered across biological taxa in all of its occurrences, colour is a heterogeneous collection of perceptual concepts generated from wavelength-sensitive data for a variety of specialized purposes by cognitive systems with different neurocomputational structures and evolutionary histories.

Philosophers are unaccustomed to such heterogeneous collections. They are more used to thinking about mental concepts as based on the duplication of information-processing function in different neural structures. They think that the function of vision pre-exists evolution, and assume that evolution worked, much like a benevolent Creator, to realize pre-existent this function in diverse animals. The truth is that such duplication of function is exaggerated. Function emerged from an evolutionary history; it is not an omega-point at which evolution aims. Hardly ever does the same apparatus emerge twice: history rarely repeats itself; apparent convergences are unlikely really to be so (cf. Matthen 2001). There are many commonalities among organisms, of course, but shared function is largely due to common descent and shared apparatus. Biological kinds are thus to be defined by evolutionary history, not just by function or descriptive essence (cf. Griffiths 1997, ch. 8; Matthen 1998). The same applies to biological information-processing kinds. Colour vision originates more than once—but colour vision performs different functions in its various incarnations. To the extent that colour vision does involve the same kind of functioning across the biological realm, there is common descent.

The Functional Definitions of colour vision and of colour accommodate this heterogeneity by defining colour vision by functions shared across all biological colour-vision systems. To recapitulate from Chapter 6, section III, they are:

Functional Definition of Colour
A colour classification is one that is generated from the processing of differences of wavelength reaching the eye, and available to normal colour observers only by such processing.

Functional Definition of Colour Vision
Colour vision is the visual discrimination capacity that relies on wavelength-discriminating sensors to ground differential *learned* (or conditioned) responses to light differing in wavelength only.

These definitions do not refer to the products of colour processing, whether these be colour classes or colour experiences—these being a heterogeneous collection. Rather, they rely on the 'front end', the receptors, which colour-vision systems share.

Colour vision comes in degrees—dichromacy and better, and varieties— differences of similarity structures, of features detected, of behavioural significance. These variations are better accommodated by a set of parameters within which variation can be measured and systematized than by some unitary framework that derives from the human case. The definitions given above mark the ground level of such a parametric approach, the weakest sense in which we can say that something has colour vision, or that a particular sense-feature is a colour. More demanding definitions, including anthropocentric definitions, mark special kinds of colour-vision systems. Such special definitions are useful in coming to grips with particular systems of colour detection. What they fail to do is provide a general account of colour or colour vision.

8

Pluralistic Realism

In Chapter 7, we argued that phylogenetically isolated colour-vision systems are idiosyncratic, each one especially evolved for a specific information-gathering purpose not shared by other such systems. Colour cannot, then, be defined as some common property delivered by all such systems; it must be understood comprehending *any* feature that needs to be processed by wavelength-differentiating light sensors. Some think that it follows from the specialization of colour-vision that colour must be a classification scheme with no external validity, a figment of colour-vision systems. As proof of this, they present evidence to show that human colour categories are a poor match with their physical counterparts—wavelength, reflectance, etc. The present chapter contests this idea: it attempts to show how even idiosyncratic sensory categories can possess external significance and validity. The argument will prepare us for the theoretical framework for sensory function and content presented in Chapter 9.

I. Hardin's Catalogue

Here is a partial list of ways that human colour experience is poorly matched with physical reality. I call it *Hardin's Catalogue* because it was first introduced into discussions of how to define and understand colour by C. L. Hardin (1984, 1988). Hardin argued that his catalogue proves the non-reality of colour.

Opponency. As we have seen, the structure of experiences occasioned by opponent processing does not match up with the physical structure that exists independently of opponent-processing perceptual systems.

(i) Because of the subtractive functions used in opponent processing (Chapter 6, section I above), some colour signals carry *negative* values. Thus, *blue* is represented by a negative value on the *blue-yellow* hue-component scale, and *green* by a negative value on the *red-green* scale.

This accounts for the intuitive feeling that *red* is opposed to, or incompatible with *green*, and cannot combine with it to make a mixed colour, i.e. that there is no such thing as a reddish green. This bipolarity is a very important feature of colour phenomenology, and constitutes a strong initial motivation for opponent process theory as presented first by Hering, and then, in its present form, by Leo Hurwich and Dorothea Jameson. But what does it mean to say that, independently of its being processed in the way that humans process it, red light is opposed to green light? Nothing, Hardin argues. If *red* is component-incompatible to *green*, then, since there are no physical counterparts of colour that are component-incompatible in this way, *red* and *green* are not identical with any properties in the physical world (see Chapter 3, section I, for the notion of component-incompatibility).

(ii) Since *violet* looks reddish, it looks more similar to *red*, with which it shares a component, than to *greenish yellow*, with which it shares no component. However, *violet* is at the opposite end of the visual spectrum from *red*, and from that perspective at least, it is as dissimilar to *red* as any colour can be (see Figure 8 in Chapter 5, section I, and Table II in Chapter 6). Nor does the similarity of *violet* to *orange* have a counterpart in the three-dimensional space of reflectances where each dimension corresponds to reflected light energy in the receptive zone of one of our cone cell types. Violet occupies a region of this space that is close to *dark blue* and further from *orange* than *green*.

(iii) *Violet* is experienced as mixed, since the experience involves a non-zero component in both hue dimensions. In this it contrasts with the so-called 'unique' colours, in which one component is null, and which are experienced as 'pure'. In the spectrum, however, *violet* simply occupies a waveband; this waveband is no more mixed or pure than any other. Spectral colours can be mixed, but the results do not parallel the mixture of hue components. The notion of a mixed colour is ill-defined in reflectance space.

(iv) Our experiences of *black* and *white* are the result of the activation of an achromatic channel, which carries the result of adding the outputs of the cones. Black-and-white 'lightness' constitutes a component of colour experience which varies independently of the hue dimensions. Consequently, one and the same hue can have variants that are more or less black. This dimension of variation has no counterpart in the visual spectrum or in reflectance space: neither makes sense of the idea that the *same* hue can have different grey values.

For these and other reasons, the quality spaces of reflectance and wavelength, as these are ordered by physical laws, are simply incommensurable with the psychological colour spaces created by opponent processing.

Metamerism. The output of the colour-vision system, and to an approximation, colour experience, depends on input to the colour sensors. (As we saw in Chapter 6, section I.2, colour experience can be modified by other factors such as contrast and adaptation, but let's put this aside.) Now, since the cone cells are sensitive to light in a rather broad band, signals of widely varying spectral composition can affect them in the same way. For example, the response elicited by a monochromatic ray of light at the peak sensitivity of a cone cell, will activate that cell the same way as a stronger ray of a different frequency, still in the cell's sensitivity range. The cone cell is simply unable to distinguish between these two rays, though they are of different wavelength. This means, other things being equal, that they will look the same colour. Thus, light signals of diverse spectral composition and of paints of diverse spectral reflectance can *look* the same colour as one another. One's first reaction to this phenomenon might be that it is simply a case of performance deficit. In the example given above, for instance, one might be tempted to say that the system simply lacks the fineness of resolution that would enable it to distinguish the strong off-peak ray of light from the weaker on-peak ray. But this is not obviously the right way to look at the matter. For metamerism is not generally a case of neighbouring frequencies being confused. Among signals that are a mixture of many different frequencies, those that evoke the same response from the cone cells can be of very different composition. It seems that the system is producing a jumble without any clear resolution.

Categoricity. The colours to which human languages give names are experienced across cultures as sharply different from one another, or at least as more sharply distinguished from one another than any *physical* difference across the divide (Berlin and Kay 1969; Rosch Heider 1972; Hardin and Maffi 1997, Introduction). This phenomenon, which explains the banded look of the rainbow, and the apparent zones of a Munsell colour chart, has no counterpart in the physical counterparts of colour. The real quality spaces which we have been considering as candidate counterparts for colour experience—wavelengths, reflectances, etc.—do not display such discontinuities.

Affect etc. Colours carry affective associations. Red has an agitating effect on people, for instance, while green is soothing. The warmth and coolness of colours, discussed earlier, also have affective associations. Some of these are strongly cross-cultural. Obviously they have no mind-independent counterpart; it makes no sense to say that red is agitating or bold except by reference to particular kinds of perceivers. Yet it seems as if these qualities are a part of how the colours are experienced and contribute to their similarity and difference. This kind of affect is thought by many to be peripheral to visual experience, but others take it to be central, for as John Dewey said, 'It is as certain as anything can be that optical qualities do not stand by themselves with tactual and emotive qualities clinging to their skirts' (quoted by Firth 1949, 448.) (Effect is perhaps more pronounced in music than in other modalities: minor keys are said to be sad, disharmonious chords displeasing, and so on. It is hard to resist the analogue of Dewey's observation when we consider music.)

II. Three Irrealist Positions

Because of such failures of correspondence between experienced colour and real properties discriminable by wavelength, a number of philosophers and the majority of visual scientists reject all attempts to associate colour with properties that exist independently of perception. This section reviews and assesses some of the different irrealist conclusions that have been drawn from the kind of evidence just reviewed.

1. *Hardin's Catalogue from the Sensory Classification Perspective*
Before we go into the details of irrealism, however, let us briefly assess Hardin's Catalogue from the Sensory Classification point of view. Recall, once again, Hayek's description of a ball-sorting machine (Chapter 1, section I.3):

We may find that the machine will always place the balls with a diameter of 16, 18, 28, 31, 32, and 40 mm in a receptacle marked *A*, the balls with a diameter of 17, 22, 30, and 35 in a receptacle marked *B*, and so forth. The balls placed by the machine into the same receptacle will then be said to belong to the same class, and the balls placed by it into different receptacles to belong to so many different classes.

The phenomena in Hardin's Catalogue seem perfectly to illustrate Hayek's principle. Take metamerism. The colour vision sorts very different spectral compositions into the same class. From the Sensory Classification point of view, there is nothing anomalous or even surprising about this. Hardin's phenomena are seen to be products of the system's classificatory activity. Thus far, Hardin would agree. What he does not see is this leaves unresolved the status of the classes that the system constructs. Should Hardin's Catalogue persuade us that these classes fail to map onto the external world? This is the moral Hardin himself draws (see also Dedrick 1996*a*). And Hayek suggests that the system is idiosyncratically sorting balls with no regard to rightness and wrongness. I shall argue in this chapter that these conclusions are unwarranted.

What *is* clear from Hardin's Catalogue is that the colour-vision system is classifying and ordering stimuli in a way that does not correspond to the wavelength-based ordering of the spectrum. But it should not, on this account alone, be reckoned to be acting with reckless disregard for the real world. After all, the system is classifying stimuli for its own purposes. The wavelength-based ordering may not, or may not uniquely, suit these purposes.

The question about the rights and wrongs of Hardin's phenomena must be assessed from the point of view of function and utility. Hardin's irrealism and Hayek's Extreme Nominalism say nothing about utility, and are thus unmotivated at this stage of the argument.

We now examine three different irrealist responses to Hardin's Catalogue.

2. *Burden Shifting: Colour as an Attribute of Sensations*

Some psychologists insist that Hardin's mismatches show us that it is *sensations* that are coloured, not environmental objects. The Commission Internationale de l'Eclairage (*CIE*) International Lighting Vocabulary, for example, defines hue as an 'attribute of visual sensation' (quoted by Byrne and Hilbert 2003, 5–6).

In the face of the evidence presented in the last section, this is a tempting move. Let us take the argument step by step. Consider:

> *(1) The colour *red* is agitating.

On the face of it, (1) attributes an objective property to the colour *red*. But surely *red* does not have any such property independently of human responses to it. Since (1) is based on a human response to *red*, it is tempting to substitute:

> (2) Humans tend to get agitated when they are in red surroundings.

(2) ascribes the emotional response that underlies (1) to the viewer, not the scene. And that is where it belongs.

By analogy, one might think that since the impossibility of mixing *red* and *green* is based on an activity of the human colour-vision system, rather than on physical reality, it would be better to shift the burden of explanation to human colour-vision processing rather than placing it on the colours themselves. Thus, one might be suspicious of:

> *(3) *Red* is opposed to *green*.

And one might want to replace (3) with something like:

> (4) When humans experience *red* they are in a visual state opposed to the one they are in when they are experiencing *green*.

Here the relationship of opposition is ascribed to the sensations that emerge from colour processing, instead of to environmentally located colour properties.

The psychologists who compiled the *CIE* International Lighting Vocabulary are influenced by the whole raft of idiosyncrasies listed in Hardin's Catalogue. They are inclined to use the burden-shifting method illustrated above to reconceptualize colour. In its most encompassing form, the argument goes like this. One is ordinarily inclined to think, on grounds of intuition, that

> *(5) Physical objects are coloured.

But, as Hardin's Catalogue demonstrates, colour experience is idiosyncratic. So these scientists recommend that we should abandon (5) in favour of

(6) Visual sensations are coloured.

This is a position known as Projectivism. The claim is that the visual system projects on to material objects properties that properly belong to sensations.[1]

Projectivism is a wrong turn: it is simply the wrong way to accommodate the system-dependence of the colours. This is so for two closely related reasons. The first is that as argued in the Afterword to Part II, the sensory ordering measured by the methods of Chapter 4, section II are relations among distal stimuli mediated by sense features that belong to these stimuli. When we report a particular sensory state by saying that x and y are similar or opposed in colour, the x and y that we are talking about are environmental objects. These are the objects that are likely to be confused with one another if they are similar with respect to colour; they are the things that become associated with one another by similarity. We are not concerned here about *sensations* getting confused with one another or *sensations* becoming associated with one another by conditioning or learning—it is not even clear what it would mean, in such a context, to say that a sensation could be confused with another.

Distal objects are thus the primary focus of our sensory awareness. We get to know these objects simply by being in certain sensory states. To illustrate: when I am looking at a red cup in good light, I get to be in a certain visual state, and as a result of being in this state I possess the knowledge that the cup looks red. It is *not* that first I scrutinize the visual state that the cup occasions in me, and using the characteristics of this state make an inference about the cup. Such a view casts me in the role of a homunculus gazing at an inner display provided by the senses (cf. Dennett 1991). A more adequate way of describing what goes on is to eliminate the homunculus: when I look at the cup, I come to be in the visual state of its looking red to me. Now, it is certainly possible to argue that this visual state is idiosyncratic and misleading. However this might be, the fact remains that visual *sensations* are not what we seem to see: that is, vision does not present us with purely internal objects and their properties. The *CIE* move amounts, unintentionally, to an attempt

---

[1] James McGilvray (1994) presents a *construction* which attempts to validate (6), and Jonathan Cohen (2003*b*) traces Hardin's Catalogue to structural properties of sensations—citing my own work in Matthen (1992) as a source. All of us would have done better to use the delineation of the three stages of the sensory process delineated in Chapter 1, section II.2, and further discussed in the Afterword to Part II. This posits a similarity structure for colour *classes*, rather than colour *experiences*. For as Alex Byrne (2003) rightly says, criticizing certain attempts to deal with the argument from Hardin's Catalogue, 'If we have opinions at all about salient similarities . . . holding between our *color experiences*, that is surely because we take such similarities to be induced by the apparent similarities between the *colors*' (645). (Unfortunately, he goes on to modify this sensible position, and to eliminate the role of the colours.)

to correct the idiosyncrasies of colour classification by denying that these colours are presented to us as belonging to material objects.

In short, going down this path is the wrong way to get to the heart of the problems posed by Hardin's Catalogue. For as Byrne and Hilbert (2003) rightly say the *CIE* vocabulary falls into an error that results from 'the conflation of the properties *of* an experience with the properties *represented by* the experience'. The proper use of the burden-shifting strategy is to replace (3) with

> (7) The human visual system represents red things as opposed in respect of colour to green things.

and (5) with

> (8) The human visual system represents things as coloured.

rather than to replace the offending sentences with claims about sensation.

(7) and (8) are still compatible with a form of irrealism, as we shall see in a moment. But at least they locate colour where it is experienced—among the things we see, rather than in sensations, while at the same time, much as when (4) is substituted for (3), allowing that it is *vision* that locates it there.

3. *Interrogating the Messenger: Error Theory*

(7) and (8) are congruent with the approach to sense perception taken in Parts I and II of the present work. The idea is that the senses assign stimuli to classes, as the Sensory Classification Thesis maintains, and arrange these classes in a similarity space. (8) arises from things being assigned to colour classes; (7) from certain interrelations in the similarity space of colour. In view of the idiosyncrasies of this data processing, one might ask whether sensory classifications reflect some truth in the real world. For instance, according to (7), the visual system tells us that *red* is opposed to *green*. And one might ask whether *red* is *really* opposed to *green*, i.e. whether there is some property that red things have which is opposed to some corresponding property in green things. We ask, in short, whether these messages from the visual system are *true*.

In a tradition tracing to the Scientific Revolution, many philosophers argue that visual representations of colour are *false*: they hold, in other words, that distal objects are not coloured, though our visual systems represent them as such. We may call this conclusion:

> **The Error Theory of Colour Perception*
> (a) Colour vision assigns (what it takes to be) distal objects to certain classes, and
> (b) Colour sensation conveys to the perceiver the message that these classes correspond to some system-independent property, and
> (c) This message is false.

The Error Theory takes the same position with respect to all of the phenomena in Hardin's Catalogue of mismatches between the categories of human colour vision and those of physics. All of these characteristics of human visual categories are held to be erroneous. Now, Error Theory typically diagnoses these errors as errors of projection. Sensory systems project their own characteristics and states out on to external objects, they say, giving perceivers a false image of external things as the possessors of qualities that they do not really have. In the previous subsection, we expressed doubts about this Projectivist thesis, and here I will treat it as an unnecessary accretion. All that we need to be concerned with now is the falsity claim, (c), above.

The problem with Error Theory lies, in the first instance, with (b) above— it relies on an extremely implausible interpretation of the *message* conveyed to us by the senses. The Error Theorist is obliged to establish two things: not just that there is no correspondence between visual categories and physical categories, but also that vision 'tells' us that there *is* such a correspondence. For instance, the Error Theorist has to show not just that there is no physical opposition between *red* and *green*, but also that colour vision tells us that there is such a physical opposition. Only then would there be a mismatch between the sensory message and reality. But does colour vision really tell us this? Does it really tell us, or purport to tell us, anything about the opposition of colours from the point of view of a *physicist*? The message delivered us by colour vision is, as Sydney Shoemaker (1996/1990, 97) has put it, a *semantic* issue, not a metaphysical one, an issue about the meaning of a particular mental state, not about what is out there in the world. We all agree that there are no relations of opposition among wavelengths and reflectances founded on physics—the question is whether some visual states tell us that there are such relations of opposition. What motivates us to construe visual states in the way that Error Theorists do?

It is hard to see how the Error Theorist will go about establishing a semantics of visual states that supports his view. Let us examine a clearer case of sensory error, the visual illusions. With respect to these illusions, it can be directly demonstrated that the perceiver makes certain comparisons: one figure will be judged larger than another, though it isn't; two colour-patches will be adjudged to be of the same colour, though they are not; and so on. In somewhat altered circumstances of viewing, the very same figures or colour-patches will present a more veridical appearance: they will look the way they are. These illusions present us with clear cases of erroneous sensory states. They do not depend on contentious interpretations of the sensory message.

Recall the Müller–Lyer diagram:

It is possible to disagree about exactly what the sensations occasioned by these lines 'tell' us. One philosopher might say that they tell us about the retinal image, another that they present us with sense-data, a third that we are offered information about marks on the paper, a fourth that we are being informed about the distance away from us of (non-existent) three-dimensional objects of which these lines are edges. These interpretations disagree as to the ontology of visual objects, but the illusion is independent of such disagreement. Wherever or whatever the seen lines may be, it is clear (a) that the bottom one looks longer, and (b) that if the arrowheads were erased or flipped over, it would not look longer. It is clear, moreover, that if you ask an observer to adjust the length of the upper line so that the two look the same length, she will make it longer than the lower line.

One might hope and expect that the Error Theorist would be able to demonstrate an equally robust perceptual error. But he cannot. In cases like that of the Müller–Lyer diagram, there is a mismatch between the visual state V_{true} corresponding to the true state of affairs—the equality of the lines— and the state V_{false} that the perceiver is actually in when she looks at the lines. As we just saw, state V_{false} makes the perceiver do certain things (including making the top line too long when asked to make it match the bottom, issuing certain verbal reports, etc.) that she would not have done if she had been in state V_{true}. Moreover, by asking the observer to adjust the length of the lines so that they look to be the same length, we can actually measure the difference between the messages delivered by V_{true} and V_{false}. Finally, in the case of the Müller–Lyer diagram, we know how to correct the perceiver and put her into V_{true}: we simply erase or hide the arrowheads.

None of this is true in the case of the opposition between *red* and *green*. There is nothing obviously wrong in the perceiver's attitude with respect to *red* and *green*, nothing functionally off-track in the way she deals with and forms beliefs about red and green things. There is also no way of correcting the perceiver and getting her to see *red* as not opposed to *green*. In fact, there is no visual state corresponding to what the Error Theorist (correctly) identifies as the physical state of affairs: that is, there is no visual state that tells us that *red* and *green* are not opposed. That there is no such visual state *shows that the visual system has no access to the kind of opposition that the Error Theorist denies for colours—i.e. physical opposition.* Physical opposition cannot be seen; it is not a visual datum—and the same holds for its contrary, physical component-compatibility. But this implies that whatever the visual system might be telling us when it makes these two colours opposed, it is not telling us that they are *physically* opposed. It can't be telling us this, because it has no way of telling us about physical opposition.

This illustrates the difficulty that Error Theory faces. In the absence of demonstrable single-perceiver errors that do not depend on a contentious interpretation of the sensory message—demonstrations like those that are available in the case of visual illusions—it is hard to see how the theory can be substantiated. As Alex Byrne (2001*a*) documents, philosophers can some-times be quite cavalier about making claims concerning the semantic content of perceptual states. Boghossian and Velleman (1997/1989) claim, for example, that 'When one enters a dark room and switches on a light, the colours of surrounding objects look as if they have been revealed, not as if they have been activated' (87). Harold Langsam (2000) says: 'Colours *do* look like dispositions, for the objective properties that are presented in colour experience are presented as dispositional properties, dispositions to present certain kinds of appearances.' Such claims are made dogmatically, as if they were obvious to anybody with vision, without even a suggestion regarding how they might be tested. Yet seemingly substantive theories—Error Theory, Dispositionalism, refutations of Dispositionalism, etc.—are based on such assertions. This is regrettable. But let us move on.

4. *The Failure of Reductivism: Colour as a Non-Physical Property*
Hardin himself approaches the issue in the terms offered by a classic delin-eation of realism concerning 'universals' or properties. David Armstrong (1989) puts the realism question like this: 'What distinguishes the classes of tokens that mark off a type from those classes that do not?' (13). According to Armstrong, the realist holds that the distinction should be 'founded on a difference in things themselves and not, say, in some different attitude that we take up to the different classes' (ibid. 14). Armstrong's form of realism conforms to what, in Chapter 5, section IV, we called *Correspondence Realism*. Applied to colour, it maintains that there is something in the colours (or in coloured things) that corresponds to our perception of them—when they look the same colour, there is some system-independent property they share; when they look different there is such a property that distinguishes them. Hardin thinks that his catalogue of idiosyncrasies shows that the colours are not founded on resemblances and differences in things themselves, but rather on an attitude that we, or rather our colour-vision systems, take up to things. This is the central message he wants to deliver.

The argument, which Hardin does not make completely explicit, goes something like this:

(9) *Red* is experienced as more similar to *violet* than to *green*.
(10) Therefore, *red is* more similar to *violet* than to *green*.
(11) The property that occasions experiences of *red* is not *physically* more similar to that which occasions experiences of *violet* than the one that occasions experiences of *green*.
(12) It follows from (10) and (11) that the physical properties that occasion experiences of *red, green,* and *violet* are not identical with *red, green,* and *violet*.

(13) In other words, colour is not the same as any of the physical properties that occasions experiences of colour.

(14) Therefore, colour is not a physical property.

(14) is taken to be an irrealist conclusion, because it denies the correspondence of colour classifications to any physical property, i.e. to any property in the external world. In the terminology of Chapter 5, section IV, (14) contradicts Correspondence Realism.

The passage from (9) to (10) may seem surprising. Just because something is experienced a certain way does not mean that the thing that occasioned the experience is the way that the experience indicates. True, but we expect sense-features like the colours to be psychologically accessible—we expect that colours will be defined in ways that preserve the instinctive grasp of colour through colour experience. Grasping the instinctive colour classification practices discussed in Chapter 1 and the sensory similarity spaces discussed in Chapter 4 should demand no more knowledge than is available through the experience of colours. Thus, colour features, like all other sense-features, are *known* or *grasped* by experience. (We will discuss this further in Chapter 11.) If this is right, and if sense-features are as they are experienced, Hardin's argument looks, on the face of it, to show that there are no properties in the real world that correspond to experienced colour.

The problem is that Hardin's (or rather, Armstrong's) construal of realism is contentious. It assumes that if *physical* similarity does not line up with sensory similarity, then irrealism is forced on us. This is a mistake. For as we can gather from Nelson Goodman's (1972/1970) 'strictures on similarity' (see Chapter 4, section II), there are *many* kinds of similarities and differences grounded on 'things themselves', not just closeness with respect to the fundamental variables of physics. One might want to say that light of wavelength 550 nm (A) is more similar to light of 560 nm (B) than it is to light of 570 nm (C), because the difference in wavelength between (A) and (B) is smaller than that between (A) and (C). One might argue that this is relevant because various laws of physics are expressed in terms of monotonic (constantly increasing or constantly decreasing) functions of wavelength, from which it follows that B will behave more like A than C will, at least in respect of these laws. From this point of view, it seems that if colour vision were to represent A as more similar to C than to B, it would be looking at things idiosyncratically. This is Hardin's inclination, and as far as it goes, it is true and correct.

However, we can look at these wavelengths from the point of view of how they affect the colour receptors of the human eye. From this alternative point of view, A and C are each 10 nm off the peak receptivity of the long-wavelength cone, while B is right at the peak. In this respect, A and C are more similar to one another than either is to B. This similarity can be specified in system-independent terms thus:

$|A - 560| = |C - 560| \neq |B - 560|$ (where $|x|$ stands for the absolute magnitude of x).

Why is this second similarity not relevant? Is it that it is not founded on characteristics found in things themselves, but depends on some attitude that *we* take up? This diagnosis would be more compelling if cone cells were epistemic organs that we were able to control, and the similarity relation shifted as we manipulated the cone cells. But we cannot control the activity of our cone cells. Colour experience is (normally) the system-processed product of light-signals received by optical receptors that happen to be located in our bodies. While the physical constitution of these receptors is not dictated by the laws of physics, they are certainly not chosen by ourselves. The interaction between cone cells and light is as objective as an interaction with a measuring instrument. The system is extracting information about the world from receptors it has. This makes it less clear why similarities in colour which are based on this interaction are not objective. True, these similarities are different from the ones on which some physical laws are predicated. But this is not conclusive. There could be *many* objective similarities, all different from one another. Physical similarity (if there is some one such thing) could be different from receptoral similarity, even though both are objective.

In the light of this consideration, let us distinguish (as we did in Chapter 5, section IV) between the physical variables that occur in the laws of physics—*physical* categories—and those which can be defined in the language of physics—*physically specifiable* categories. Clearly, the former constitute but a tiny subset of the latter: the similarity that unites A and C above is physically specifiable, but has no significance for physical laws. If we reflect on the multiplicity of objective similarities, we can see that Correspondence Realism faces an unpalatable dilemma. Hallucinations and illusions aside—and these are not what Hardin's Catalogue is about—it is always possible to describe what a sensory system detects in physical terms; i.e. it is always possible physically to specify the response conditions of its various states. Now if the response condition of a perceptual state is physically specifiable, then (as Alex Byrne once pointed out to me in conversation), it carries information about the physical state of the world (where 'the world' includes the perceiver's sensory system). So it is hard to see why we should not regard *any* physically specifiable perceptual classification scheme to be 'founded on a difference in things themselves'. Under this construal, Correspondence Realism, far from being demanding, is actually vacuous. A sensory category will qualify as real as long as its internal states have physically specifiable distal response conditions—and most sensory categories do. The demand for correspondence with *physical* categories is, of course, much more difficult to satisfy than this: indeed, it makes it virtually impossible for *any* sensory system to tell the truth. But it is unclear what the motivation for such a demand would be. It is hard to see why vision should represent the categories of physics, and only these categories. After all, life is not a Physics midterm.

But this raises the question: What sort of categories *should* a sensory system represent?

III. Enter Pluralism

The question what vision should represent is complicated by the kind of sensory specialization we encountered in Chapter 6. Different kinds of organisms represent different visual objects. Already this makes it unlikely that all aim to represent the quantities of physics. Putting this aside, we ask: What would make an organism right in its representational strategies? What would make it wrong?

This question arises with considerable urgency in connection with an argument put forward by David Lewis (1997). In Chapter 6, section II, we saw that Lewis believes that (paradigm) colours are surface reflectances, which exist independently of humans. What then is he to make of Hardin's Catalogue of the oddities of human-colour categories? What is he to make of the fact that these oddities have no counterpart in the world of physical quantities like reflectance? Lewis's response is surprising: he disarmingly concedes Hardin's points about the psychophysical origins of colour similarity, simply allowing that the similarity space of colour—call it S—might originate in colour *experience*. But this point about origins is all he concedes. He does not think that his concession implies irrealism.

Lewis argues that the psychophysical origins of the colour similarity space S should not lead us to conclude that reflectance properties *fail* to be ordered in parallel with S. The pairing that he establishes between colour properties and colour experiences 'yields relations among colours *in the image of relations among colour experiences*', he says (330). Hardin assumes that S must parallel quantities that occur in *physical* laws. Lewis demurs. Stripped of the unwarranted assumption that colours are always surface reflectances, his position amounts to this: experiential relations *are* real. If two properties are *experienced* as opposed, or *experienced* as pure or mixed, that is evidence enough that they are really so. Experiential similarity is *constitutive* of the similarity of colours.

The similarity space of colour experience is created by the brain's encoding of colour-signals. (Please note that this statement does not imply irrealism. The Mona Lisa was created by Leonardo da Vinci; this does not imply that it fails to portray its subject realistically. The *CIE* scientists of section II.2, but not Hardin, make the mistake of inferring realism just from the fact of the brain's involvement. Hardin relies on non-correspondence with physical quantities.) In effect, Lewis constructs the similarity space of colours in parallel with the brain's activity. Take each colour and plonk it down, according to how it is experienced, in the Hue-Saturation-Brightness space of red-green, blue-yellow, and black-white. Gather metamers together. Introduce the sharp boundaries of categoricity, perhaps by stretching the space in between adjacent categories—i.e. by rescaling just-noticeable-differences at the breaks. Account for the commonalities of affect and the like by introducing extra dimensions to the space. Take account of the fact that at the ends of the spectrum, light affects only one receptor, and that these colours are consequently very dark and difficult to differentiate. There you have the real similarity space of colours. It looks somewhat like Figure 5 (Chapter 4).

Lewis's *force majeure* is tempting. Why are *red* and *violet* similar? Because they are both experienced as reddish. Why is this so? Because the opponent-processing system happens to calculate the strength of the ends of the spectrum relative to the middle. Isn't this all that there is to the matter? Why should we refuse to certify this similarity as objective? Because it does not correspond to similarity of wavelengths? What difference does that make? There are many kinds of objective similarity. The linear similarity ordering of the spectrum is just one. The similarities that experience betokens are others.

This is an elegant proposal, but sensory specialization spawns complications. Lewis's path to realism is laid down on a base of commonsense metaphysics.

An adequate theory of colour must be . . . commonsensical. [This] can be compromised to some degree . . . . But compromise has its limits. It won't do to say that colours don't exist . . . [I]t is a Moorean fact that the folk psychophysics of colour is close to true. (1997, 325; cf. Boghossian and Velleman 1997/1991: 'Your knowledge of these matters is such that nothing would count as evidence against it' [117].)

This assertion puts Lewis into a difficult position with respect to specialization. The trouble is that the 'folk psychophysics of colour' is not just different from pigeon colour psychophysics, but, superficially at least, incompatible with it. Folk psychophysics does not just tell us that every reflecting surface is *experienced* as reddish or greenish or bluish or yellowish; it insists that every chromatic surface *is* so. (This is the sort of claim that can be elicited from 'folk' in a psychophysics lab.) If these propositions are close to true, what of pigeon psychophysics? It proclaims the existence of hues unknown to humans, and asserts that ultraviolet is a colour. Perhaps this is not so bad by itself: perhaps, the pigeon's seeing ultraviolet is similar to some animals seeing finer grain than we do, or like the difference between the sharp-eyed lynx and the blind mole. But what about the experiential similarity relations that Lewis wants to preserve? The pigeon makes hue comparisons in a dimension orthogonal to *red-green* and *blue-yellow*, denies that every colour is reddish or greenish or bluish or yellowish, and finds among its colours similarities and dissimilarities that we do not experience. Pigeon psychophysics must, then, be largely *false*. Is this not an objectionably anthropocentric conclusion? If human experiences determine the truth about colour, why should pigeons not be regarded as similarly authoritative? Would a G. E. Moore of the pigeons not take umbrage if we did not so regard them?

The only plausible way out of this difficulty is to capitulate: we must accord to pigeon colours exactly the same authority as we have just ceded to the colours that humans experience. This need not violate logic. Properties—even physically specifiable properties—are infinitely numerous; in a situation of unlimited supply, we do not need to squabble over the division of the loot. It is possible for different colour perceivers to fasten on different properties, or even different property structures; apparent variations in colour reports need not be taken as conflicting with one another—they can be explained by the fact that perceivers are not really talking about the same thing. The pigeon's way of classifying stimuli is simply different from ours: just because we both have colour vision, we should not conclude that we both have the same colour classes or properties. Why then can both not be correct? Let's call this extension of Lewis's proposal *Pluralism*.

The question that jumps out at us at this juncture is: What exactly does it mean to say that the colours *really* have these properties? Pluralism is not meant to be a 'relativistic' proposal. The suggestion is not that the colour properties need to be relativized to observers, that truths about colour exist only relative to how particular species experience colour. It is rather that different species might be converging on different properties of distal stimuli, though since they all use information gathered by wavelength-sensitive receptors, they are all fastening on colour properties, as defined by the Functional Definition of Colour discussed in Chapter 6. This leads us back to the question posed at the end of the previous section. How can very different sets of experiences be authoritative with respect to colours? What does it mean to be *right* in this context?

IV. Standards of Correctness

We will now reconsider the question of realism by reference to two significant idiosyncrasies of colour vision. Do these idiosyncrasies have a representational function? If so, what standards of *correctness* or *truth* is it appropriate to apply to them? We will find that though it is initially implausible that either of these aspects of colour vision could be interpreted in a realist fashion, the criterion that we shall propose differentiates them, and makes it at least plausible that one denotes a real category.

The first phenomenon to consider is the perception of certain shades of the Hering primary colours—*red, green, blue,* and *yellow*—as 'focal' or 'unique'. Every trichromatic person can be brought to recognize a certain shade of *green* as containing neither any *blue* nor any *yellow*, and to do this with a fair degree of reliability. The trouble is that there is substantial variation among humans concerning which shade is *unique green*: what some observers see as *unique green*, others see as distinctly bluish. Now let us suppose that one observer, *O1*, finds light of 520 nm to be uniquely green, and another, *O2*, finds light of 525 nm to be so. Who (if either) is right? The problem with saying that *either* one is right, is that this seems to imply that the other one is wrong. But there seems to be no reason to choose between them: why should one of these observers be in a privileged position over the other? Is this a case where both can be right, in the Pluralist manner? Or does our inability to choose show that everybody is wrong?

In a strongly realist manifesto, Alex Byrne and David Hilbert (2003) suggest that there is an absolute right or wrong about this—either 520 nm is unique green, or 525 nm is, or some other wavelength is, but not more than one.

From the fact that we have no good reason to believe, of any chip, that it is unique green, it does not follow that we have no good reason to believe that there are any unique green chips. That would be like arguing that we have no good reason to believe Professor Plum has been murdered, on the ground that there is no particular person who is clearly the culprit. (17)

We are prepared to countenance 'unknowable color facts'—that a chip is unique green, for instance. (21, n. 50).

C. L. Hardin (2003, 200) protests: 'No scientific sense can be attached to the claim that some of the observers are perceiving the color of the stimulus correctly and others not.' Hardin worries that we are just not sure what objective fact we are to check to determine the rightness: it is one thing for a fact to be unknowable, another for the truth conditions of a supposed fact to be unknowable. Jonathan Cohen takes a similar line: 'The failure of several hundred years of systematic efforts directed at articulating standards [of correctness] establishes a presumptive case *against* their existence' (2003c, 26).

Byrne and Hilbert treat Hardin's and Cohen's position as merely a form of verificationism, an instance of the position that if one cannot determine whether *p* is true or false, then *p* is neither true nor false. This, however, underestimates the strength of the objection. In our discussion of the Error Theory, we saw that in order to determine whether a sensory state is accurate, it must first be determined what message it conveys, and then whether this message is true. One sort of problem of verification arises when, because of some limitation of our investigative or measuring faculties, we are unable to determine whether a sensory message is true, though we are quite clear about what the message is. And it is surely reasonable in this kind of case to allow that the message might be true (or false) though we can never find out. But *this* is not the problem with unique colours. The problem here is that we have no idea what the message is. What does a colour have to be in order to be *unique green*? There is a glib answer to this question, of course: it has to be unmixed with blue or yellow. But what is it for a colour in the real world to be unmixed in this way? We do not know. This is exactly the point made by Hardin's Catalogue: this kind of colour mixing has no counterpart in the real world. It follows that the real world is not available to adjudicate the squabble between perceivers who disagree about *unique green*. We must, therefore, entertain the possibility that uniqueness is not a signal of classification at all, but just a non-representational feature of certain colour experiences.

The second phenomenon I want to consider is the 'categoricity' of colour perception (see section I above): the perception of sharp breaks between named colours like *red* and *orange* where physically the transition is quite smooth. Our colour vision system tells us that

(15) There is a sharp qualitative difference between *orange* and *red*.

But as far as physical reality is concerned there is no such sharp difference. Wavelengths, reflectances, etc. all vary smoothly over the perceived categorical divide. In what sense, then, can we concede to our colour-vision systems the reality of the sharp break asserted by (15)? In what sense can the system be *right* about this? In what does this sharp qualitative difference consist? This is a problem even if humans cannot generally agree where the divide occurs. In fact, the divide is fuzzy; humans only agree within certain limits as to where it occurs. The question still is: What does the break tell us? Why would it be wrong for an individual perceiver to place the break outside normal limits or even to deny that such a break exists?

I will now present a proposal to adjudicate such cases. It rests on two propositions.

The first proposition is that the categories posited by perceptual states such as the above (and others) can be *physically specified*: for the break between *orange* and *red* to be even a candidate for reality, we should be able to say in terms of physics where the break occurs (i.e. roughly at 600 nm). Consider, then, the proposition:

(16) Light of 598 nm is more similar to light of 594 than it is to light of 602 nm.

(16) is a physical specification of an experiential fact that arises from (15): there is a greater dissimilarity across the categorical break between *orange* and *red* than there is on one side.

We saw earlier that physical specifiability is quite a weak condition. The point of insisting on it here is that if there were no physically specifiable fact corresponding to the perception, then there would be no consistent basis for the qualitative break between *orange* and *red*, and then it would seem to be based simply on a situationally determined response. Here is a parallel case: one might experience pleasure when one takes one's first sip of coffee, and then experience much less or even no pleasure when one takes another sip from the same cup. Clearly, this is a case where the experience of pleasure does not tell us anything informative about the coffee. Descriptive content in perception must (as the Sensory Classification Thesis tells us) have a consistent basis, and we are insisting here that this consistent basis should be physically specifiable. Insisting on physical specifiability helps us exclude cases like this—perhaps there are other ways of achieving the same end, but physical specifiability will do for present purposes.

On the other hand, the criterion of physical specifiability is clearly not sufficient for saying that there is a right and wrong about how vision represents the world. The wavelength of the light I perceive as uniquely green is physically specifiable. Similarly, categoricity may be physically specifiable in an individual or in the entire species. But why should we say that I would be error if I perceived light of some other wavelength this way? Why would the system be *in error* if, either on some specific occasion or always, it made a break at 595 instead of 600 nm? The criterion of physical specifiability is not sufficient to answer these questions. Another condition is needed.

By way of an introduction to what is needed, let's consider a problem that is closely related to the one about the validity of (15). Normally, dogs are dichromats; normally, humans are trichromats. Dichromatic humans are colour-deficient. Does this mean that dogs are colour-deficient? Pluralism forbids us to take such a position since it denies dog colours the same validity as human colours. Dogs are not in error because their vision blurs colour distinctions that humans can easily make. To say that dogs are deficient on account of their failure to compute human colours would be like saying that trichromatic humans are colour-deficient since they fail to compute tetrachromatic pigeon colours. But if dogs are not to be regarded as colour-deficient, what about dichromatic humans? Why should *they* be stigmatized as colour-deficient when they perform as well as dogs?

An adequate answer to this puzzle depends on a proper understanding of specialized functions. Most perceptual categories are put to some use with regard to our functioning in the external world. Now, the *utility* of a perceptual category may be disrupted if the organism fails to respond to its customary delineation. Trichromacy is no exception. Roger Shepard (1997/1992) and Lotto and Purves (2002) claim that trichromacy is required for certain sorts of comparisons between spectral distribution curves. If they are right, then both dichromatic humans and dichromatic dogs are unable to make the comparisons in question. The difference (I am claiming) is that while there are innate, i.e. genetically or developmentally specified,[2] *human*

---

[2] How is it possible to distinguish developmentally specified activities and categories from learned ones? A distinction of degree can be made in terms of two criteria. Development, on the one hand, is 'canalized', i.e. the same outcome will come about in environments that differ markedly from one another, and as a consequence outcomes will be relatively independent of

capacities that depend on such comparisons, there are no such innately specified *canine* activities.

Let us assume that *most* species are in evolutionary equilibrium *most* of the time—call this the Punctuated Equilibrium assumption. Punctuated Equilibrium implies that for most species now there is no mismatch between sensory capacities and innate sensorily guided activities. On this assumption, it would be reasonable to think that dogs must have evolved to get by without the spectral comparisons enabled by trichromacy, while humans, by contrast, have evolved to exploit them.[3] Dog colours are adequate for dog activities; human colours for human activities. An individual is deficient—for example, colour-blind—only if there are innate activities specific to that individual's species that the individual cannot properly perform. A human dichromat fails with respect to human activities: this is why she is colour-deficient. (This species-specific conception of normality and deficiency is congruent with Karen Neander's 1983 conception.)

With this in mind, we can now introduce our proposal concerning realism. The fundamental idea can be put like this. In pursuing specialized functions, the sensory systems of each species engage with certain stimuli, organizing them into physically specifiable classes. An act of classification is *wrong* if it disrupts a specialized function that this act of classification is supposed to aid. Thus:

Action-Relative Realism

Sense experience E (or neural state N) represents distal feature F in the action-relative sense for a member of species S if

(a) F is the physically specifiable response condition of E (or N), and

(b) misclassifying things as F disrupts some innately or developmentally specified use to which E (or N) is put by members of species S.

To summarize: If the occurrence of a state in violation of its normal response condition disrupts some innate activity, then we say that there is an environmental feature represented by that state, and that this representation is real in the sense that it is subject to error. (This will be elaborated further in the Theses of Primary and Secondary Content in Chapter 9, section III.) But if the occurrence of this state in violation of its normal response condition leads

the specific events that occur in a developmental history (see Ariew 1996). Learning, on the other hand, is an outcome that is more specifically matched to the input; in other words, it is quite path-dependent. If a newborn kitten is completely deprived of horizontal lines in its visual field, it may ultimately lack a response to horizontal lines. This does not mean that generally speaking kittens *learn* about horizontal lines. For they will have perceptual grasp of horizontal lines in a large number of situations: grasp of horizontal lines is highly canalized.

[3] This is not an 'adaptationist' assumption, though to establish this would take us very far afield. It assumes that adaptation is a species-relative, not an absolute, standard, and I have argued elsewhere (Matthen 2001a) that this is exactly what is needed to avoid adaptationism.

to no disruption, then we will say that this normal response condition is not represented, and that there is no question about right or wrong in this case.

This gives us a better idea of the status of the Moorean intuitions to which Lewis appeals. When I notice that a banana is marked with black spots I conclude on the basis of past learning that it is getting ripe. If this impression is based on error, my inference about its ripeness will be unfounded. Such patterns of learning, inference, and confirmation or disconfirmation are what I intuitively use colour for. It is extraordinarily unlikely that such a pattern of use could be shot through with error. It is, if you like, a Moorean practice, and thus it generates Moorean facts. To the extent that the inference rests on the supposition that colour vision sorts and classifies distal stimuli such as bananas, this supposition is deeply engrained in our innate practices, and thus constitutes a Moorean fact. Thus, as Lewis says:

> It won't do to say that colours do not exist; or that we are unable to detect them; or that they go away when things are unilluminated or unobserved; or that they change with every change in the illumination; or with every change in an observer's visual capacities; or that the same surface of the same thing has different colours for different observers. (1997, 325)

These are the propositions presupposed by our inferential practices concerning colour; as such they should not be denied.

At the same time, other species may not see in colour, and even if they do, they may not use colour for this kind of learning and inference. For this reason, they may fasten on to a cross-cutting scheme of colour classes and a different set of Moorean facts. Thus:

The Thesis of Pluralistic Realism
In general, organisms from different biological taxa may represent different distal features, and all of these features may be real in the action-relative sense.

Returning now to the comparison between humans and dogs, we note that the human trichromatic scheme of colour classification has action-relative representational significance for humans because the failure properly to classify distal stimuli by this classification scheme will disrupt some human activity. To say this is compatible with allowing that for the (tetrachromatic) pigeon or the (dichromatic) dog, *our* colour categories have no significance. None of the pigeon's activities are disrupted (one might assume) by the pigeon's failure to follow human colour classification schemes. The world is classified one way by humans, and in other ways by these creatures. A human's colour-vision system will be in error if it were to classify things the way dogs do; a dog's would be if it followed human ways.

The Thesis of Pluralistic Realism focuses on *species* activities, but it does not have to deny that some members of species might construct idiosyncratic sensory classification schemes based on sensory capacities that outstrip other members of the same species in representational significance. An example (suggested by Nola Semszycyn) is that of perfect pitch. Some humans can identify a note absolutely, and not relative to other notes: they can for instance distinguish between a middle C of 512 hz and one of 515, even if these tones are played on their own. Most humans are unable to do this. By the Punctuated Equilibrium assumption offered above, we should conclude that no human-species activity is disrupted by the inability to recognize a single tone as the 512 hz middle C. Does this mean that we should dismiss the fine-tuned auditory experience of an individual *with* perfect pitch as non-representational? No, because not all representation emerges from subpersonal sensory systems. The individual with perfect pitch has learned to identify and use certain aspects of her experience; these aspects of her experience have physically specifiable response conditions. Thus, these aspects of experience have action-relative representational significance in her acquired representational scheme, though they may lack it in the innate perceptual representational scheme that she possesses qua human.

We can distinguish now between how *individuals* and *species* make errors.

An *individual* goes wrong in a case like this. Suppose colour vision is used for making generalizations about the world—suppose, in other words, that we are accustomed to making inferences about unobserved properties of things on the basis of their colour. Suppose that fruit of a certain type are ripe when they are yellow. By encountering several such fruit, an individual forms the expectation, before she has tasted it, that a yellow fruit of that type is ripe. *Yellow* is a physically specifiable category that serves some species-specific practice; *normally*, the system will put a thing into this category only if satisfies the physical specification associated with it. Now suppose that because of unfavourable lighting conditions, or because something is internally wrong, this individual misclassifies a particular fruit as pale green, though in fact it meets the physical specification of the sensory category, *yellow*. That is, these unfavourable conditions lead her to put something into the category which does not satisfy the associated physical specification. The consequence is that the perceiver forms the false expectation that the fruit is not ripe. We say that she has committed a perceptual error because her inferential activities were disrupted by her classifying the fruit as green in violation of her normal practice.

A *species* goes wrong in a case like this. Primates use colour vision to identify fruit against a background of leaves. Suppose that a particular primate species constructs a colour space that fails to maximize the difference between fruit and foliage, so that the search task is difficult from a distance. This species possesses a wrong classification scheme (or more accurately, a wrong similarity ordering); the scheme does not serve its function adequately. The assumption of Punctuated Equilibrium suggests that most species get things right most of the time.

Returning now to categoricity, in order to answer the question whether there *really is* a sharp break between *red* and *orange*, we must ask whether the sharp perceived break between *red* and *orange* is functional or simply a 'spandrel'—i.e. a non-functional byproduct of opponent processing. This is, of course, an empirical question; not every feature of human colour classifications needs to be certified Moorean (as Lewis admits). As philosophers, all that we need to take on board is that it is at least possible that categoricity is functional. For example, the categoricity may enhance the utility of colour constancy by making object-identification easier in varying conditions of illumination; it may figure in the semantics of colour terms, thus aiding signalling by colour, and so on. The point is that *if* categoricity does these things, then getting the breaks between colours physically wrong in a particular situation may disrupt the tasks that categoricity aids. If for some reason my visual system makes the break at 595 nm rather than 600 on a particular occasion, then, even if it correctly classifies a 598 nm stimulus as redder than one of 595 nm, it will still classify this stimulus as red rather than orange. Thus it may misidentify some object, or miss some induction about it, or simply miscommunicate its colour to another human observer. (Would it have been a joke to say: 'Ronald Reagan's hair is prematurely red' instead of 'prematurely orange'?) In view of such disruptions, we would acknowledge that the physically identifiable categories spawned by categoricity have objective validity, even though they are (as we might say) evolutionarily constructed. (Cf. Hacking 1999, 6: X is a *socially* constructed category if it is not 'determined by the nature of things', but only by social convention, that X should be 'all as it is'.)

On the other hand, it seems likely that the perception of certain hues as unique *is* non-representational for humans as a species. At least this is strongly indicated by the high degree of variance that humans exhibit with respect to the perception of hues as unique: if uniqueness fed into some innate activity that the species shares, then there would not be a great deal of variation with respect to what distal stimuli are perceived as unique. We conclude that this perception is a feature of experience, and is physically specifiable, but it has no representational significance. Note, however, that this is empirically falsifiable. Some such innate activity could be discovered.

To summarize: Action-relevant realism allows that different species engage with different characteristics of the environment, using idiosyncratic schemes and methods of classification. Pluralistic Realism is simply the thesis that there are lots of seemingly heterogeneous physical characteristics brought under the umbrella of colour by the fact that they are detected by the processing of differences of wavelength in the visible-range electromagnetic signal reaching the eye—many of these characteristics are objectively verifiable, and associated with functional, species-specific, standards of correctness and the possibility of error.

PART FOUR

Content

9

Sensing and Doing

In the Cartesian tradition, a sensory system does little more than capture and deliver to conscious awareness the state of its receptors. Since these receptors are affected by the signal impinging from the environment, their state is assumed to reflect certain limited properties of the proximal environment—the values of some small number of physical variables at the surface of these receptors. These variables are thought to be brightness and colour in the case of vision (since they are the properties of light that affect the retina), pitch and loudness in the case of audition (since they affect the vibrations of the basilar membrane), hardness and warmth, in the case of touch (since there are receptors in the skin that are sensitive to these), and so on. The sensory image is conceived of as a kind of inward *projection*, something like the image thrown by a lens.

Now, lenses differ from one another with regard to their resolution, breadth of sensitivity, width of field, depth of focus—these affect the extent of the image, how well it is projected, and account for the 'imperfections' mentioned above. Because the Cartesian paradigm concentrates on the receptoral image, it explains sensory variation in terms of such variations in the properties of receptors and departures from performance ideals. Within the bounds of such variations, the Cartesian paradigm implies that sensation must be invariant across species. Accordingly, it is committed to:

Universalism
Since sensation consists in a more or less faithful projection of the state of the sensory receptors, it is the same across species, except for imperfections.

Action-Relevant Realism departs from the Cartesian paradigm in two ways. First, it assumes that sensation consists in awareness of physically specifiable, functionally relevant features in the distal environment beyond the sensory receptors. Secondly, since there are plenty of such features to catch, Universalism is no longer well motivated. It seems entirely plausible that different kinds of organism should seek out different features to suit informational needs for their own unique styles of life. This is confirmed by the specialization of sensory systems, for example, in the niche-adapted colour-vision systems discussed in Chapter 5. Specialization challenges Universalism: in its place, we have proposed:

Pluralistic Realism
In general, organisms from different biological taxa may represent different distal features, and all of these features may be real in the action-relative sense.

Sensory systems have functions that are peculiar to a particular evolutionary group or taxon. They deliver information in a form particularly relevant to specific behaviours.

Pluralistic Realism focuses on feature detection beyond the sensory image, on the detection of different features in different species. Part IV aims to present and argue for a general account of sensory function within Pluralistic Realism, a framework in which realism and sensory specialization can be properly motivated and understood. What features of the distal environment does sensory consciousness present, and how, in evolutionary-functional terms, did it come to fasten upon these? What is the nature of an organism's grasp of the features its sensory systems capture? These are the sort of questions to which we now turn.

I. The Motor Theory of Speech Perception

The 'motor theory of speech perception' is a beautiful example of a realist account of a perceptual capacity. It ties the human perception of phonemes not to a *general* ability to receive and discriminate among the sound patterns that occur in our proximal acoustic environment, but to a *specific* sensitivity to sounds that the human articulatory tract is able to produce. It hypothesizes a species-specific connection between human speech perception and human voicing capabilities, and thus supports Pluralistic Realism. It is worth recounting in some detail, not so much because it is true in all of its details—it probably is not—nor because its species-specificity is in principle different from the colour vision systems considered in Part III, but because it brings out with special clarity how perceptual systems converge upon distal features. In addition, considering a new modality is useful, to prevent us from becoming overly focused on the case of vision and colour, where our intuitions are overburdened by four centuries of receptor-focused analysis. The motor theory will help in the formulation of a new account of the function of perception.[1]

---

[1] For my account of motor theory, I rely mainly on Liberman, Cooper, Shankweiler, and Studdert-Kennedy (1991/1967), and Liberman and Mattingly (1991/1985). I am very much indebted to Bryan Gick, Joe Stemberger, and Janet Werker for discussion of these points. It is worth mentioning that I first heard of the motor theory in a conversation with Ignatius Mattingly, one of the pioneers, at a non-academic social event.

A *phone* is the smallest perceived part of spoken speech. [d] is a phone: it is clearly heard as a temporally distinct part of such syllables as 'dig', 'deg', 'dog', 'dag', 'dug', 'bad', 'bid', and so on, and perceived, moreover, as (a) qualitatively invariant in these occurrences, (b) possessing a definite temporal position in the sequence of sounds heard in these syllables, and (c) having itself no heard temporal parts. A *phoneme* (marked by slashes, rather than square brackets) is a class of phones that are considered to be equivalent with respect to their contribution to meaning bearing units within a certain language. The phones [t] and [tĥ] are both considered to instantiate the phoneme /t/ in English; that is, we regard the utterance of either phone as an utterance of /t/. Thus, [t] and [tĥ]—the latter is the aspirated 't' that occurs in most West and South Asian languages—are what are known as 'allophones' in English, i.e. distinct phones recognized as instantiating the same phoneme. Allophony is a language-specific phenomenon: that [t] and [tĥ] are allophones is a phenomenon of English—they are not equivalent in most Asian languages—but many phonemes are universal, i.e. cross-linguistically recognized as a unit comprising phonic variety. The grouping of phones under phonemes represents a second level of categorization in spoken sound: sound patterns of various types are co-classified as phones, and phones are grouped together as phonemes.

Now, in virtue of the fact that /d/ is an identifiable part of the above-mentioned syllables—'dig', 'dog', etc.—one might wrongly conclude that there is some kind of acoustic pattern that various occurrences of phones possess in common, and that this pattern occurs as a distinct component of the acoustic patterns corresponding to the syllables in which it occurs, in the temporal position in which we hear the /d/. This intuition is strengthened by the fact that when we *produce* a /d/ in speech, we seem to be (and really are) always doing the same thing—roughly speaking, we press the tips of our tongues against our palates and produce a noise by releasing the pressure built up in this way. We feel as if we produce a predictable sound by doing this thing (the different *allophones* that fall under a /d/, or /t/, or /n/ constituting variations of the same predictable sound). Thus, we tend to think that, as Aristotle put it, we are able to produce and discriminate 'spoken *sounds* [which] are symbols of affections in the soul' (*De Interpretatione* 1, 16a4).

Early spectrographic investigations of the acoustics of speech proved, however, that the Aristotelian intuition is mistaken. (A spectrograph separates a sound into its component frequencies; an oscilloscope simply records the total resultant frequency over time. The advent of spectrographic analysis marked a revolution in the analysis of spoken sounds.) In the first place, we produce, and are able to discern, something in the neighbourhood of 10 to 20 phones per second, and as Liberman et al. (1967) point out, it is simply impossible either to produce or to perceive discrete *acoustic patterns* at this rate. So sounds, or acoustic patterns, cannot *temporally* correspond one-to-one with phones: many phones have to be packed into a single articulated sound. Liberman et al. suggest that the speech production system solves this problem by evolving a *code* in which a single sound contains information about a *sequence* of phones, rather than a one-to-one substitution scheme where a single sound stands for a single phone—the latter constituting what cryptologists call a 'cipher'. Thus, the sounds—identifiable acoustic patterns—produced by the human articulatory tract encode units larger than phones. The acoustic pattern corresponding to an action like putting the tip of your tongue against the palate and releasing the pressure that builds up in this way corresponds to something like a syllable, a succession of phones.

This leads to a second point. Liberman et al. show by means of the spectrographic analysis of consonants, that there is a large contextual variation depending on the phonemic sequence in which something like a /d/ occurs. The identifiable acoustic patterns within which a phoneme like /d/ occurs are what we might call 'brief syllables' like 'di', 'da', 'du', and so on—units in which /d/ is followed by a vowel. As we remarked before, /d/ is heard as a qualitatively invariant part of these syllables, but in fact *it takes a different acoustic shape in each of these different contexts.* A brief syllable containing a 'voiced stop' like /d/ contains a fairly steep transition of frequency lasting a little longer than 50 ms.; the vowel consists of a longer steady tone, the whole combination lasting about 300 ms. However, the character of the transitional part—the slide or change of frequency to the steady vowel sound—varies quite markedly with the vowel that follows: 'di', for example, is marked by an upward transition at two *widely* separated frequency ranges, whereas /du/ is marked by an upward transition in the lower one of these, and a downward slide in another *closely* neighbouring range. (See Figure 11 it should be noted that the data are not quite as clean for all consonants.)

There is no acoustic pattern common to these and other productions of /d/ that mark them as such, Liberman et al. (1967) say—in each brief syllable

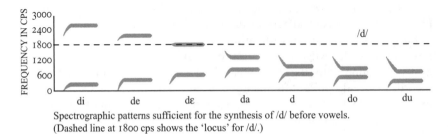

Spectrographic patterns sufficient for the synthesis of /d/ before vowels.
(Dashed line at 1800 cps shows the 'locus' for /d/.)

FIG.11 Contextual Variation in /d/.

Source: Liberman et al. (1967) with permission of the American Psychological Association.

the /d/ is marked by a different acoustic pattern. (This is what constitutes the system as a code rather than a cipher.) Thus:

The [acoustic] speech signal typically does not contain segments corresponding to the discrete and commutable phonemes . . . . We cannot cut either the /di/ or the /du/ pattern in such a way as to obtain some piece that will produce /d/ alone. If we cut progressively from the right-hand end, we hear /d/ plus a vowel, or a nonspeech sound; at no point will we hear only /d/. This is so because the [acoustic signal] is, at every instant, providing information about two phonemes, the consonant and the vowel— that is, the phonemes are being transmitted in parallel. (436)

To find acoustic segments that are in any reasonably simple sense invariant with linguistic (and perceptual) segments . . . one must go to the syllable level or higher (451).

When someone says 'di' or 'du', we clearly *hear* /d/ followed by a vowel. But there is no common acoustic element corresponding to the heard /d/ in both—or at least none that is coincident in time with the apparent length of the /d/. Moreover, when we attempt to cut the signals into temporal bits, we find no segment of either which sounds like /d/ by itself—the initial segment sounds like a whistle, or some other meaningless sound. We have, then, a classic locked-room mystery: how did /d/ get in and out of 'di'?

The answer proposed by Liberman and his colleagues at the Haskins Laboratories is brilliant and surprising: *speech perception does not consist in perceiving sounds*. Rather, 'the objects of speech perception are the intended *phonetic gestures* of the speaker, represented in the brain as invariant motor commands' (Liberman and Mattingly 1985, 2, my emphasis). Of course, the perception of these objects proceeds by means of sound; thus, the *proximal stimulus* of speech perception is sound, but the claim is that its *distal objects* are intended gestures. An early hint of this lay in the fact that the transitional parts of the brief syllables containing [d] 'point back' to a particular frequency, 1800 hz—that is, there is one component transition (the 'second formant') in each of these syllables, such that if you extend it backwards in the time dimension, all intersect at 1800 hz. (see Figure 12). However—and this is the important point—the backwards-extended portions of the spectrographic lines that diverge from this frequency are actually silent for periods lasting for about 50 ms—if they were not, they would not sound like /d/. This silence corresponds to a feature of how the voiced stops are produced: 'the resonant frequency of the cavity at the instant of closure [of the articulatory tract] is approximately 1800 hz, but since no sound emerges until some degree of opening has occurred, the locus frequency is not radiated as part of the acoustic signal' (Liberman et al. 1967, 438).

When you press your tongue against your palate in order to produce a /d/, you thereby create a resonant frequency in the articulatory tract. This resonant frequency is *silent* because the tract is closed. You then open the tract; how you do so depends on the *following* vowel—the shape of your lips is

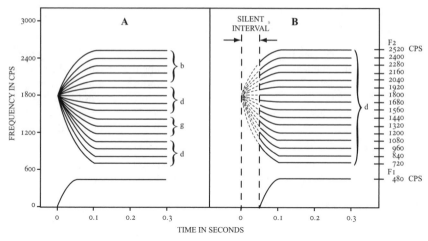

A   Second-formant transitions that start at the /d/ locus and
B   comparable transitions that merely 'point' at it, as indicated by the dotted lines.

Those of **A** produce syllables beginning with /b/, /d/, or /g/, depending on the
frequency level of the formant; those of **B** produce only syllables beginning with /d/.

Fɪɢ.12 The Silence of /d/

Source: Delattre, Liberman, and Cooper (1955), with permission of the *Journal of the Acoustical Society of America.*

different for an /a/ and for an /u/. Consequently, the sound you produce is different; 'da' and 'du' correspond to different acoustic patterns. The only hint of the silent frequency is the starting point of the rapid transition to the steady vowel frequency. It appears, in other words, that the perceptual system is *retrospectively* reconstructing ('decoding' as Liberman et al. say) the 'gesture' by which the speaker produced the sound—i.e. the closure of the articulatory tract in order to produce the stop—from sound received 10 or so milliseconds subsequent to that closure. To put it dramatically, the speech perception module 'infers' the silent 1800 hz resonance from the 'shape' of the sound produced subsequently, and provides you with the experience of hearing /d/ to mark this 'conclusion'.

One could pose the same problem for the perception of phonemes as Dan Dennett (1991, 114) (following Nelson Goodman) does for the *phi*-phenomenon (see Chapter 11, section II below). *When* does one perceive /d/? When somebody says 'dig', the /d/ seems to *precede* the vowel. Now, as Figure 12 shows, the vowel occurs about 100 ms after the speaker began the articulatory 'gesture'. The first 50 ms or so of that gesture are actually silent, so that cannot be when the /d/ was heard: the hearer had no acoustic clue about what sound was going to emerge from the speaker's mouth when it opened. Nor does the slide to the vowel portion of the syllable, lasting another 50 ms, sound like a /d/, as noted above. The claim is that the system cannot have known that a /d/ had been uttered until *after* it seemed to have been heard, i.e. until the entire brief syllable had been received and decoded. How can this be? The answer has to be that the signal does not encode the /d/ separately, but it appears to us that it does. Why does the articulated brief syllable sound like a succession of sounds though it is in fact unitary?

The answer offered by the Motor Theory is that we are reconstructing our own voicing gestures: the *act* of producing a /d/ does precede the act of producing the vowel, though the former act is silent. When we encounter the pattern corresponding to 'da', we perceive a sequence of phonemes timed by the articulatory 'gesture' of producing this syllable. This lends credence to the claim that we are hearing voicing gestures not sounds: for it is voicing gestures not sounds that occur in the temporal order that we attribute to 'dig'.

The Motor Theory conceives of speech as a kind of semaphore—a series of gestures, some actually silent, that are cumulatively responsible for the sounds we produce. The idea is that we communicate by producing a series of bodily gestures which can be reconstructed by the sounds that result from them. Any given brief syllable is a structured group of such gestures, and presented in the form of a single long acoustic pattern. What is available to auditory awareness in the form of the distinct *phoneme*—/d/ or whatever—are the decoded parts of the message conveyed by this long pattern. This theory is quite likely false in its details. The data are not so beautifully unified with regard to sibilants and fricatives as they are in the case of dental stops. Moreover, the variance in sounds that fall under a single phoneme is quite likely different from that predicted by the Motor Theory, and there are probably ways of learning phonemes other than the nativist paradigm suggested by the tight pairing of phonetic gestures and phonemes.

Nevertheless, we can take two lessons from the theory advanced by Liberman and his colleagues.

First, the spectrographic analysis on which the theory rests is on the right track. It suggests a speech 'code', a sequence of several distinct phones contained in the same acoustic pattern. It has been suggested that *pace* Liberman there actually *is* an acoustic pattern characteristic of /d/—see Stevens and Blumstein 1978. However, this pattern is, as these authors say 'global'—a common characteristic of whole brief syllables starting with /d/, not a characteristic of a part of them, *as we hear it*. So it is essentially correct to say that the /d/ is contained in the entire sound, not in a part.

Second, the connection between speech production and speech perception suggested by the Motor Theory is also on the right track. The acoustic patterns decoded by the speech perception system are those produced by the speech production system. The speech perception module is specialized for the detection of sounds that in nature emanate only from the human articulatory tract.

The second point above—the tight association between speech perception and speech production—is supported by the following findings.

The co-classification of phones under a single phoneme varies according to the language spoken. Newborn babies can recognize the whole range of phones produced by the human articulatory tract, but this fine differentiating capacity collapses as they adapt to and learn a language. For it turns out that 'learning' the phonetic structure of a language actually amounts to 'forgetting' or losing the ability to hear certain phonic distinctions, to match the coarse allophonic structure of the language these babies hear and are learning to speak (Werker and Tees 1984, 1999). The result of this 'learning' process is that phones are grouped together as phonemes: adult English speakers fail to hear clearly the difference between [t] and [tĥ] (or register it only as an artefact of accent), though speakers of Hindi, Arabic, or Farsi can, and the difference between the four different r-sounds that speakers of Hindi distinguish; similarly, native speakers of Japanese have difficulty discriminating /r/ and /l/. It is presumably not coincidental that [tĥ] is not a distinct phoneme in English, and that /r/ is similarly not one in Japanese.

The perception of consonants is 'categorical', i.e. there is a sharp distinction between neighbouring phones even though *acoustically* they shade into one another—a sharp perceived dividing line between [b] and [p], for instance, even while the acoustic pattern is being continuously varied from clear instances of one to clear instances of the other. Significantly, when produced by humans, the transitions between perceptual categories correspond to changes of gesture, rather than to changes in acoustically defined parameters. (This phenomenon was cited as a counter-example to the mistaken principle of Similarity of Effect in Chapter 5, section I.)

Speech perception occurs in parts of the brain physiologically distinct from those devoted to the general perception of sound.

Speech perception is bimodal, involving visual input regarding facial gestures as well as auditory input, as is shown by the fact that the visual perception of certain gestures of the lips can overwhelm evidence from the sound (McGurk and MacDonald 1976), while visual perception can improve intelligibility under adverse auditory conditions (Sumby and Pollock 1954). There is evidence that the visual information read from people's mouths and faces and auditory information concerning their voices is integrated in a part of the brain's temporal lobe (see the citations in Callan et al. 2003).

Callan et al. (2003) produce evidence to show that, as expected for a part of the brain devoted to multisensory integration, this part of the temporal lobe is especially active when the output from either of the separate modalities is degraded and indistinct. For instance, when the spoken sound is indistinct or cloaked by noise, this module will pay special attention to facial gestures and semantic context, and thus it becomes active. In addition, there is a so-called 'mirroring' phenomenon at work here: when we hear somebody speak, areas of the brain involved in speech *production* become active (cf. Zatorre et al. 1992).

That speech perception decodes sounds into discrete phones, which are individuated by speech production 'gestures', strongly suggests that there is a match between the quite contingent particularities of human speech production and the decoding capacities of human speech perception. Provided that humans fail to be able to decompose arbitrary sequences of sound, this point is valid even if the nativist overtones of Motor Theory are mistaken. It could even be that, *pace* Zatorre, and Callan et al., there is no localized brain module dedicated to the decoding of phonemes: it could nonetheless be true that the brain comes with specialized decoding heuristics for phonemes which are not applicable to arbitrary sound patterns.

It is thus the nature of speech *production* that constrains the range of sounds we discriminate as distinct meaningful sounds, not the nature of ambient acoustic information. A differently designed communicative species might have evolved to produce rapid sequences of phonemes that sound to us like barks, grunts, and whistles (like the sounds of dolphins?)—but such an evolutionary development would be useful only if members of the species could also *hear* these noises as meaningful sounds. Much of the speech code of this species would not be accessible to our ears: we would hear the barks and grunts, but not as sounds that make meaningful contributions to language—we would be unable to gather these together into *phones* or *phonemes*, classes of sounds that are equivalent with respect to how they are produced or their contribution to meaningful communication. Speech production in its turn is constrained by what can be heard. There would be no advantage in designing an articulatory tract to produce phones that other members of the species cannot hear, either because they are outside the range of auditory sensitivity, or because decoding them would be very difficult or impossible. We cannot work backwards from the nature of *sound* to the nature of speech production and of speech perception; the cooperative character of communication by speech serves as a constraint on speech production and speech perception.

We are proposing, in short:

The Codependency Thesis for Phonemes
We perceive phonemes because humans produce them. We produce phonemes because humans perceive them.

Summarizing the motor theory in the terminology of the Sensory Classification Thesis of Chapter 1, we may say that the speech perception module sorts diverse acoustic patterns (distinct phones, the same phone spoken by different individuals) into phonetic categories, and a further category of meaningless sound—a whistle, grunt, or hum would be assigned to the latter. (The over-activity of speech perception leads to meaningless sounds being heard as phonemes: this is probably how schizophrenics come to be troubled by non-existent voices.) These sensory classes correspond to articulatory gestures of the human speech tract.

II. What Are Sensory Systems for?

With the codependence of speech perception and speech production in mind, let us turn now to the function of sense perception. What is it for? Put into an evolutionary context, the question amounts to this: In virtue of what advantage to organisms were our sensory systems selected? (cf. Matthen 1988; Millikan 1989). Universalists assume that the function of sensation is definable with no essential reference to the species of the perceiving organism and its species-specific activities. There are physical qualities that impinge on our bodily surfaces, the Universalist says: regardless of what it does, it is useful for an animal to be well-informed about these. What needs explanation, the Universalist figures, is an organism's *failure* to capture ambient information—for instance, colour in the case of dichromats such as dogs and cats (as compared with human trichromats), or high-pitched sound and a variety of odours in the human case (compared with that of a dog). Making the further assumption that natural selection has an optimizing thrust, the Universalist concludes that such failures must be explained by the fact that a kind of organism has simply not evolved the receptors to pick up proximal information, either because it has taken a evolutionary path that led in a different direction, or because the information comes at too great a cost given the benefits that the deficient organism would have derived from it.

The realization that sense perception is concerned with the capture of *distal* features that exist beyond the proximal world of the sensory image leads to a change of perspective. As far as the classic paradigm is concerned, it is plausible to think that sensory receptors yield a determinate set of measurements shared by all who share the receptors themselves. Once we shift to the view that sensory systems reach out into the world beyond the receptors, the Universalist can no longer rely on receptors to make his argument. There are lots of features out there, and we sense only some of them. The question that immediately arises is one of choice: why does evolution lead to the choice of one rather than another such target? A reasonable way to address this question is to focus on why it is advantageous to an organism to capture a particular feature. In line with the argument presented in the previous chapter, we will assume that each new information-processing capacity serves some new activity that helps an organism create a new niche for itself. The incremental value of each addition to a sensory system is assessed not merely in terms of which features it captures, then, but in terms of the activities that the capture of this feature enables. The Codependency Thesis for Phonemes suggests a particular investigative strategy.

Looking back at the Motor Theory, we observe that speech consists of a number of coordinated systems. All subserve a single goal—verbal communication. The output of the speech perception module is taken up by parts of the brain that analyse the syntax and semantics of the string provided. If the speech perception module has done its job properly, these units will be able to decipher the incoming message. If not, they will be unable to perform their task; consequently, they will not be able to play a useful role. Conversely, if the syntactic and semantic modules are absent or deficient, there will be no point to the activity of the speech perception unit: decoding the phoneme will yield no advantage if they cannot be assembled into a coherent message. Further, the phones and phonemes heard by a species must correspond—if not exactly, then at least roughly—to those that the species can produce. Now, the mechanisms of speech production, speech perception, syntactic coding, and semantic coding are anatomically distinct. They do different things. But if any *one* of them failed to perform its task properly, *all* would fail. If speech perception failed, for instance, the communicative function of speech production would be thwarted, and the syntactic and semantic decoders would be for naught. This interdependence of all on all is the clue to a proper identification of function.

The hypothesis on offer here is that *all* perception should be understood along similar lines. All animals possess systems that classify incoming information. How they organize the incoming signals into classes depends on what they do with the information. Take the visual perception of colour or shape. It would do an organism no good to perceive distal features if it had no use for information about these features. Conversely, it would have been unable to develop whatever activities depend on the capture of specific information if it didn't have adequate means of gathering this information. It is this interdependence of perception and use that explains the specialization of perception dealt with in Part III. All that we need to add is that different organisms have different environmental needs, and hence engage in different activities requiring information about different environmental variables.

The coordination of activities to produce an end is reminiscent of a mathematical structure in the Theory of Games known as a coordination problem. Here is David Lewis's (1969) description of this problem:

Two or more agents must each choose one of several alternative actions. Often all the agents have the same set of alternative actions, but that is not necessary. The outcomes the agents want to produce or prevent are determined jointly by the actions of all of the agents. So the outcome of any action an agent might choose depends on the actions of the other agents. (8)

There is a special class of coordination problems in which the interests of the agents more or less coincide with one another. A well-known example is that of two people who want to meet somewhere, to go on to dinner together. It is of little interest to them, let us suppose, *where* they will meet, so long as they do. There may be two places they can meet: P_1 and P_2. If both go to P_1 or both go to P_2, both are happy; if one goes to P_1 while the other goes to P_2, both are unhappy. It is in the interest of both parties to develop an agreement to go to P_1 or to go to P_2. Once such an agreement is established, it is in the interests of each party to go to the agreed upon place, since it is likely that the other one will do the same, and each, finding the other there, will then be happy. A *coordination equilibrium* (also known as a Nash equilibrium) is a combination of actions in which nobody would have been better off if she had chosen a different action, assuming that the actions of all the other players remained fixed. The combination of both agents going to the same place—say P_1—is a coordination equilibrium in this problem. Both players would have been worse off if they had chosen to go somewhere else, i.e. P_2, keeping fixed where the other player has gone, i.e. P_1.

Suppose that the interests of the agents *exactly* coincide, for instance, that meeting each other is the only thing that matters to them in this situation—both value meeting equally, and there is no divergence of interest at all about where to meet. Then, we get a situation as shown in Table 3. This is called a *game of pure coordination*. Games of pure coordination always have a coordination equilibrium. For there is at least one outcome that is best for R in every such game, and that outcome is best also for C (since their interests coincide exactly) and any other players. A state that is best for all players is clearly such that nobody could have done better if any player had chosen differently.

Let us look now at a coordination problem in an evolutionary setting. Let us suppose that we have two interacting subsystems of the same animal. A simple example is the frog's visual so-called 'bug detector' and its tongue. When a spot of a certain size moves across the frog's retina, its tongue lashes out. This helps it catch bugs, because in its habitat most moving spots are caused by bugs flying past its nose. The problem posed is this: what size should the moving spot be to trigger the tongue-lash? Clearly, this depends

TABLE 3 A Game of Pure Coordination

	C goes to P_1	C goes to P_2
R goes to P_1	1, 1	0, 0
R goes to P_2	0, 0	1, 1

TABLE 4 Evolutionary Game of Pure Coordination

	Tongue is long	Tongue is short
Small spot triggers tongue-lash	1, 1	0, 0
Large spot triggers tongue-lash	0, 0	1, 1

on the length of the tongue. Suppose for the sake of simplicity that there are only two possible lengths, long and short. If the tongue is long, an in-range bug will project a small spot on the frog's retina; if it is short, an in-range bug will project a large spot. The frog is at an advantage, from an evolutionary perspective, if the length of its tongue coordinates with the size of the spot that triggers the tongue-lash.

Now suppose that the following independence condition obtains: the genes that encode visual control of the tongue-lash and those that control the length of the tongue can mutate independently of one another. *Since both derive their fitness from the organism, the value of every outcome is equal for both genes.* For this reason, these genes are playing a game of pure coordination. There is an equilibrium point in all such games, as we have seen. In the simple game that we have been describing, the equilibria formally coincide with the simple game of meeting described earlier, as shown in Table 4. Here as before, the actions performed by each player are different, but certain *combinations* of actions are more beneficial to both parties. Movement between the two equilibria is unlikely. Changing just one of these actions will be bad for the organism; thus two changes are the minimum required to maintain the fitness levels assigned above. Assuming that the two genes will very rarely mutate together, a mutant will very rarely win. Thus, the two equilibria are, in the sense of John Maynard Smith (1982), evolutionarily stable strategies. That is, the system will be resistant to evolutionary change when the coordinated solution is achieved, i.e. where the tongue is long and the retinal spot is small, or vice versa.

Obviously, coordination equilibria in evolution are not maintained by *agreement*, as in the game described earlier, which is played by two people wanting to meet somewhere for dinner. Here, the coordination equilibrium states are explanations of the outcome without the intentions of the agents figuring into the equation. The coordination points are arrived at by natural selection—i.e. by the accumulation of chance. The process by which the equilbria are reached is stochastic—it is an outcome of random events— but one should not conclude that it is *unlikely* that systems will arrive at them. For as Brian Skyrms (1996) demonstrates by the use of computer simulations, the emergence and stability of a coordinated solution is a virtual certainty in cases like this. Skyrms assumes that all the *phenotypes* mentioned above are available in the population—the long and short tongues, the small-spot reacting and the large-spot reacting motor systems—his simulations consist of each of these types competing with every other pair-wise. This is an idealization: what is required is the assumption that these phenotypes are *genetically accessible*. That is, we need to assume that the genetic modifications required for these phenotypes to be expressed can be achieved by mutation. If this is the case, then the Skyrms round-robin tournament becomes a reality.

In a case like this, natural selection is not working backwards from the properties of bugs to the properties of the retinal spot. Rather, the tongue and the retina are working together with the properties of the bug serving as a background constraint or 'boundary condition'. By analogy, imagine two people who evolve a strategy for meeting in strange cities. Let's suppose they always go to the cafeteria in the biggest local art gallery at 6 p.m. These people always find themselves in a certain sort of restaurant, but that was not the point of the strategy. However, the fact that most cities have an art gallery and most art galleries a cafeteria ensures that their strategy suc-ceeds. As it happens, art gallery cafeterias are all pretty much the same. But it can be imagined that they knew nothing about this. These facts form the background constraint of the search for a strategy. In a similar vein, it seems appropriate to say that the retina is not providing the tongue with informa-tion about the bug *per se*, but about the appropriateness of lashing out in the circumstances. Since an animal with a short tongue and large triggering spot has the same advantages as one with a long tongue and a smaller trig-gering spot, we cannot say that the frog possesses information about the size or distance of the bug except in tongue-relative terms. For this reason, any explanation of the environmental significance of the retinal spot must refer to how the frog uses the information provided, rather than simply to the environmental feature itself. Equally, any explanation of the tongue's role in catching flies needs to refer to the kind of information that is available to the tongue.

In the case described, evolution arrives at a sensory classification. In the case of frogs with long tongues, it co-classifies small spots as lash-worthy; in the case of frogs with short tongues, large spots are so classified. Notice that in the case of frogs with long tongues, the large spots are left unclassified. They have no special significance; they are just lumped into the class of non lash-worthy things along with many other items.

The example given is, of course, highly schematic and simplified. Here are just a few considerations that might complicate the picture.

> Generally speaking, there may not be a plurality of equilibria in a game like this. It may be that the historical situation permits of only one solu-tion; however, as long as there is a perfect coincidence of interests, the existence of a solution is guaranteed—in a game of pure coordination,

there must be at least one outcome that is best for both players. Since subsystems inherit the fitness of the organisms they inhabit, there is a perfect coincidence of interests.

One cannot in any case assume (as we have been assuming) that the organism has *no* interest in which of two equilibrium points is chosen. It might well be, for example, that for reasons unrelated to the game of coordination described above, it is advantageous for the frog to have a long tongue—perhaps bugs rarely venture very close to a frog's mouth. This will mean that one of the above equilibrium points will be better than the other.

It is a slight idealization to claim there will always be a perfect coincidence of interests. The argument used above was that genetic units inherit their fitness from the organism they serve, with the consequence that the fitness of all genetic units is equal. However, it is well known that genes can enhance their own fitness at the expense of the organisms on which they rely to propagate themselves (Dawkins 1976). Thus in general the fitness of genetic units need not be exactly the same as that of the organisms in which they reside. So we cannot always be sure that there will be even one equilibrium in games of coordination. But this probably does not affect the case of perception.

One should not assume that the interests of the players are fixed in advance. The interesting situation from an evolutionary point of view is that interests may change as new possibilities become available. For instance, the frog's retina would not have had any interest in recording moving spots of any size until the tongue-lashing behaviour started to be expressed; equally, the tongue-lashing behaviour would have lacked value until the possibility of retinal guidance became possible. Moreover, the interrelationships of interests may change as further developments occur. Suppose that a mutant frog is able not only to snap at spots of a certain size, but develops the disposition to move towards out-of-focus spots that happen to be somewhat smaller. Then, it will have gained the beginnings of a visually guided pursuit ability; this demands a richer range of visual information and new visual classification systems. A pursuing frog must, for instance, discriminate between bugs that are in range and worth lashing out at, and those that are out of range and must be pursued further. When they arrive at ways of making these discriminations, they will be constrained by characteristics of the bugs in the environment and of the other systems.

The hypothesis being offered here is that *generally speaking* the evolution of sensory systems should be regarded as the solution of a coordination problem of the above sort. A sensory system should be regarded as one of a suite of systems that determines how an organism will interact with the world. The problem that evolution solves is that of coordinating sensory classifications with the activity of the other systems (and vice versa). Environmental properties serve as boundary conditions on solutions to this problem: that is, the existence of bugs, their size, the speed with which they move, etc., determine how the problem can be solved. The sensory system does not converge, as the Universalist believes, on properties of the proximal stimulus regardless of the activities of the organism. Sensory systems are not for the capture of universally available ambient properties. They are to provide specific information to specific effector mechanisms—information that serves the actions of these effectors, actions which are themselves possible only because certain sensory discriminations are possible. The human colour-vision system evolves in directions determined by what humans do with colour information; what we do with colour information evolves according to what information is available. The same holds for pigeons. Since the pigeon's needs are different from ours, and since its eyes have a different evolutionary history, the pigeon's colours are different from ours.

This is not to say that the pigeon will share nothing with us. We argued in Chapter 7 that the raw material of colour vision, the opsins and the cone cells in which they are located, are of ancient origin and shared by all organisms with colour vision. New colour receptors are not easy for evolution to construct, and so cone cells form the shared foundations on which colour-vision systems are built. A similar remark can be made about the processing systems close to the retina. The modification of an evolved complex system is difficult because so many systems have to be tinkered with at once. Opponent processing is a useful way of extracting information from the retinal array; moreover it is flexible, easily adaptable to the emergence of additional cone-cell types that carry new information. Information flows to other colour-data streams through opponent processing cells. Thus, it is not easy to replace the opponent-processing mechanism: changes have ramifications downstream, and require extensive engineering as a result. For reasons like this, most specialization must occur fairly far downstream, where it demands the fewest changes. In humans, the earlier stages of visual processing—right up to the primary visual cortex—is shared with a large number of other animals, including birds and all other mammals. The differences come later, in the ramified stream that emerges from the primary visual cortex. The pattern of development in perceptual specialization recalls Haeckel's remark: here, it is the flow of information along perceptual pathways that recapitulates phylogeny. Information flows first along ancient highways and is then channelled down modern distributor routes.

Our proposal, then, is this:

The Coevolution Thesis
Sensory systems coevolve with effector systems. Their function is to provide effector systems with information specific to the performance of

the behaviours produced by the effector systems, much as it is the function of effector systems to use the information available to them to do things that are advantageous to the organism they serve.

The Coevolution Thesis is non-universalist in its thrust: the Phonetic Codependency Thesis stated in section I is a special application. Different kinds of organism inhabit different ecological niches, that is, they interact with their surroundings in different ways. The Coevolution Thesis suggests that sensory and effector systems evolve together to create such niches. Note that we are not simply saying that perception evolves in order to serve an organism's activities. The claim is rather that there is coevolution here: if the activity did not emerge, the perceptual subsystem that would serve it is of no advantage; if the perceptual system did not emerge, the activity would be impossible.

The Coevolution Thesis is foundational with respect to the specialization evident in speech perception and speech production; it explains the principles of specialization deployed in Chapter 7 with regard to the thesis of Pluralistic Realism. Incidentally, the Coevolution Thesis should not be taken to imply that each of the coordinated systems in a given perception-action nexus must actually have changed in order to participate. Coevolution occurs in a strong sense where *all* the coevolving systems have undergone coordinated evolutionary change. Here, we can work with the weaker assumption that the evolutionary *optimum* is specified by reference to a number of different systems because all these systems jointly contribute to the successful activity of the organism. It is not necessary to assume that all the systems have changed in response to this demand: it may well be that one or more is resistant to change, and that all the others have had to change in order to arrive at the optimum implied by the immovability of that one. In the case of the frog, for example, tongue-length might be fixed, and the size of the triggering spot may have evolved to match. Even if this were so, we will still not say that evolution was working backward from the size of bugs, but that it was working to establish a coordinated equilibrium.

The idea that sensory systems furnish information of specific utility to effector activities is realist, in two ways. First, it implies that the features of concern are located in the space where effector organs work, and hence in the distal environment, not just a feature of the receptoral image. Secondly, it conforms to the principle of Action-Relative Realism propounded in Chapter 8, section IV. Moreover, this conception of the function of sensory systems is pluralist in its implications—different organisms take advantage of different external properties for different purposes.

III. Epistemic Action

The Coevolution Thesis is implausible if one thinks of effector systems as *motor* systems. It is absurd to think that colour perception, for instance, could be dedicated to the guidance of bodily motions, or that this exhausts its significance. And though it is true that speech perception is *connected* to speech production, which is a motor action, our perception of phonemes does not guide us in *performing* any particular action, but simply to our having reason to believe that someone else has performed it.

The connection with effector systems becomes more inviting upon the introduction of a supplementary hypothesis. The 'actions' to which feature-attributing sensory states are connected are not *motor* actions, i.e. actions achieved by moving parts of one's body. Rather, they are *epistemic* actions, for example, coming to believe that a speaker has issued a certain gesture. When an auditory pattern sounds to us like a /du/, it is because the speech perception module has classified it as apt for believing that the /du/ gesture has been performed by a speaker: as a consequence, the perceiver takes the speaker to be conveying a message about a *dupe* rather than a soup, or about a *duke* rather than a toque.

By the same token, there is a set of instinctive epistemic practices in which colour-experience enables us to participate. Human visual systems instinctively use colours in at least the following ways:

> to co-classify things for purposes of induction, for example, to make generalizations concerning the ripeness of fruit, or the health of one's conspecifics;

> to re-identify things on different occasions, for example, one's car in a crowded parking lot;

> to segment the visual scene into figure and ground, adjacent things of similar colour being both assigned to the figure or both to the ground;

> to find things by visual search, for instance red or orange fruit against a background of green foliage; and

> to match and differentiate things by the colour-looks they present, in order to be able tell, for instance, which part of a uniformly coloured lawn is shaded by trees.

The thesis is that we instinctively use colour-looks in order to group things together for the above-mentioned tasks. Colour-properties are equivalence concepts. Things grouped together by colour are treated in the same way for the purposes mentioned above. Or to put this in terms appropriate to the Sensory Ordering Thesis, rather than the cruder Sensory Classification Thesis: things that are found to be more similar with respect to colour are treated in proportionately similar ways. (Given sensory ordering, colour concepts are not strictly speaking equivalence classes, since sensory similarity is not transitive. But as stipulated in Chapter 1, section I.6, we generally ignore this complication in this book.)

Sensory classifications feed via sensory experience into the epistemic faculties of classical conditioning, inductive learning, signal decoding, and inference based on all of the above. Once epistemic actions are included in the mix, this way of looking at sensory content becomes much more plausible.

The Coevolution Thesis yields individuation conditions for sensory concepts. For if the Thesis is correct, there can be no difference between sensory states that does not express itself in terms of some action-related difference. That is, any point of discrimination between two sensory states, however fine, corresponds to some difference between what each represents. That we can discriminate between two phonemes—a relatively crude distinction—enables us to differentiate words with these phonemes as components. That we can discriminate the allophones grouped together under a phoneme—a much finer distinction—potentially enables us to differentiate conditions of utterance, accents, and to identify a voice as belonging to a friend, and feeds into associations useful for determining where somebody comes from.

Thus, we have:

Three Principles of Sensory Equivalence
(1) *Resemblance* x and y sensorily appear (on a particular occasion) to resemble each other if there is some epistemic action E, such that the sensory experience of x and the sensory experience of y (on that occasion) suggest that x and y be treated similarly with respect to E.
(2) *Non-resemblance* x and y sensorily appear (on a particular occasion) *not* to resemble each other if there is some epistemic action E, such that the sensory experience of x and the sensory experience of y (on that occasion) suggest that x and y *not* be treated similarly with respect to E.
(3) *Indiscriminability* x and y are indiscriminable (on a particular occasion) relative to a particular sensory modality or submodality if the sensory experience of x and the sensory experience of y in that modality (on that occasion) suggest that for *all* epistemic actions associated with that modality or submodality, x and y should be treated exactly the same.

See Chapter 11, section IV.1 for the application of such principles to the case of colour.

These considerations connect with the mutual involvement of sensory classification, sensory consciousness, and memory sketched in Chapter 1, section II. Sensory classification does not merely assign present stimuli to classes that connect with immediate bodily action. It also builds up a continuing record of what actions are appropriate given sensory appearance. That is, it learns how things that possess certain sensory properties are in other respects—for example, that fruit of a certain colour are ripe. For both applications—that is, both for associating properties with one another (induction) and for assigning particular occurrent stimuli to classes (classification and inference)—the sensory system needs to issue an internal symbol of its determinations. This symbol does not compel any particular action, but it is available to be considered by other systems in the light of other concurrent information, and also to be compared with other occurrences of things in this sensory class in the past. This signal serves, in short, as a trigger of a particular range of epistemic actions. This is the role of sensory experience: it is an occurrent and stored signal of sensory classification.

IV. Sensory Content

Alva Noë and Kevin O'Regan (2002) propose an account of visual consciousness that parallels the account of sense features offered here in certain respects, but having limited the relevance of sensory states to *motor* action, they explicate sensory consciousness in terms of such action.

Consider the experience of driving a particular kind of car, say a Porsche. In what does this experience consist? Notice that, in one sense, there is no *feeling of driving a Porsche*. That is, the character of Porsche driving does not consist in the occurrence of special sort of momentary flutter or bodily sensation. What defines the character of driving a Porsche, rather is *what a person does when he or she drives a Porsche*. There are characteristic ways in which the vehicle accelerates in response to pressure on the gas pedal. There are definite features of the way the car handles in turns, how smoothly the gears shift, and so on. What it is like to drive a Porsche is constituted by all these sensorimotor contingencies and by one's skillful mastery of them. (571)

Noë and O'Regan go wrong at a crucial point. They purport to be explicating sensory experience in terms of 'sensorimotor contingencies'. In fact, they are talking about the feeling of *doing* something, namely driving a car. This is different from the sensory experience to which one *responds* while driving. It certainly is not right to say that the sensory experience that one enjoys when one drives a car is constituted by the feeling of driving the car. That is, it does not seem right (or even coherent) to say that the sensory experience that prepares you to shift gears—perhaps the auditory experience of the engine revving too high—is a recreation of shifting gears, a mental simulation of the associated action. (Incidentally, they are also wrong about there being no bodily sensation associated with driving a car: there clearly is a bodily sensation of changing gears, for example.) There is obviously a big difference between the experience of the characteristic engine sound that leads you to shift gears and the experience of shifting the gear. Thus it is a mistake to say that 'the character of seeing, like that of driving, is constituted by the character of the various things one does when one sees (or when one drives).' It is true, as we have argued, that there is an intimate connection between the character of seeing and the character of the associated epistemic actions.

But seeing a colour does not feel the same as performing an induction based on colour, no more so than hearing the high-pitched whine of an engine revving too high feels the same as shifting gears. Rather, to sense something is to be given information that prepares one for that action.

Taking this into account, and also broadening the purview of the Noë and O'Regan thesis to include epistemic action, we now propose the following definition:

Primary Sensory Content
The primary content of a sensory state is that the situation is right for a certain action or actions, these actions having been associated with this state by evolution. These actions may include epistemic actions.

If we extend J. J. Gibson's notion of an *affordance*—an object or situation apt for certain actions—to include epistemic actions of co-classification and the like, then the thesis is that perceptual states offer information about affordances, including—crucially—epistemic affordances.

In Chapter 8, section IV, we suggested that representational states are associated with predictable physically specifiable states of affairs. Thus, there are two associated ways to express the message carried by a sensory state. From the point of view of the perceiver, a sensory state signals the appropriateness of certain actions. This is its primary sensory content as defined above. However, it is also possible *physically* to characterize the distal situation in which a particular sensory state normally occurs. Presumably, there is a connection between these two characterizations: in evolutionary times, a situation of that physical type must have been right for the associated action. In other words, that a situation is appropriate for a particular response was extensionally equivalent in evolutionary times to its being physically so characterized. This leads to the following:

Secondary Sensory Content
The secondary content of a sensory state is the physically specifiable environmental situation in which it is functionally correct to perform the associated action.

Given different physiological realizations, evolutionary histories, and different states of the world, the same primary content of a sensory state could go with different secondary contents. Recall, for example, that any given colour consists of a set of metameric spectral profiles grouped together by colour vision (Chapter 8, section I and II.1). Had our colour receptors been slightly different with regard to their sensitivity to various parts of the spectrum, these sets of metameric profiles would have been differently grouped. The colour would then have had the same primary content, but different secondary content. Similarly, if the physiology of our vocal tracts had been slightly altered, different acoustic patterns would have been grouped together under the phones. But the *primary* content of these phones need not have been any different. The relation between primary and secondary content is thus analogous to that between meaning and extension.

Secondary sensory content is the primary focus of psychophysical invest-igation. Suppose for instance that two things look exactly alike in colour. Or suppose that two phonetic utterances are exactly alike. We can ask in what *physical* respect they match. This is the kind of task that psychologists of perception undertake in their laboratories. The spectrographic analysis of phonemes discussed in section I is an example of this. This spectrographic analysis does not tell us, and does not purport to tell us, the significance of phonetic perception *to the perceiver*, that is, the perceiver does not come to know, by hearing a /d/ that the second formant of the speaker's utterance conforms to such and such a spectrographic pattern. The brilliant contribu-tion of Motor Theory was to go beyond the spectrographic analysis of phonemes and to connect this to the articulatory gestures of human speech. By means of such analysis one comes to see how the physical characterization of a phoneme marks that the situation is right for a certain epistemic action.

Physicalist theories of sensory properties identify sense features with physical properties. Physicalist theories of colour, for instance, identify colours with surface spectral reflectances or something similar. (See Hilbert 1987; Matthen 1988; and Byrne and Hilbert 2003 for physicalist accounts of colour.) The theory being offered here is that while physicalist theories cap-ture the *secondary content* or extension of sensory states, they do not capture the primary content or meaning of sensory states from the perceiver's point of view. In Chapter 11, we will return to a further consideration of this claim, and to a more detailed account of sensory content.

10

Sense Experience

So far we have been discussing sensory classification and sense-features. We come now to sense experience. Sense experience signals sensory classification. That is, many organisms come to know that a stimulus has been classified a certain way because they find themselves in a conscious state with a certain qualitative character. For instance, I come to know a certain stimulus has been classified as round, or as red, because I find myself in a characteristic conscious state—the state, that is, of that thing looking round, or looking red. What is the role of sense experience in this connection between perceiver, object, and classification? How does consciousness contribute to the perceiver's state of knowledge? This is the question addressed in the present chapter.

I. Coercive Content

We have been supposing that the function of a given sensory system coordinates with that of an effector system. The effector system has several actions within its repertoire, $A_1, A_2, \ldots, An$, and these are appropriate in circumstances $C_1, C_2, \ldots, Cn$ respectively. The job of the perceptual system is to determine which of these circumstances obtains.

In order for the organism to prosper, two things must happen:

a. The sensory system must accurately determine which of $C_1, C_2, \ldots, Cn$ obtains, and
b. The effector system must reliably do $A_1, A_2, \ldots,$ or An depending on which of $C_1, C_2, \ldots, Cn$ (respectively) obtains.

This raises a question. How is the coordination of sensory determinations and actions achieved? It is not enough that the sensory system should *determine* which of the circumstances obtains. This determination has to be made available to the effector system. Otherwise, we are no further ahead: the effector system would be on its own as far as 'deciding' what to do.

In certain cases, it is quite sufficient that once the sensory system has determined which of C_1, C_2, etc., obtains, it should simply cause the effector system to perform the associated action. This is plausibly the case with respect to the frog: once the frog's eye has determined that the frog's tongue should lash out, it might simply issue a neural impulse that makes the tongue lash out. Similarly, in the case of the human immune system. This system has the task of determining when a foreign 'antigen' has entered its host environment. Once it determines that a particular antigen is present in the system, it simply 'turns on' the production of a matched antibody in large numbers. The antibody is specifically shaped so as to match the antigen, to bind with it to form an immune complex which is then flushed from the body by a separate part of the system. In these cases, the sensory system acts directly on the effector system. Thus, its output must be causally apt for bringing about the matched action. If the immune system were to react to the presence of antigen A by producing an antibody that does not match A, it will not succeed in flushing A from the system. If the system consistently issued a different antibody in response to A, one would be able to deduce when it had detected A. This, however, would not be good enough for such a system, since the requisite effect would not ensue. It is not enough then that the immune system should (a) determine that A has entered its environment, and (b) do something that shows that it has so determined. It must also (c) issue an impulse that brings about the right action. The condition (c) is a constraint on the nature of the system's output, for it implies that the output must be causally apt for the action in question. I'll call response-apt output 'coercive' in recognition of the fact that it brings about a system response directly.

It is possible to discern coercive output even with regard to familiar sensory classification functions in humans. Consider the phenomena of *habituation*, *priming*, and *classical conditioning*. In each, the state of the system changes without the perceiver's intervention. In the case of habituation (or 'adaptation'), a perceiver's attention more easily wanders from a stimulus if stimuli of the same kind have been presented repeatedly just before. For instance, if an organism is presented with a flash of red, it will pay attention. After a series of red flashes, it will stop doing this. A blue flash will, however, rekindle its interest. Sensory classification, indeed sensory ordering, is involved in perceptual habituation: the effect depends on the sameness or similarity of the stimuli that were presented before. Priming is another phenomenon that is sensitive to sensory classification. Here, the perceiver is hypersensitive to a particular occurrence, having experienced it before. For example, a previously ambiguous and illegible pattern might pop out at you if you had been shown it before in clearer form. Again, you might easily recognize a word which is presented partially obscured if you had encountered that word in a list a little earlier. Here the classificatory system is 'primed' by a previous act of classification to recognize the word on the basis of inadequate and incomplete information. All of this happens without the perceiver's awareness or intervention. Its response patterns have been coercively changed by the sensory system.

II. Non-Coercive Content

Not all the cognitive effects of sensory classification are so determinate. In sophisticated organisms, the one-to-one match between triggering circumstance and associated action is considerably loosened. For the system may be so organized as to react to a particular circumstance in different ways on different occasions, depending on what else obtains in the environment. Here is a realistic example:

When the phone rings—a stimulus—people normally pick it up. But if the phone rings at a friend's house—that is, in a different context—people let it ring. However, if the friend, before hopping into the shower, asks a visitor to pick up the phone if it happens to ring . . . the visitor answers the phone. (Helmuth 2003, 1133)

Here, many different considerations are contributing to the eventual outcome. As we shall see in a moment, this complicates the question of how the effector system is to be manipulated.

A further complication arises when a sensory system's determination that a particular circumstance obtains feeds in to a number of different actions. Speech perception and colour vision, for example, have a number of different consequences for action. The perception that a particular phoneme has been uttered results in our recognizing that a particular articulatory gesture has been performed; it also contributes to the decoding of the *word* uttered by the speaker, to the recognition of the speaker's mood, of his accent, and so on. Similarly, the perception that something has a certain colour leads to our registering a number of different epistemic affordances, as we saw in Chapter 9, section III—induction, figure-ground segregation, object-identification, and so on. In such cases, the output of the sensory system cannot consist of a direct manipulation of *all* the different effector systems, unless each effector system is so organized that what it takes to manipulate them is exactly the same, or the sensory system is so organized as to issue a plurality of manipulative outputs—both surely cumbrous arrangements. A solution is for the sensory system not to manipulate the effector systems directly, but simply to issue a signal that a certain situation obtains, leaving it to the effector system to do what is appropriate and necessary. Kim Stereny (2003, ch. 3) calls such signals 'decoupled representations'.

In both kinds of situation—a single effector system taking input from more than one sensory system, and a single sensory system sending output to several effector systems—it will be advantageous for the sensory system to issue a *non-coercive* message, a message that does not directly manipulate the operation of the effector system. Having issued this non-coercive message, it leaves it to some other system—perhaps the effector system itself, or perhaps another intervening system (cf. Koechlin et al. 2003)—to sort out what must be done in the light of the context and the multiple affordances open to the system. This non-coercive output is not tailored to the workings of the effector system, though the effector system or its intermediaries should be capable of changing their own states in the appropriate way when the output indicating a particular circumstance is issued. The claim here is *not* that in these cases deterministic causation breaks down, or that in these situations there is some mysterious determinant known as 'free will' or the like. The claim is simply that the sensory system does not push the effector systems around, but rather simply posts a message as regards its determination of circumstances. There is a similar contrast between getting you to go through the door by pushing you, and getting you to do the same thing by saying 'Go through the door'. In the former case, my action has to be causally just right in a physical sense: I can't push you leftwards if the door is towards the right. In the second case, the utterance has to be correct in a different way—it has to carry the right meaning. Similarly, in the case of sensory output. Non-coercive output has to be semantically right, but is not subject to a physical-aptness constraint on its form.

We are subjectively well aware of the difference between coercive and non-coercive output in our own experiences. The startle reflex and feelings of sleepiness or hunger are initiated by determinations that certain circumstances obtain: a sudden change in the nearby environment in the case of the startle reflex, the passage of time in the case of hunger and sleepiness. The systems that make such determinations are coercive in their output: they do not offer us a great deal of choice regarding the action to be taken. When we are startled, we jump; when we feel sleepy, we go to sleep: though we might fight such impulses, it costs us discomfort, or even pain, to do so. On the other hand, the sensation as of *red* does give us a great deal of choice: we do not *have* to believe that a thing that looks red is red; there are many circumstances in which it would be inappropriate to do so. We may have a strong urge to believe that a thing is red when it looks red (or we may not, depending on the circumstances), but there is, in any case, no literal *pain* or *discomfort* involved in maintaining scepticism or disbelief. Moreover, this kind of sensation feeds into many different actions—inductive learning, object identification, figure-ground segmentation, etc.—as sleepiness and startle do not.

Let us then differentiate two types of states: we call startle and sleepiness *drives* or motivational states, and sensations, such as of red, *sensory* states in a stricter sense than we have been using so far. The former sort of state is normally accompanied by some sort of hormonal or endocrinal secretion apt for causing a particular response, the latter consists typically in a neuron or neurons firing, apt only for creating a record. The former typically have mid-brain involvement; the latter are primarily cortical. Philosophers are wont to say that the sensation of red has a 'feel': it is a self-identifying conscious state. Hunger and sleepiness have a conscious feel in a much stronger sense—we can recognize the growling stomach, the slight faintness of hunger, the torpor, the tingling of one's limbs, the urge to close one's eyes in sleepiness. One might say that while there is something it is like to be sensing red, there is something it *feels* like to be hungry or sleepy. The latter conditions are, so to speak, characteristic *feelings*.

III. Convention

There is no physical-aptness constraint on non-coercive output. Since this output does not have to be causally apt for bringing about appropriate behaviour, it is important only that the systems that use this output should be able to recognize the different sensory signals and match these to the appropriate action. Thus, it is a matter of indifference to the utility of the sensory system which output gets matched to which circumstance-determination.

David Lewis (1969, ch. 4) and Bryan Skyrms (1996, ch. 5) each have seminal accounts of how *meaning* emerges in situations like this. Lewis considers a plan arrived at by a sexton and one Paul Revere. (Apparently, this alludes to an incident in an eighteenth-century North American rebellion.) Simplifying the story somewhat, the sexton looks out for one of two situations:

R_1. The redcoats set out by land.
R_2. The redcoats set out by sea.

Once the sexton has ascertained which of the two situations has occurred, he does one of two things:

S_1. Hangs one lantern in the belfry.
S_2. Hangs two lanterns in the belfry.

Revere for his part looks to see how many lanterns are displayed in the belfry. Depending on how many he sees, he performs one of two actions.

A_1. Warns the countryside that R_1 has occurred.
A_2. Warns the countryside that R_2 has occurred.

Now, plainly the sexton can adopt one of two action plans. They are:

X_1. If R_1 then S_1, and if R_2 then S_2.
X_2. If R_1 then S_2, and if R_2 then S_1.

Similarly, Revere can adopt one of two action plans:

V_1. If S_1 then A_1, and if S_2 then A_2.
V_2. If S_1 then A_2, and if S_2 then A_1.

Given that both the sexton and Revere want it to be the case that A_1 if and only if R_1 and A_2 if and only if R_2, they must coordinate action plans. This is the *signalling coordination problem*. Either the sexton should adopt X_1, and Revere should adopt V_1, or the sexton should adopt X_2, and Revere V_2. When one of these combinations of action plans is achieved, Lewis says, S_1 and S_2 are *signals*. In Lewis's case, the requisite combination is achieved by agreement. Here, as in Chapter 9, section II, we assume that the coordination equilibria have an 'attractive force' of their own; organisms arrive at them by courtesy of natural selection, and there is no need for explicit agreement. As Skyrms (1996, 103) says: 'Signaling system equilibria . . . *must* emerge in the games of common interest that Lewis originally considered.' (Skyrms was considering signals between organisms. The idea of signalling between subsystems of an organisms is original here.)

Notice that if there is to be a possibility of signalling in such a situation, the sexton has to have at least as many putative signals available to him as there are circumstances that demand different actions on the part of Revere. But neither cares at all which communicative action plan is adopted, as long as the mutually desired result ensues. There is always more than one situation that can be signalled: there is no point in signalling if things never change. It follows that there is *always* a choice as to which signal is associated with which circumstance. In Chapter 9, section II, we proposed that sensory systems co-evolve with effector systems. There may not be a choice of solutions in such a case, though in the simple example considered, there were two equally valuable solutions—long tongue-small spot, short tongue-big spot. As far as *signalling* is concerned, we have just argued, there is *always* a choice. Thus, the association between signal and circumstance is a matter of convention: there is no intrinsic match between them, only an interest that they be matched up in such a way as to bring about the requisite signalling coordination.

Notice also that here, as we have been urging all along, there is a distinction between the sensory classification state itself and the signal sent to the effector. The human colour-vision system is so organized as to be in a particular state when and only when red things are present (ideally speaking—we are not worrying about perceptual error here). In some systems, such a state is directly and seamlessly linked to the effector system, but not in non-coercive systems. In such systems, the output is merely a 'display' or 'read-out' of the sensory system's state that is evaluated in the light of other considerations. This read-out is inert, but the effector system has access to it when it makes its decision.

Now, one might ask: What is the message conveyed by the *red*-signal, i.e. the sensation of something as red? Does it say: '*Red* there'? Or does it say: 'Perform the epistemic operations appropriate to *red* being there'? Is it *indicative* or *imperative* in content? (Ruth Millikan 1995 has an interesting discussion of states that show this kind of ambivalence.) Discussing the case of the sexton–Revere coordination problem, Lewis (1969, 144–7) insightfully remarks that this depends on who retains the discretion regarding the action to be carried out. If the agreement between the sexton and Revere is that when one lantern is hung in the belfry, Revere will do whatever he thinks best given that the redcoats have set out by land, then the signal is indicative: it means that they have set out by land. If, on the other hand, the arrangement is that the sexton will hang a single lantern in the belfry when he, the sexton, deems it appropriate that Revere should do whatever they have agreed he should do in those circumstances, then the action of handing the lantern in the belfry is a command not a message with informative content—an imperative, not an indicative. Lewis's insight is good here as well. Since the sensation of something as red is non-coercive with respect to the epistemic effector system, and since the effector system's action depends on context, the sensation is deemed indicative. A non-coercive signal says: 'Situation S obtains: do what you think best.' However, it was argued in Chapter 9, sections III–IV, that this situation is characterized in terms of a canonical response, often or usually an epistemic response. Thus the non-coercive signal says: 'The situation obtains in which you would normally do A: do what you think best'. This is still not a completely satisfactory account of sensory content: contrary to this account, sensory content does not seem make reference to the perceiver. We shall modify the account slightly in Chapter 11.

IV. Sensations as Conventional Signals

Sensory experience is a conventional sensory signal in indicative mood which signifies an epistemic affordance. The indicative mood is characteristic of *sensory* as opposed to *motivational* states. Thus, we propose:

Sensory Signalling Thesis
A sensory experience is a signal issued in accordance with an internal convention. It means that the sensory system has assigned a stimulus to a certain category—the same category as when other tokens of the same signal are issued.

The link between the experience of red and the occurrence of red is, as we said, *conventional*. A sensation as of red is a conventional sign that the situation is ripe for certain epistemic actions. It is an indicative sign of an epistemic affordance.

Some philosophers are inclined to think that it makes sense to ask why a particular experience is linked with a particular sensory classification. Joseph Levine (1983), for example, complains that materialism leaves us with an 'explanatory gap':

Let us call the physical story for seeing red 'R' and the physical story for seeing green 'G'. My claim is this. When we consider the qualitative character of our visual experiences when looking at ripe McIntosh apples, as opposed to looking at ripe cucumbers, the difference is not explained by appeal to G and R. For R doesn't really explain why I have the one kind of qualitative experience—the kind I have when looking at McIntosh apples—and not the other. (357–8)

Levine's complaint obviously implies that there is something that needs to be explained about why a particular sensory classification leads to a particular experiential signal. Along similar lines, David Chalmers (1996, 5) asks (echoing Locke): 'Why is seeing red like *this*, rather than like *that*? . . . [Why is it not like] some entirely different kind of sensation, like the sound of a trumpet?'

If sensory experience is a *conventional* sign, however, the spirit in which such questions are asked is misguided. They are no different from asking why 'bat' stands for *bat* rather than *mat* or *cat*. There is only a *historical* expla- nation for why 'bat' stands for *bat*. Seeing red is like this—not the result of a historical act of agreement or legislation as in the case of 'bat', but a chance arrival by natural selection at one equilibrium point rather than another. There is no appropriateness of signal to property beyond that which is endowed upon it by historical accident. Levine's question is ill-posed because it assumes that there is some such natural match—what else could bridge the supposed explanatory gap?

Exactly the same mistake lies behind attempts to define sense-features like *red* in terms of the experience of red. Most philosophers of perception are convinced that experience constitutes the identity of sense-features. They are convinced of this because we seem to possess an intuitive grasp of sense- features—they seem to be directly and immediately *given* to us merely in virtue of experience. If you accept the Sensory Signalling Thesis you will be inclined to think that this is a wrong turn. The experience is not constitutive of the quality; it is merely a signal of the occurrence of this quality, according to an internal convention. The Sensory Signalling Thesis implies that the experi- ence of red is no more constitutive of *red* than the utterance of 'bat' of *bat*.

Gathering these threads together, we may summarize the thesis of this chapter as follows. First we define a sensory state (in the strict sense, intro- duced at the end of section IV) as follows:

> A sensory *state* is
> (a) a classificatory state (in the sense of Chapter 1),
> (b) formed by a process of sub-personal automatic data-processing on neural records (transductions) of ambient energy patterns,
> (c) which evolved for the purpose of guiding epistemic actions.

> A sense *experience* is
> (a) a signal issued according to a convention developed during an evolutionary game of pure coordination,
> (b) in order to inform an effector system of the guidance for action provided by a perceptual state,

(c) in such a way as not to coerce action in the way that drives or feelings do: sensory experience is not intrinsically, i.e. outside the context of the system, causally apt for ensuring a particular epistemic action, and hence it should be possible for such experiences to have been deployed as signals of different sensory determinations.

We note that sensory experiences have *indicative* content because of clause (c) above, but at the same time that their content is specified by the message that the current situation is such as to make appropriate the action that is associated with them.

V. Action-Relevant Categories and Teleosemantics: A Retrospective Assessment

There are some clear drawbacks to treating of perception as action-relevant, even when the actions in question are taken to be epistemic in character. But before we address these, let us note some strengths. Let us start with this: the Thesis of Primary Sensory Content articulated in Chapter 9, section IV, falls into a class called *teleosemantic* theories of content. Such theories attempt to define the content of a sensory state in terms of its evolutionary function. The theory that has been presented in Chapters 9 and 10 has all of the strengths of teleosemantic theories, and avoids some of their weaknesses. (The present section is an attempt to contextualize my position in the recent debate; readers may skip it if this does not interest them.)

Teleosemantic theories were first posited to avoid some of the pitfalls of classic *indicator* theories. Let us say that

An occurrence of type S *indicates* the presence of a thing with property F (or more briefly S indicates F) if occurrences of type S are so dominantly caused by F-bearing things that it is reasonable to infer the presence of an F-bearing thing from the occurrence of type S.

Indicator theories of perceptual content state (in one form or another) that

A. A perceptual state S has content F if S indicates F.

Indicator theories fail for three reasons. First, not every indicator state has content. It might be, for instance, that the chemical composition of my blood indicates that I have had more than one alcoholic drink, but the chemical composition of my blood does not have this *content*: my blood has no content at all; it delivers no message to my epistemic faculties. Second, it is not strictly true that perceptual states indicate their content. We are prone to misperception, and this shows that it is not always reasonable to infer the truth of what an occurrent perceptual state tells us. Third, not everything that a perceptual state indicates is included in its content. That one sees something as blue indicates that a certain region of the visual cortex is excited: but this is not part of content of the sensation.

Now, various forms of indicator theories can avoid these difficulties. Without going into these, let us just consider the following teleosemantic theory:

B. The content of perceptual state S is F if the biological function of S is to indicate F.

This removes the difficulties mentioned above. First, though the chemical composition of my blood does in fact indicate how many drinks I have had, it does not have the biological function of so doing. Second, even if something has the biological function of doing some particular thing, it does not follow that it will always do it: certain perceptions of brightness may therefore possess the biological function of indicating the reflectance of a stimulus, even though in certain circumstances they fail to do so. Thus, it is possible for a sensory state to be in error. Finally, since not everything that indicates F was, as it were, 'designed' to indicate F, we need not say that a blue sensation gives us a message about everything it indicates: it does not inform us about the state of the visual cortex, for instance, though it contains information about this. In these ways, teleosemantics improves on simple indicator theories.

Now, there are two major difficulties that teleosemantic theories face. The first is that they often manifest adaptationist thinking. That is, they think of evolution as solving a 'pre-existent' 'problem' that the environment sets the organism. (For this interpretation of adaptationism and a critique see Lewontin 1985/1980 and Matthen 2001a.) In Matthen (1988), I defined perceptual content pretty much along the lines of B above, and said that this definition 'provides a justification for expressing the content of colour vision in distal terms' (23) and that 'distality implies that perception purports to be of features of the world which are independent of perception itself' (24). Now, this implies that perceptual content is as specified in the Thesis of Secondary Sensory Content in Chapter 9, section IV, However, my 1988 proposal neglects species-specific Primary Sensory Content. Much the same is true of other teleosemantic theories, for instance, that of Ruth Millikan (1984, 1989). The thought was that (for instance) detecting surface reflectance was *the* problem of colour vision, and that various different organisms solve this problem by independent evolutionary paths. This view is adaptationist: it posits a single pre-existent ecological problem that is independently solved by several organisms, a single source of environmental information pressed into service by all organisms able to take it in. It is rebutted by the Thesis of Pluralistic Realism offered in Chapter 7.

The present version of teleosemantic theory does not take this stance. It specifically treats of the adaptation of perceptual systems as specialized.

Perceptual systems subserve specific actions; their content is differentiated by the action they serve. It can happen, and often does happen, that in order to serve *different* ends, a system has to do some of the same things. And it does seem that animals in very different phylogenetic classes detect surface reflectance and show colour constancy (Neumeyer 1998). But the Thesis of Primary Sensory Content implies that even where this is true the *content* of different detections of surface reflectance will be different if the actions subserved by these detections are different. Suppose for instance that the colour vision of primates evolved in order to discriminate fine details of foliage and fruit, and the colour vision of honey bees evolved to detect pollen in flowers. The thesis is that despite overlaps with regard to the detection of surface reflectance, the content and phenomenology of colour visual states will be very different in the two species (see Chapter 6, section VI above). It is not that human colour vision should be interpreted as conveying a *frugicentric* message as such: rather that it is sensitive to certain contrasts relevant to foraging for fruit, integrates colour information with surface and relief categories (rather than with polarization and directional categories, for instance), and is sensitive to fine detail, while that of the bee may well be different in these respects. The colour classifications that humans use are adapted to different epistemic tasks and display different connections to sensory classes in other categories than those of bees. Human colours are, in short, different from those of bees in ways that the Thesis of Primary Sensory Content accommodates, but most standard teleosemantic theories do not—at least, not as originally conceived and articulated. (Neander 2002 has a sensitive discussion of how to repair and rehabilitate these standard theories—but I do not think that she succeeds in addressing the fundamental difficulties of organism-independent specifications of function and content.)

A second major difficulty that traditional teleosemantic theories face is that they cannot account for the unmediated character of our knowledge of sensory properties. In 1988, I claimed that teleosemantic theories justified expressing the content of colour vision in distal terms, and suggested that colours were (a generalized form of) reflectances. This seems to imply that one would need modern physics—at least enough of it to understand what a reflectance is—in order to grasp the content of colour visual states. Surely, this is false: Aristotle and his trichromatic contemporaries possessed exactly the same sensory grasp of colours as we do, though they knew nought of wavelengths and reflectances (cf. Peacocke 1989; Boghossian and Velleman 1997/1991; Braddon-Mitchell and Jackson 1997). Here again, the present version of the theory does better. Since it defines perceptual content in terms of innately specified epistemic affordances, and since these were shared by trichromatic humans in Aristotle's time, the Thesis of Primary Sensory Content better accounts for the instinctive character of sensory knowledge. We return to this topic in Chapter 11.

11

The Semantic Theory of Colour Experience[1]

We have argued that sensory systems evolve to coordinate with epistemic effector systems. Such effector systems are responsible for classical conditioning, inductive learning, signal decoding, object differentiation, linguistic and non-linguistic communication, and inference. Sensory experience has a special role in what we called the 'non-coercive' use of sensory classification. It signals, in accordance with internal conventions, that an object or a situation is such as to make certain instinctive epistemic actions appropriate. This 'epistemic affordance' constitutes its *primary* content.

As we saw, there are certain background ecological conditions that dictate the terms in which the problem of coordination between sensory and effector systems is solved. Taking these background conditions into account through scientific inquiry, the secondary content of a sensory state can be equated with the occurrence of a certain physically specifiable state of affairs. Normally, a sensory state indicates the occurrence of this state of affairs. Had the evolutionary history or the physiology of sensory systems been different, the same primary sensory content might have been associated with different secondary content. In this respect, the secondary content of a sensory state stands to its primary content much as extension or reference does to meaning.

Now, the secondary content of sensory experience is not immediately available to us: it takes empirical investigation to discover the physical specifications of situations in which particular instinctive epistemic reactions are appropriate. However, the *primary* content of a sensory state *is* immediately available to us, at least in the form of an urge or disposition to perform certain epistemic actions: when we are in a sensory state, we are implicitly aware of the epistemic actions that such a state recommends, whether or not we are

[1] This chapter derives from parts of Matthen (2001 *b*) which appeared in a collection edited by Jill MacIntosh. Such overlaps as there are with this article appear here by the kind permission of the *Canadian Journal of Philosophy*.

inclined, all information considered, to do it. Thus, the Thesis of Primary Sensory Content goes some distance towards accounting for the subjective significance of sensory experience.

Not far enough, however. For by itself, this account of primary content still does not seem to capture the intuitive content of sensory experience correctly. Such experiences *seem* to tell us that external objects or states of affairs possess certain properties categorically, not that they make some action of our own appropriate. True, a perceiver does feel an urge to make certain inferences about stimuli because she experiences them a certain way. But this seems to her to be a *response* to the knowledge that sensory states afford her, not what that knowledge amounts to in itself. In short, sensory information about stimuli seems to contain no self-referential element, as the Thesis of Primary Sensory Content implies. This clash with naïve intuition leads to a pressing problem. In what form do sensory states yield information about the external world? How is their message translated into a categorical utterance about external things?

This is the problem addressed in the present chapter. We will deal specifically with colour experience here because, as we shall see, it brings special problems: an adequate account of the content of colour experience will apply smoothly to other sense modalities, but not necessarily the other way around. We shall see how the primary content of colour experience can be used to construct a categorical notion of colour as a sense-transcending property of things without the need to invoke the secondary content of colour states. In order to prepare ourselves for this task, let us first resurrect some traditional problems about the nature of colour (and of sensory properties, more generally).

I. A Problem Concerning the Ontology of Colour

1. *Conflicting Intuitions Concerning Colour Ontology*

Colour appearances are highly variable with illumination, contrast, adaptation, and the perceiver's individual physiological constitution, much more so than philosophers have traditionally allowed. For example, *black* and *white* are contrast colours. The very same thing can look black when placed next to things much more reflective than it, and white when placed next to things that are much less so. (If X reflects 30 times as much light as Y, then X will look pure white and Y pure black when placed together in a black and white photograph: Y can be made to look pure white by placing it in a surround 30 times less reflective than it.) A relatively unappreciated consequence of this contrast phenomenon is that colours like *brown*, which have *black* as a component, and colours like the pastels, which contain *white*, are seen only when there is a contrast available. Thus, an object that looks brown when you look at it surrounded by certain other objects might look orange when you isolate it by looking at it through a reduction tube or surround it with darker objects that make it look less dark by contrast. Now, what colour is such an object, *really*? Is it brown because it looks that way in a *normal* multi-coloured scene (however 'normal' is to be understood)? Or is it orange because it looks that way when we remove the highly variable influence of contrast? Are we to discount its glowing appearance when it appears next to things much darker than it, and the black that is more often present in it turns to white?

There seems to be no principled way to decide in favour of one of these appearances. All of these viewing conditions have *some* claim to metaphysical privilege—the first because it marks a necessary condition for seeing anything as brown, the second because it removes the distraction of contrast, the third because there is no obvious reason to discount it as abnormal or misleading. Moreover, all are within the range of conditions that could be considered 'normal' in evolutionary terms. Thus, the variation in appearance seems nothing more than that. It seems that the best one can say is that the object is brown when the appropriate contrast is provided, orange when contrast is removed, and neither colour independently of viewing conditions. On this account, colour is 'response-dependent', or even 'subjective', in the sense that it is the product of an interaction between a perceiver and the distal environment, and cannot absolutely be attributed to things in that environment: it is, according to this view, a property that things have only relative to certain conditions of viewing, not a property they have in isolation.

Now, the idea that colour is 'response-dependent' sits uncomfortably with the approach taken in this book. We have been urging that colour and other sense-features are markers for the appropriateness of certain epistemic operations we perform with regard to distal stimuli. The point of these epistemic operations is to build up a stable record of the properties of these environmental objects, a record, that is, which does not fluctuate with ephemeral conditions. If colour is response-dependent, how can it be a part of this kind of stable record? Of course, the subjectivists have an answer to this question. They say that how something interacts with you in different circumstances *is* an enduring characteristic of that thing, even if it interacts with you differently in different kinds of circumstances. For example, somebody might be quiet and unassertive in certain kinds of circumstances, bold and commanding in others. This would not prevent you building up a record of what this individual is like. It is the same when an object looks one way in certain circumstances, another way in others. In this vein, colour could be held to be a disposition to present different appearances in different circumstances.

This defence of response-dependent theories of colour does not, however, fully square with the phenomenology of colour. Colour appearances are much more constant than one might expect given the variability of the light array that reaches the human eye. For example, human faces look normally coloured even under heavy leaf cover, even though the light they reflect in such circumstances shows distinctly green in colour photographs. Colour vision seems, then, to extract and separate the underlying determinants of colour appearance, and runs to *correct* and *standardize* the fluctuating appearances that things present in changing circumstances. This kind of constancy suggests to many philosophers, and to some colour scientists, that colour vision is about *real* properties of things, properties they have independently of any appearance. This would make colour 'objective', an absolute characterization of things. It implies that we cannot just leave the variability of colour appearance unresolved, as the subjectivist and the relativist would urge.

Which should we take more seriously, the variability of colour appearance or its constancy? Should we say that colour vision converges on certain invariant distal properties, and leave variation as an anomaly? Or should we say that colours are appearance-relative, and hold that our epistemic operations are based on enduring dispositions to present varying appearances in different circumstances? Should we dismiss constancy as a useful oddity—merely a byproduct of certain properties of colour-sensitive cells in the retina?

2. An Epistemological Constraint on Theories of Colour

This dilemma is sharpened by a recently articulated epistemological constraint on colour. Mark Johnston (1997/1992) phrases the constraint this way:

*Revelation The *intrinsic nature* of canary yellow is *fully revealed* by a standard visual experience as of a canary yellow thing (and the same goes, *mutatis mutandis*, for the other colours). (138)

What do we know solely in virtue of experiencing a colour? In accordance with the *Sensory Signalling Thesis* articulated in the previous chapter, a 'standard visual experience as of a canary yellow thing' is a signal that it is functionally appropriate to co-classify whatever we are seeeing along with other things that present a similar canary-yellow appearance. When a thing is assigned to this sensory class, the sensory system takes it to be epistemically equivalent to other things that look canary yellow—apt for the same inferences, generalizations, object-identifications, and so on.

Presumably, animals enjoy the same kinds of knowledge. They use colour in comparable ways without the aid of linguistic concepts—a honeybee identifies flowers by their colour, an old-world monkey identifies fruit, and so on. (See the criterion of perceptual grasp in Chapter 3, section VI, and the Meta-Response Schema of Chapter 6, section III.) Colour categorization is a primitive ability we share with these animals. Revelation would be plausible if we construed it as asserting that this kind of categorization is unlearned and unconditioned, or at least learned in predictable ways invariant across individual experience sets and across culture. Colour experience may or may not 'fully reveal' everything constitutive of colour but at the very least, it does give us the instinctive *know-how* that follows in the wake of colour categorization.

With this in mind, let us consider the following version of the condition stated by Johnston. This version of the condition invokes primary content only—that is, it alludes only to the epistemic action-priming content of colour vision.

Transparency A visual experiences as of a canary-yellow thing is

> (a) sufficient for knowing how to classify canary-yellow things for the purposes of inductive inference (etc.), and
> (b) sufficient together with experiences as of lime-green things to know how to differentiate canary-yellow things from lime-green things with respect to inductive inference, etc.

This form of Revelation must surely be true.

Imagine, then, that you have never experienced *canary yellow*. A colour scientist arranges for you to have this experience by artfully arranging for you to have an after-image of the opposed shade—he asks you to stare at a certain shade of blue for thirty seconds, and then to look at white paper, at which point you experience *canary yellow*—or, more diabolically, by electrically stimulating your brain in such a way as to produce in you a sudden flash of canary yellow, floating free of any object or shape. You do not form any belief about the external world because of this self-evidently ephemeral experience. You do not attribute the colour to any external thing. Properly understood, *Transparency* implies that even this experience is somehow sufficient to demonstrate what kinds of things are apt to be treated as outlined above.

The puzzling question: what kind of classification is this that its entire basis can be fully revealed by a mendacious experience? Moreover, how can such a classification be useful for externally validated practices such as object-identification and induction? This sharpens the conflict of intuitions noted earlier. If colour experience fails to correspond to an independently existing thing, then how will we reconcile Transparency with colour constancy, and with the instinctive belief that the senses put us in touch with objective properties of things? If, on the other hand, colour is objective, then how can it be so easy to know, in contrast to so many other objective categories, like mass or electrostatic charge?

3. *The Contrasting Case of Musical Harmony*
From what we have said so far, one might think that if Transparency poses a problem for colour, then it would pose a problem for other sense features as well. To an extent this is right. That is, it must be the case that if we participate in instinctive classificatory practices that involve these other qualities, these practices too must be appearance-based. Nevertheless, Transparency is more puzzling when applied to colour than, for instance, to musical harmony. The reason is surprising, and worth examining in a little detail.

Before we get to that, however, we need a preliminary observation to avoid confusion. With *any* sensory modality, the novice observer requires training in order to be sensitive to the character of her experience. That is, it takes practice (and possibly some instruction) to recognize the presence of yellow in lime green, the taste of raspberries in wine, the component structure of a musical chord, and so on. However, the need for this kind of 'training' does not compromise Transparency. True, one might not appreciate all that is present in an experience of canary yellow *immediately* upon having an experience as of it. One may need to be trained by an expert who exposes one to relevant contrasts, teaches one colour vocabulary, and so on. After one has been so trained one might become much better at discriminating, remembering, and naming colours than one had been before. Still, the single untrained experience may implicitly have contained everything needed to grasp the ways in which we classify things as canary yellow. By training the eye, the palate, or the ear, one does not come to have *new*, more complex experiences. Rather, one gains more reliable discriminatory capacities and sharper awareness of the components already present in the old experiences. Or so I shall assume for the sake of simplicity.

Now, we have seen that colour experience leaves us in doubt about the nature of colour properties. Are these properties tied to ephemeral responses that objects momentarily and relationally evoke in us, or are they signs of persistent and stable properties of objects? It seems that in the experience of musical harmonies there is less room for this kind of puzzlement: these experiences *do* 'reveal' something about the 'intrinsic nature' of musical harmonies.

Consider one's auditory experience of a minor third. After a period of ear training, one begins to recognize such things as the interval heard when the constituent tones of this chord are played in sequence, its relationship to other chords, the musical character of chord progressions in which it figures, and so on. Now, it turns out that what one cognizes in this way has a counterpart in objective reality. An ear-trained listener will find that her discriminations are confirmed by certain tests on a piano or other musical instrument; for instance, she will find that she hears a minor third just when one is played. If not, she is simply in the wrong. That is, something is wrong with a listener who has an auditory experience as of a minor third when we sound C and E together. Such a listener experiences a minor third when she hears the components of a major third. Her ear training (or just her ears) is shown to be deficient by her failing this objective test. From these facts, we may conclude that

(1) there is a structure to one's experiences of a chord, and
(2) this structure corresponds (perhaps imperfectly and incompletely) to objective structural characteristics of the chord itself.

The correspondence between the structure of one's auditory experience and the sound one hears goes some distance, at least, towards explaining the counterpart of Transparency for the auditory grasp of chords. It is legitimate to project certain structural characteristics of the auditory experience on to the distal stimulus.

However, this conjunction of conditions does not hold of colour experience. The difference between the two cases does not lie in condition (1) above. There is, as we saw in Chapter 4, section II and Chapter 6, section I, a structure in our experiences of colour, for these experiences order colours in the dimensions black-white, red-green, blue-yellow. The difference lies rather in (2): the experienced component structure of colour does not correspond to the intrinsic character of coloured objects and lights. For as we saw in Chapter 8, section I, the physical counterparts of colour experience do not share the component structure of colour experience—for instance, there is no physical counterpart of the opponency experienced between red and green, no counterpart of experienced colour components, and so on. Moreover, the experienced similarity of the colours is misleading as to the physical similarity of the stimuli which occasion colour experiences: the ends of the visible spectrum are experienced as more similar to each other than either to the middle, colour space is experienced as consisting of distinct regions rather than varying smoothly, and so on. The lack of match between experienced colour space and physical colour space is how colour differs from musical harmony: a chord *physically* contains its component notes; listeners can be right or wrong about what they hear in this respect. Thus, *there is no transfer, as in the case of music, from the structure of colour reality to the structure of colour experience.*

We can now say what is especially puzzling about Transparency. Sensory categories, including colour, underwrite induction and other epistemic practices. In order to be useful in these epistemic roles, one would think that they must correspond in some way to objective characteristics. It seems to follow that colour experiences must correspond, somehow, to objective colours. But, on the face of it, they do not, at least not in any obvious way. It is unclear how colour gives us knowledge about real things and their properties.

II. Two Approaches to Defining the Colours

1. *Defining Colour Looks*

We now introduce the convenient notion of a *colour-look*. Recall first that colours can be arranged in a multidimensional psychological similarity-space by systematically collating the similarity and discrimination judgements of observers presented with colour samples (Chapter 4, section II). Colour-looks can be identified with minimal regions in this similarity-space, that is, regions so small that the colours they contain are all *indiscriminable* from one another. (This is a simplification, I repeat: see Chapter I, section I.) Thus:

> Stimulus x presents observer O with colour-look $\mathscr{L}$ at t if and only if x occupies region $\mathscr{L}$ in O's colour similarity-space at t.

Colour-looks are how objects are subjectively experienced by observers, and derive from these observers' abilities to match and discriminate objects with respect to colour. Because they are subjectively determined, these looks are transparent to the perceiver. As we shall see in a moment, philosophers, especially empiricists, standardly define *colour-attributions* in terms of *colour-looks*. They suppose that that this ensures Transparency: if we define colours in terms of colour-looks, we gain some hope of piggybacking our knowledge of colour on our knowledge of colour-looks. This supposition is another reason these philosophers embrace a subjectivist view of colour.

There is, however, an obvious difficulty in basing colour-attribution on colour-looks. The look that a particular object presents to an observer varies with viewing conditions, while colour seems to be an enduring and non-relational feature of objects. So unless we are simply going to give up all hope of making sense of our instinctive attributions of enduring colours to objects, we need some device to construct stable and enduring colour properties out of colour-looks.

Philosophers tend to approach this problem by relativizing colour-looks to various viewing conditions. Let us suppose that the following statement is *fully specified* in this respect:

> Stimulus x presents colour-look $\mathscr{L}$ to observer O when x is illuminated by light of spectral distribution S of luminance L, with surround colours C_1–C_n, when O is adapted to light of spectral distribution S' and x is displaced from the centre of O's retina by $\theta°$.

Fully specified colour-looks are invariable because all the relevant variables are fixed. The thought is that we can use an appropriately chosen fully specified colour-look in our definition of object-colour. Now, there is a proposal (Jackson and Pargetter 1987; Cohen 2000 and 2003*b*; McLaughlin 2003*a* and *b*) that simply identifies colours with fully specified colour-looks. Briefly:

> **Colour Relativism*
> x **is** *Col* (where *Col* is a colour term) to observer O in circumstances C if and only if x **looks** *Col* to observer O in circumstances C. (Note here that the expression 'looks *Col*' alludes to a colour-look by means of the same colour term as is used on the left side of 'if and only if'.)

Or more fully:

> x **is** *Col* to observer O when x is illuminated by light of spectral distribution S of luminance L, with surround colours C_1–C_n, when O is

adapted to light of spectral distribution S' and x is displaced from the centre of O's retina by $\theta°$

if and only if

x **looks** *Col* to observer O when x is illuminated by light of spectral distribution S of luminance L, with surround colours C_I–C_n, when O is adapted to light of spectral distribution S' and x is displaced from the centre of O's retina by $\theta°$.

The authors of this relativizing proposal claim to be objectivists—they argue that they have relativized colour—made it relative to the circumstances in which it is observed—while leaving it objective.

Now, it is certainly right to say that a fully specified colour-look is an objective fact. But it is strange to appeal to this highly ephemeral fact to support objectivism with respect to colour: any form of objectivism that comes at so small an epistemic cost ought to make one suspicious. There is no question of transcendence or error here—what you see is what you get when you get it. It is odd to call this *colour* objectivism; it is at best colour-*look* objectivism. A deeper problem with the relativizing proposal is that it confuses a signal with the fact signalled. Colour experience is a signal the system issues when it has determined that something is of a certain colour. What does this underlying determination signify? This is the issue that the relativizers simply evade. They stick with the look as constitutive of colour itself.

Now, with the exception of the relativizing proposal, no *other* proposal based on colour-looks helps us with our problem of how we come to know colour—the problem posed by Transparency. The problem with all the others is that colour experience does not, in general, tell us how to choose among fully specified colour-looks. Consider the appeal to 'standard observers' and 'standard conditions' to provide the needed specifications, as in the following principles of colour-attribution.

> *Dispositional Principle of Colour Attribution
> 'x is *Col*' is true if and only if x has the disposition to look *Col* to a standard observer in standard conditions.

> *Counterfactual Principle of Colour Attribution
> 'x is *Col*' is true if and only if x would look *Col* to a standard observer in standard conditions.

These principles become fully specified by providing details of standard observers and standard conditions. Such a specification might go something like this. A standard observer is one who has non-anomalous trichromatic vision—that is, the observer must possess three cone types in the 'standard' proportions, with their peak sensitivity frequencies at the 'standard' wavelengths. This observer must be white-light adapted, and fixating x in the centre of her retina. x must be presented to such a viewer in a surround of neutral grey, illuminated by white light to luminance 10 millilumens. The problem with this specification is obvious: even if the viewer knows, by visual experience, what the colour-look mentioned in the above attribution-principles is, she has no perceptual grasp (see Chapter 3, section VI) of these 'standard conditions'. (There are many other problems with specifying standard observers and standard conditions, as Hardin 1988, 67–82, has painstakingly detailed.)

Think again of the shimmering canary-yellow film floating in the air. Transparency implies that this ephemeral experience is enough to reveal the primary content of a canary-yellow experience. However, this visual experience contains *no* information about standard viewers and conditions, *no* means of determining to whom and in what circumstances a thing must look like this if it is to be canary yellow. Indeed, your experience of the film does not contain any allusion to viewing conditions at all: we just do not know how the film would look in 'standard conditions' or what standard conditions are for it. The advantage of appealing to colour-looks was thought to be that experience gives us direct knowledge of them. This advantage is negated when this appeal is relative to viewing conditions other than those present to the viewer.

2. *Introducing the 'Semantic' Account*

Colour-looks seem to give us direct knowledge of colour-classes or colour-properties, but we are finding it difficult to understand how this can be so, given the failure of the standard viewing conditions approach to defining colour-properties. At the risk of repetition, let us summarize the difficulty. The colour-look that an object presents varies with conditions of viewing. While colour constancy is an indication that the system is capable of compensating for this variability to some extent, there is still a range of circumstances, all 'normal' in evolutionary terms, in which the same object will present a different look. Thus, despite constancy, colour-looks do not vary one-to-one with any object-property. The standard-conditions approach seeks to negate variability by focusing on the conditions under which a colour-look reliably indicates what colour-property an object has. However, since the colour-vision system does not automatically signal whether or when it is operating within this range of conditions, the perceiver requires empirical knowledge to grasp and apply this definition of colour-properties. This is the problem. If one wants to preserve the instinctive grasp of colour implied by Transparency, one needs a connection between colour-looks and colour-properties that demands less empirical knowledge.

Luckily, there *is* a relation between colour-looks and colour-properties available to help us. Suppose that somebody shows you a coloured object, and asks you what colour-property it visually *appears* to have. You need no collateral information about viewing conditions in order to answer this question. You need such information only in order to know what colour something *is*, not to know what colour it *looks*.

Consider the following propositions:

(3) *x* presents a red look. (Or more simply: *x* looks red.)
(4) *x* is red.

Now, it is clear that (3) does not imply (4). For it makes perfectly good sense to suppose that something that is not red could present a red look. On the other hand, it seems obvious that there is some logical connection between (3) and (4). Subjectivists think that one can cash out this logical connection by defining a colour property in terms of reliable indications of when a thing actually possesses that property. The problem that we have noted is that this goes beyond our perceptual grasp of *red*: we lack the information needed to assess when looks are reliable. The theory presented in the previous chapter is more promising. Let us suppose that the red-look is a signal, in accordance with internally established system of conventions or rules, of the occurrence of *red*. This would account for the direct knowledge that we seem to possess of what colour-property a thing looks when it presents a given colour-look.

These considerations suggest the following schema:

Look Exportation
Col is the colour-property something visually appears to have when it looks *Col*.

It must be emphasized that in the above schema, 'looks' does not betoken a tendency to believe. (There is a difference between saying '*x* looks canary yellow' and '*x* looks as if it *is* canary yellow'. The former does not imply any tendency to believe that *x* is canary yellow; the latter does.) That is, Look Exportation does not say what would clearly be false: that canary yellow is the colour you automatically attribute to *x* when *x* presents you with the canary-yellow-look. All that Look Exportation says is that you instinctively know the meaning of the internal signal. Thus construed, it is a consequence of Transparency.

An analogy with linguistic communication is helpful in understanding Look Exportation. Suppose somebody says to you, 'I make one hundred thousand dollars a year.' It takes quite a lot of empirical knowledge to figure out whether this statement is a reliable indication of the speaker's income. Moreover, determining the likelihood of the speaker's truthfulness depends on divining the context. Is she negotiating a salary offer? Is she negotiating a divorce? However, it takes only *semantic* knowledge, and no knowledge of either background or present conditions to determine what the speaker is telling you. The semantic link between utterance and meaning bypasses the evidentary link between an utterance and the real state of the world.

The connection between colour-looks and visual appearance is just like this. We said earlier that when we undergo a colour-experience, we may not know what colour the thing presenting that experience is, but we do know instinctively what colour classifications the experience conveys. Look Exportation is a consequence of this instinctive link. The fact that somebody can teach you the meaning of a colour simply by producing an after-image or by stimulating your brain shows that we have an instinctive grasp of Look Exportation.

Look Exportation gives us a quite direct way of defining what it is for something to be canary yellow. A thing is not canary yellow merely because it presents a canary-yellow look. Something is canary yellow if it *really is* the way such a thing looks. This gives us:

> *Fundamental Principle of Colour Attribution*
> 'x is *Col*' is true if and only if x really is the colour something visually appears to be when it presents the *Col*-look.

The Fundamental Principle introduces a 'Really is the way it looks' operator. This operator takes colour-looks as arguments, and yields colour-attribution conditions as values. Its logical force is different from the 'would look that way in standard conditions' approach considered earlier, which requires that we know how something would look in specified or standardized conditions. It is a look-to-property operator, while the 'would look' operator goes from looks to looks.

The Fundamental Principle of Colour Attribution parallels the Disquotation Principle enunciated by Alfred Tarksi (1944). Tarski observed that the removal of the quotation marks from 'snow is white' gives us a way of asserting what would be the case if 'snow is white' were true. This observation led him to his famous principle:

> The sentence 'snow is white' is true if, and only if, snow is white (343).

Tarski's Disquotation Principle takes advantage of our semantic grasp of the sentence 'snow is white' to convey the truth conditions of this sentence. In much the same way, the Fundamental Principle of Colour Attribution takes advantage of our perceptual grasp of colour-looks to specify the colour-property that this look presents. Tarski entitles his conception 'the semantic conception of truth', explaining that

> Semantics is a discipline which, speaking loosely, deals with certain relations between expressions of a language and the objects (or 'states of affairs') 'referred to' by those expressions. As typical examples of semantic concepts we may mention the concepts of designation, satisfaction, definition. (ibid., 345)

Following him, we say that colour-looks designate colour-properties, and entitle this conception the 'semantic' account of colour.

The semantic account points to a very different way of thinking about colour-attribution than that which is implicit in the 'standard conditions' approach, which looks for conditions in which colour-looks are especially reliable or in some other way privileged. This difference is analogous to that between an epistemic theory of truth, like Epicurus's, and a semantic theory of truth, like Tarski's. Epicurus proposed that 'true opinions are those attested and uncontested by self-evidence.' He meant this as a 'criterion', a theory that (a) tells us how to test an opinion for truth-value, and (b) defines the truth of an opinion in terms of a positive test outcome. Tarski's theory does not aspire to give us this kind of 'criterion'; it simply identifies the fact that would make the sentence true without telling us how to determine whether that fact obtains. In exactly the same way, the standard-conditions approach to colour-attribution attempts to tell us how to test a colour-look for truth-value. The Fundamental Principle does not do this: instead, it reorients our attitude towards the look-property relation away from epistemic criteria, emphasizing instead the signal-properties of colour-looks.

The 'semantic conception of colour' implicit in the Fundamental Principle is insufficient by itself actually to provide us with a philosophical account of the look-property relation. All it does, as we have seen, is take advantage of our instinctively implicit knowledge of colour-attribution. In order more fully to understand the relationship between colour-looks and colour-properties, we need to undertake two further tasks. We must

> First: explicate the nature of the semantic relationship between colour-looks and colour properties.

and

> Second: give a more explicit account of which property each colour-look designates; in other words, make our implicit knowledge of colour-attribution more explicit.

Given the demands of Transparency, we need to do this in a way that excludes collaterally acquired knowledge.

III. How Colour-Looks Function as Symbols

1. *Property-Designation in Measuring Instruments*

Fred Dretske (1994) offers us a metaphor that proves useful in explaining the semantic character of the connection between colour-looks and colour-properties. He likens sensory systems to measuring instruments. Every measuring instrument is associated with a measurement function, m, which connects its measuring states—its pointer readings, for instance—to measurement values, properties of the object being measured. Sensory systems seem to be similar: the colour-vision system has states that seem, as we saw in the last section, to designate colour-properties. Transparency implies that we are instinctively able to use the measurement function associated with sensory systems.

How are we able to use the measurement function of measuring instruments? How do we know (a) what state the instrument is in, and (b) what property corresponds to that state?

(a) *Identifying the measuring state* Measuring instruments are designed in such a way as to enable us easily to identify their measuring-states: for instance, they might have needles that point to markings on their faces or some other type of display. Each position of the needle marks a different measuring state. Imagine a pressure gauge that has lost its needle. Such a gauge too has measuring states, but these are now impossible to read. We are in the same position with regard to this gauge as an effector system is with regard to a perceptual system when the latter registers a particular state of affairs but *fails to signal it*. A read-out display is needed.

(b) *Knowing the measurement value of each measuring state* In order to use a measuring instrument, we need access to a key that tells us how to specify the values of various measuring states. Often, we can read a linguistic expression of the object property off a *transparent* notation expressed by the gauge-display. For instance, we might find numerical expressions like '14' written on a pressure gauge, with a notation 'pounds per square inch' written across the bottom. When the needle points to '14', the notation on the dial enables us to express the object property as 'fourteen pounds per square inch'. (A notation in newtons per square metre would express the same property but in a different language.) Notations that are more opaque are also possible. A graphic notation would be an example. A square might indicate 14 psi, but you would need to consult a look-up table to discover this. When such a key is provided, whether transparent or not, we say that the instrument is calibrated.

The relationship between measuring states and object-properties, i.e. the measurement function, is semantic in exactly the same sense as demonstrated in the case of colour-vision in the last section. That is, given that the instrument is in a particular state, the thing it is measuring appears, as far as the instrument goes, a certain way. The calibrated notation on the face of the gauge gives us a way of expressing this property. This connection persists even when a particular instrument is broken, out of range, or improperly connected. Even when the gauge ceases to be a reliable indicator, it is still clear what *description* it yields—what it 'says' may be wrong in these circumstances, but it is still clear what it is saying.

In the transparently notated gauge, we get to say that the atmosphere is at 14 psi by recognizing that the instrument is in the '14'-pointing state. This is an epistemic connection, not a constitutive one: it is not that the atmosphere is at 14 psi because the gauge is in the '14'-pointing state; rather, the fact that the gauge is in this state gives us a defeasible reason for thinking so. Even when the instrument is malfunctioning, the atmosphere continues to be at 14 psi, whatever the gauge might indicate. Thus, it makes perfectly good sense to allow that the atmosphere *might not really be as the gauge indicates*. In this sense, the state measured by an instrument transcends the state of the instrument itself. This is the crucial feature of Dretske's metaphor, and central to understanding the case of colour. It shows why it is not trivial to say, as we do in the Fundamental Principle, that something *really is* as the machine says it is when the machine is in state such-and-such. This recognizes that there is more to the atmosphere being at 14 psi than an instrument indicating that it is so. We must not confuse the machine-state, or the pointer-reading, with what is being measured.

The parallels between the measuring instrument and our sensory systems ought to help us understand the semantic character of sensory states. However, there is a problem here. Apparently, our sensory systems do not come marked in a convenient notation that we can use to describe the world: 'this is not a courtesy that nature extends to us', Dretske says (1994, 47). So how are we to concoct a notation that gives us a way of expressing their measurement functions? This is the problem Dretske tries to address when he asks us to imagine what would happen if we are given an instrument, as before, but find that 'there is nothing there (or the numbers are no longer legible) to tell a curious onlooker what the pointer positions mean.' This approximates the task of someone trying to discover what his own sensory systems measure. Dretske says (ibid., 48) 'if we know the instrument was working properly, we can find out what the pointer's present position means simply by finding out what the pressure is.' In other words, if the markings needed to translate a gauge-state into a description of the world are absent, we recalibrate the instrument. If the unmarked instrument is connected to the atmosphere, and we find that the atmospheric pressure is 14 psi, then we can paint '14 psi' on the face of the gauge right where the pointer is.

The idea of recalibrating the gauge is disarmingly simple. But it demands that collateral knowledge be available to the pressure gauge user, and puts her under too heavy an epistemic load. How is the user to determine the pressure of the atmosphere in pounds per square inch simply by looking at states of an unmarked pressure gauge? How is she even to know that it denotes *pressure*? Yet, that, by analogy, is what the naïve perceiver is trying to do with regard to his own sensory systems. A philosopher who represents the naïve perceiver's sensory concepts in scientific notation exceeds the epistemic capabilities we can expect of unaided perception. Similarly, 'physicalist' specifications of colour-properties, in terms of reflectance etc., fail properly to capture the content of colour vision as it presents itself to the naïve observer, to an animal, young child, or adult untutored in physics. Such specifications may capture the *secondary* content of colour vision, but not its transparent primary content.

2. *Auto-calibration*

Consider now an approach to calibration epistemically less committed than Dretske's. Suppose that we paint arbitrary symbols on the blank face of the gauge— 'A', 'B', 'C', etc. Each such mark helps us identify a measuring state of the gauge. Now, by analogy with the 'transparent' gauge markings described in the last section, we can simply use the marks we have painted to express object-properties. Where before we said 'The air is 14 psi' when the instrument is connected to the air and the needle pointed to '14', now we say 'The air is A' when it points to 'A', or 'The tyre is B' when it points to 'B'. (Notice that 'A' and 'B' could have been switched. The notation is conventional.) These marks give us a way of identifying and reidentifying the instrument's measuring-states, and at the same time, a way of describing objects connected to the instrument. The marks on the instrument are used to designate object-properties, and to compare objects used at different times. They constitute what we may call an auto-calibrated system of signs. In such a system, easily accessible marks of an instrument's measuring state are used to generate descriptions of the things that the instrument measures. It is an implicit assumption of such a system that the instrument does measure things external to itself. This assumption could be mistaken, but it is testable—if it causes problems, it can be abandoned.

The insertion of conventional auto-calibrated signs give a user of the illegible gauge a way of describing the world. And just as before, the properties described by these signs transcend the gauge-states themselves. It still makes sense to say, in general, that the gauge could be wrong. Suppose the needle points to 'A'. Then the gauge indicates that the thing being measured is A. Suppose that the user gives the gauge a sharp tap, and finds that it goes to 'B'. Now the user has evidence that the earlier reading was in error. Thus, when the needle points to 'A', the user has only defeasible evidence that the measured object is A. This evidence does not compel him to describe it in that way. When he does in fact do so, he is endorsing what the gauge says. So we could say:

> The air is A if it really is as the instrument makes it appear when it points to 'A'.

This would be analogous to the observation on which the Fundamental Principle of Colour Attribution rests: something has a particular colour-property if it really is the way it looks when it looks that colour.

In order fully to understand an auto-calibrated sign, we need an explication of what it designates. Now, there is a very simple way that such signs can acquire meaning. Imagine a naïve person using the auto-calibrated pressure gauge for various everyday purposes, for example, for checking tyre and balloon pressures and the like. The marks on the face of the gauge allow her to identify and compare readings on different occasions of the instrument's use. Thus, they furnish her with signs that she can use in generalizations. For example: 'When the bicycle tyre is pumped up only to A on the gauge face, it goes bump when you ride over a kerb, but when you pump it up to B, kerbs are no problem.' Or, in our auto-calibrated notation: 'A tyre at A will go bump, but a tyre at B will not.' These inductive generalizations are based on co-classifications—the gauge-user co-classifies things by means of the values of gauge markings registered by such objects, and uses such classifications as the basis for future induction. The suggestion is that auto-calibrated signs can acquire meaning by being associated with such a taxonomy. With respect to these signs, *meaning* consists, as Wittgenstein insisted, in *use*. (Note that if all such inductions fail, one might conclude that the instrument was not actually measuring the properties of the things to which it is connected. This would be strong evidence for a 'subjectivist' reading of the instrument's states. Similarly, if induction with respect to colour-properties was always unreliable, we would be right to conclude that colour vision measures nothing but the state of the perceiver.)

3. *Colour-looks as Auto-calibrated Signs*

The thesis is that colour-looks (and, more generally, sensory experiences) are auto-calibrated signs. Just as the marks painted on the dial allow us to identify measuring-states of the gauge, so colour-looks have the function of serving as easily accessible marks by which states of the colour-vision system can be identified. Like the 'A' on the dial, they also yield a conventional notation for the things that this system 'measures'. When a perceiver S looks at a wooden tabletop, she is in visual state B. In virtue of being in this visual state B the thing that S has in view looks a certain colour, say *brown*. S uses this colour-look, her own measuring state, to designate an object-property of the object at which she is looking. In this sense, the designator is categorical. It makes no explicit reference to anything other than the object to which colour is attributed. Though the use that S instinctively makes of B is a contributor to the meaning of this state, this action-category is buried in S's use of the look.

What is the property designated by a colour-look? In addressing this question we have appealed, in Chapter 9 and at the end of the previous subsection, to the uses to which we instinctively put colour-information. What we have just encountered is an account of how we use colour-looks as analogous to the meaningful terms by which we designate properties. Earlier, we found Dretske making the claim that our sensory systems do not come marked with a convenient notation which we can use to describe the objects they measure—'this is not a courtesy that nature extends to us', he said. We see now that this is wrong. Colour-looks are auto-calibrated, and thus they *are* associated with a transparent system. There was no need for Nature to be more courteous than this.

IV. Colour-Properties

1. *Task-oriented Taxonomies*

It is one thing to say that the signs that a sensory system uses are categorical. It is another thing to say that they are grasped without reference to other things. Our account of the semantics of colour-experiences vindicates the categorical character of colour-experiences: they are simply auto-calibrated marks applied to stimuli by virtue of the *Fundamental Principle*. But this is quite compatible with the suggestion that we might endow these signs with meaning by means of the uses to which we put them.

This is how the teleosemantic theory of the previous chapter should be understood. Colour-visual states get their meaning from their genetically or developmentally specified uses. Here is an example. An association *base* is a class of things which, because they share some feature, are expected to be similar in other ways—thus, when one member of an association base is observed to have property *F*, this affects the subjective probability of other members of the association base having *F*. Colour-vision constructs association bases using colour-looks. Two things *share* a colour-property if they are assigned, because of colour-looks, to association bases within which objects are expected to have further features in common. They are different with respect to a colour-property if colour-vision assigns them to different association bases corresponding to different expectations. Colour-categories form equivalence groupings not only for association, but also for the other epistemic practices listed above. Things of the same colour might tend to be assigned to the same figure against a ground of a different colour. One uses colour when one is trying to decide which of several Hondas in the parking lot is one's own—it can only be so if it belongs to the same colour-equivalence class. And so on. (Remember, though, that we are presented with a sensory ordering, not a field of discrete sense-features: talk of equivalence classes is a simplification. This sensory ordering is constructed from *degrees* of association.)

Following Principles of Sensory Equivalence (1) and (3) in Chapter 9, section III, we offer, thus, the following definitions:

> *x* and *y* resemble each other in colour if there is a colour-based epistemic practice *E* such that the colour-looks presented by *x* and *y* signal that *x* and *y* are to be treated as equivalent with regard to *E*.

x and *y* are *exactly* the same colour, if *x* and *y* are to be treated as equivalent for all colour-based epistemic practices.

Consider, then, a case like this. In the supermarket, a particular mango looks reddish-orange. I infer that it is ripe. I take it home, and it looks more yellowy-green than it had before. It turns out not to be ripe. I conclude that in the supermarket it looked different from the way it really was. My assumption here is that though the mango presented different colour-looks in different conditions, it retained the same enduring colour-property. And I might well conclude that in the supermarket, my senses told me something false: they assigned the mango to a category—the category I use for ripeness-inferences in mangoes—to which it did not in fact belong. In the supermarket, I attributed to the mango the colour-property designated by the look it presented there. At home, I came to realize that I was wrong to do so. At home, I realized that it *really had*—remember the Fundamental Principle of Colour Attribution—the property designated by the yellowish-greenish look it presents here, not the property designated by the reddish-look it presented in the supermarket.

What then does our grasp of canary-yellow consist in? It is

> *first*, that there is a region of colour space—the canary-yellow region—within which each minimal region designates a colour-property, and that canary-yellow is the union of all of these properties, and

> *second*, that the colour-vision system instinctively groups things with this property together and treats them as similar for *some* colour-based epistemic practices.

What is it to grasp a different colour, say *lime-green*? That *lime-green* has a look defined in the same fashion as above, but that lime-green things are not equivalent to canary-yellow things with respect to at least some of the tasks mentioned above. (There could be, of course, a broader colour category that includes both as subcategories, but this broader category would be distinct from both *canary-yellow* and *lime-green*.)

The proposal is that we should construe the meaning of colour-looks by reference to the equivalence classes defined by instinctive use. What do colour-attributions say about external things? Many philosophical theories of colour seek for the answer to this question by considering the *information* carried by colour-looks. These theories concentrate on world-to-sensory-system links, in the hope that an adequate account of these will tell us what we can infer about the condition of the world from the states of our colour-vision system. However, because such inferences generally depend on information about distal conditions that is not available in colour experience alone, they end up offending against what Boghossian and Velleman call the 'naïveté of vision'. The suggestion being made here is that sensory systems organize the information they get from the world in classes and categories designed for the *down*stream connections between sensory-system states and the actions to which they are linked. We know these connections implicitly and instinctively: we do not gather things together by learning and reasoning, but unreflectively. Consequently, we know implicitly what our colour-attributions mean.

The task-oriented conception of colour captures the intent of *Transparency* in section I.2 above. Since colour-properties are identified by colour-looks, it only takes experience 'as of a canary-yellow thing' *plus the task-oriented knowledge instinctively implicit in colour vision* to know the conditions under which two things are to be co-classified for purposes such as those mentioned above, and only this experience together with one as of a lime-green thing to know when canary-yellow things must be differentiated from lime-green things for those purposes.

2. *The Superficiality of Colour*

We are now ready to revisit the difference between musical harmony and colour. Why is there information transfer from reality to experience in the case of harmony, but not in the case of colour? The crucial point is the difference in what we may call the 'ergonomic significance' of the two modalities. We have been arguing that in order properly to understand the significance of colour experiences, one needs to consider what one does with them as a matter of instinct. The same is true for other sense experiences. The difference between harmony (as well as speech) and colour is that one of things that we do with harmony is manipulate our own voices to produce harmonies, but we do not know by instinct how physically to manipulate colour.

Like phonetic perception, the significance of musical perception is probably derived from the way that we *produce* musical sounds. A string produces sound by vibrating; if it is pegged at both ends, its amplitude will be zero at each end and maximal in the middle, and it will approximate a wave of length equal to the distance between the pegs. Since the heard pitch of a sound depends on its wavelength, the primary tone that a pegged string produces will depend on its length (among many other factors). Now, the main constraint on the vibration of a pegged string is that the amplitude must be zero at the pegs; all sorts of vibrations are possible in between, provided they are consistent with the tensile strength and elasticity of the string. Thus strings produce subsidiary waves; the string will vibrate as a whole with the maximum amplitude at its mid-point, as described above, but it will also vibrate, at the same time, like two pegged strings with a zero point in the middle, and like three such strings, with two zero points evenly spaced along its length, and so on. The lengths of these subsidiary waves, or overtones, will be in whole number ratios to the primary wave; generally speaking, the smaller the whole number, the more prominent the overtone. The human voice produces sound by driving columns of air; these columns behave somewhat like pegged strings. This accounts for the timbre of the human voice: the musical sounds it produces are not pure, but a mixture of waves in (small) whole number ratios.

Now, when we sing a note, and at the same time, somebody else sings a note that stands to ours in a whole number ratio, the second person's sound resonates with and reinforces an overtone in our own voice. This phenomenon gives us pleasure, and is at the centre of our appreciation of harmonies. Consequently, one of the ways in which humans can give one another pleasure is by singing together in the Pythagorean ratios. Because this is so, musical expression depends not only on the capacity to hear these ratios in a particular way, but also on that of adjusting one's own voice in such a way that it harmonizes with that of another. These two things are closely linked. The auditory experience of musical harmonies is generally associated with the innate ability to adjust one's own sound production to conform to external constraints. Since this is so, there is some sort of connection between how we produce and adjust musical harmonies and how we perceive them. This would explain why there is a transfer of structure from waveforms to auditory experiences.

Colour experience is completely different in this respect. The causal connections here are outside-in, but not inside-out; the experience of colour gives us information that enables us to undertake epistemic activities concerning external things, but it is not innately associated with the ability to produce or adjust the colour values of the things one sees. This is not because colour experience is, as it were, 'purely descriptive', and lacks all significance for action. It is, as we have seen, significant for epistemic actions. However, epistemic actions take place 'inside the head'. If colour experience is useful for influencing the world, it is so only by the intermediary of acquired generalizations. An artist can reproduce her colour experiences in paint. But she has to go to Art School to learn enough about paints to do so. When we identify the external properties correlated with the experience of colour, we go beyond untutored vision, reconstructing the external reality of colour with the help of information additional to that which is available in colour-experience alone. The reader might have supposed that this is a point that applies to all sensory experience. Not so. It applies only to those modalities, which, like colour, are associated primarily with epistemic, that is, internal, actions. Sense experience in modalities like musical audition and speech perception is associated with the ability to produce or influence external things, and hence they have tacitly to contain (at least some) information about those external things, information that goes beyond how these features are encoded in experience.

However, this does not dissolve the puzzle—it only tells us why there is no transfer from the structure of colour-appearance to the structure of colour-reality. We have noted that the similarity space of colours is different from the similarity space of external properties like wavelength and reflectance.

This implies that the similarity that we experience as between two colours does not guarantee real similarity. But induction and other epistemic practices are founded on similarity. Why does induction based on colour work if the similarity on which it is founded is not real?

We can partially address this puzzle by noting that in fact nature is sparing in the inductive inferences it attaches to colour. Suppose that as an extremely naïve individual in a brand new culture you sample a canary-yellow confection and find it pleasingly tart. If there is another confection of the same colour on the same tray, you might well choose it, expecting that it too will be pleasingly tart in taste. Later in the day, you are served a dish of rice that closely resembles the confection in colour. Do you have any tendency at all to assume that the rice dish will be pleasingly tart? Not usually. This reflects the conservatism of colour-based inductions in nature. Birds identify edible fruit by colour, but they do not extend the edibility inference to other things, for instance to houses or hoardings painted the same colour, or even to fruit of different shape and size. If they did, they would waste a lot of time and perhaps get sick a lot.

Generally speaking, then, colour is a last differentia. We tend not to make inferences of the form: 'This *Col* thing is F, so all *Col* things are F.' Rather we make inferences of the form: 'This Col thing of kind K is F, so all Col things of kind K are F.' In other words, it is only within specific kinds that we will allow colour to ground inductive generalizations. Within such kinds, colour reliably matches up with underlying unobservable properties; across such kinds, it does not. If we were to make general inferences based on scarlet alone, it would be astounding if we came up with reliable results. But we do not, and this increases the chances that our generalizations will be correct. This defuses the puzzle.

Finally, then, how is it possible to know something about the properties of external things through experience alone, as *Transparency* requires? Our account demands that the similarity space of colour be tied to similarity of response with regard to instinctive, non-optional operations such as priming, habituation, and association. More explicitly, two things are similar in colour to the extent that they are treated similarly with regard to the sub-personal operations into which colour processing feeds. Now, colour similarity is at least partially determined by the utility that flows from these sub-personal operations: in other words, two colour-properties will tend to be close together in the colour-similarity space of a given kind of organism, O, if, given O's style of life, it is useful for O to treat these colour-properties similarly. Generally speaking, physical similarity and receptors shared with other organisms will also be a constraint on such similarity spaces, but the latter factors are not sufficient to account for O's classification scheme, either singly or jointly. In short, the colour classification schemes used by biological organisms correspond to some extent to the external boundary conditions that governed how their epistemic action-relevant categories were constructed.

Colour *experience* reflects the shape of colour-similarity space because its function is to be an internally available designator of this space. That two things *seem* the same is a sign that they are being treated similarly, a sub-personal action validated by evolution. This is why even a mendacious experience of a colour, of *canary yellow* for example, is sufficient to reveal something about the external world. Now, it is true that we and other animals may construct post-perceptual categories, categories for the purposes of learned or acculturated epistemic or other purposes. Such groupings are for acquired, personal, and optional operations such as aesthetic appreciation or induction. Why does the external utility of sub-personal operations transfer to these? Here, the superficiality of colour is key: the similarity space of sub-personal operations is used simply as an index of colour-related properties. Precisely because colour is superficial, this index can be used for many different purposes. Since the utility of sub-personal colour categories does not depend on their structural correspondence to physical colours, these categories are transferable to other uses that similarly do not depend on physical correspondence.

PART FIVE

Reference

12

Visual Objects

Parts I—IV of this book were concerned with sensory *classification*, the subsumption of perceptual stimuli under classes for what we termed 'epistemic' purposes. This is the *descriptive* aspect of perception. It is the focus of most empiricist conceptions. The defining characteristics of descriptive perception are that

(1) it involves *classification* in terms of categories that can be applied to a plurality of objects—much like *general terms* in language, and
(2) it makes us aware of affordances with regard to epistemic operations like induction, object recognition, and object comparison, and
(3) it is consciously presented and recorded in memory in a way that makes it possible to recall the experience to consciousness.

Descriptive perception is organized within a spatial structure. In the case of vision, features are presented as *contained*—they do not occur diffusely. Thus, a visual presentation of *blue* has a definite size: generally, it does not occupy the whole of your visual field. Because this is so, any such feature is seen as located relative to other visual features. Suppose that you visually experience *round* and *blue* at the same time. These two descriptive percepts must be experienced as standing in some spatial relation with respect to one another. Vision takes, Austen Clark (2000, 75) has argued (acknowledging P. F. Strawson as the source of his terminology), a *feature-placing* form of sensation. In virtue of their connectedness, visual features are organized and arrayed within a spatio-temporal matrix or 'manifold': they have spatial position and temporal order.

It is widely held that the spatial structure of vision helps us see *things*. A particular occurrence of *blue*, in *that* place *now*, is part of an individual that we might identify by tracing the boundary of this occurrence of *blue*, or, more generally, by distinguishing figure from ground. Thus, one might think that while feature detection enables us to *describe* stimuli; the spatial structure of vision is bound up with the ability to *refer* to individual objects. Clark and John Campbell (2002) both suggest that spatial locations are (in different ways) the ultimate referential indices in vision, that the bearers of sense-features are identified by these spatial locations. Part V, which is an investigation of visual reference, reverses their order of priority: it concludes that material objects, not locations, are the first referents of conscious visual states.

Taken as whole, Part V is a defence of the claim made in Chapter 1 that consciously available sensory states classify distal stimuli—they do not, as we shall see, simply place features in spatial locations.

I. Visual Places

Vision represents space three-dimensionally. A dog is seen *behind* a picket fence: we do not see pickets with dog-slices interlaced; rather we see a single dog behind the fence, partially occluded by it. This is how it appears to us visually: we instinctively expect the head to bark when we twist the tail. This simple observation is sufficient to refute the notion of a two-dimensional 'visual field', which used to have considerable currency among both psychologists and philosophers largely because it was thought necessary to posit a retinotopic field—the counterpart in consciousness of the two-dimensional image on the retina—as an epistemic intermediary between visual stimulus and visual percept. This notion, which is closely tied up with the idea that sense-data are the objects of vision, is now discredited, largely by visual experiments in the *Gestalt* tradition. As Austen Clark (2000) points out, it is impossible to code, within such a field, even so commonplace a visual phenomenon as that of a reflection in a window through which we see something outside.

Perhaps you see a green pine tree though the window and, overlapping it, a red reflection in the glass. How exactly do we describe this in a two-dimensional visual field? With three dimensions it is easy: the green appears at a different depth from the red. (100)

A compelling argument against the notion of a two-dimensional visual field, but Clark misses its full significance. What happens if the red happens to be at the *same* (virtual) depth as the pine tree? This is a case of incompatible features in a single three-dimensional location. How will we describe this in a *three*-dimensional visual field? We'll return to this further problem a bit later. For the moment, let us simply note that the representations of incompatible features in the same location have to be insulated from one another.

An additional problem for the traditional conception is that visual features are not presented as located in subjective coordinates: when we turn our heads or move our eyes, things are generally seen as stationary. Though objects acquire new positions in the retinotopic field, most stationary objects do not appear to move. Thus, though *some* of the feature maps referred to in Chapter 1, section VI may be retinotopically arranged—those in the primary visual cortex, for instance—conscious vision places features in objects that appear to reside in three-dimensional space, not in a two-dimensional egocentric projection thereof.

How are the locations of things presented to us in sensory awareness? This is the question Clark asks in his highly original treatment. Do we become aware of sensory locations through special spatial qualia, much as we become aware of sense-features through descriptive qualia? Clark does not think so. There are no qualia of location, he argues.

Not all of his reasons are persuasive.

Qualitatively the same A flat or red spot can be presented on the left side or the right. The timbre and pitch of the note need not change simply because one turns one's head. Similarly, red on the left need not differ qualitatively from red on the right. If it did, a split-field test could not show that the two stimuli present the same quality. Even as the apparent border between the two halves of the field vanished, one would have to say, 'No, they are not the same colour, since one has a definite leftish quality, and the other rightish.' (ibid., 58–9)

This seems to beg the question. Why should positional difference, qualitative or not, affect sameness in colour? Suppose that the left field were rough-textured and the right smooth. Would this force one to deny that they are the same colour? Obviously not. Clark says:

Whatever properties of sensation account for differences in apparent location, these properties of sensation are not among those counted when we consider the question of whether those two sensations are qualitatively identical. (ibid., 58)

It is hard to see why this is relevant: it seems to have no more force than saying 'Whatever properties of sensation account for differences in apparent texture, these are not among those that count towards sameness in colour.' Whether or not both of these stimuli have a 'definite leftish quality' has nothing to with whether they will be seen as possessing the same or different colours.

Nor is the non-qualitative character of spatial location proved by another characteristic of visual representations of space that Clark brings out. He claims that while visual sense-features like *burgundy* may sometimes fail to be instantiated in a scene, every distinct location *must* be instantiated in every scene. And this shows, he says, that there is a functional difference between visual locations and visual features. A nice argument, but is the premiss relevant? Perhaps it is true in some fashion that every possible visual location is present to the eye. It does not follow that one *sees* every location. It is true that there is a colour in every *direction* of the visual field. But it does not follow that every *location* is seen unless we take the visual field to be two-dimensional. Clark himself does not take it to be so: as we saw earlier, he thinks that vision represents space three dimensionally. It seems false that every *three-dimensional* place is always seen. One does not *see* empty locations: it is unclear even what it means to say that one does. Possibly, you see *that* there is nothing in between yourself and the wall, but what does it mean to say that you *see* every location between yourself and the wall.

Some visual locations house incompatible features, and are thus represented twice over; some are not represented at all. In these ways, at least, places seem to behave just like features. This said, one might concede some kind of difference. When one sees a filled location, it is because one sees some feature in it. Conversely, one fails to see empty locations precisely because they contain no feature to be seen. This seems to show that features and locations complement each other in vision: no location is seen without a feature in it; no feature is seen except in a location. This in itself shows that there must be some difference in the way features and locations function in vision. Moreover, it *is* true that there is a colour in every visual *direction*—that is, for every azimuth-elevation pair (ϕ, θ), there is some three-dimensional location (ϕ, θ, d), in which something can be seen, where d is distance away from the perceiver, i.e. depth, including where d is effectively at infinity. So every visual direction is represented in every scene. These observations will allow us to recast Clark's argument.

There is a Kantian argument that can be constructed from the propositions we have just validated—that there is complementarity between features and locations and that there is a filled location in every direction. This argument shows how our awareness of visual location has a different origin than our awareness of sense-features like *red*.

It is a necessary and invariant feature of visual experience that no direction ever occurs twice in any scene, whereas descriptive features like *red* and *glossy* may—this is 'necessary' in the sense that one cannot even visually imagine what it would be like for a visual direction not to occur in a scene, or for it to occur twice. Thus, the appearance of a visual direction is not empirically ascertained; it is a priori. (The term 'necessary' is used this way by Kant: *Critique of Pure Reason*, A 24.) This contrasts with the case of 'descriptive' sensory features—there is no guarantee that any one of these will be instantiated in every scene, no guarantee that at most one will be. There are many scenes without *red*, many with multiple instances.

Consider, then, the following propositions concerning the visual field:

> *Feature Alone: Red* occurs now (somewhere or other).
> *Feature Multiple: Red* occurs twice in this scene.
> *Feature with Place: Red* occurs in direction (ϕ, θ) or in place p.
> *Place alone*: Place p is seen.
> *Direction alone*: (ϕ, θ) is represented once and only once in this scene (with some feature or other in it).

That there is an occurrence of *red* in a scene, or that there are two or none: these are things you did not know before you looked. But the occurrence of a feature in every direction is not given by the on-occasion determination of vision. This is a structural fact that does not distinguish one scene from another.

There is an analogue to such uninformative statements in the realm of descriptive features. We know that there cannot be instantiations of both *burgundy* and *scarlet* in the very same part of an object. Clearly, this is not an empirically determined fact. Rather, it is a consequence of how the brain represents colour. In Chapter 4, we saw that the colours are arrayed in an integrated similarity space: each determinate colour corresponds to a different point in this space. Since every (spatially minimal) stimulus is assigned definite coordinates in this space, never assigned two different sets of coordinates, it cannot have two different colours at the same time. This relation of incompatibility among determinate colours thus arises out of how they are ordered internally (see also Hardin 1988: 113–34). The mutual exclusion of determinate sense-features is, in Kant's terminology, a question of *form*, not of empirical information. The incompatibility of colours is not, to paraphrase Kant, 'an empirical concept which has been derived from outer experiences' (*Critique of Pure Reason* A 23).

Exactly the same considerations apply to uninformative statements about location, for instance *Direction alone* above. In the early stages of visual processing, the system arrays features in two-dimensional retinotopic maps—the colour map, the map of oriented line-elements, the map of motions, and so on. As we saw in our discussion of Feature Integration Theory (Chapter 2, section III), these maps are indexed by a 'master map of locations'—two-dimensional locations, since these maps are two-dimensional. In these maps, just as in similarity spaces, each location occurs once and only once. Moreover, visual processing ensures that there is a feature at every such two-dimensional location, even the location corresponding to the retina's blind spot, in which there are no receptors. The uninformativeness of *Direction alone* is a remnant in conscious vision of these two-dimensional maps in early vision.

In later visual processing, the system tries to import a third dimension, depth or distance, by estimating the distance of the feature that occurs in each direction. Directions (ϕ, θ) are no longer the locators for features; they are now replaced by place: (ϕ, θ, d). But the earlier two-dimensional maps continue to have an influence on the form of representation: this is why there is a feature at some distance in every direction. From this story, one may conclude that the role of visual locations is different from that of features: visual *directions* constitute an omnipresent grid that overlays every scene, indexing the features represented in it. This is an updated version of Kant's argument about space: direction is part of the *form* of visual representation— this aspect of form arises from the feature maps of early vision—whereas features like *red* are part of the informative content. The uninformative propositions above are artefacts of the visual system's representational scheme, artefacts of the *form*, not the content, of vision.

Now, what is one to make of the fact that

> *Place alone*: Place p is represented in this scene (with some feature or other in it)

is informative? There is an informative discrimination of depth along every direction: in every direction, at some depth (or depths)—possibly at infinity when nothing material intrudes—there occurs some feature. It is a variable, hence informative, aspect of scenes *where* in any given direction a feature occurs. Here it seems intelligible to say that just as there is some colour in every direction, so also there is some seen place in every direction. Note, further, (a) that not every distance may be instantiated in every scene (there is nothing that I see 15 feet away from me at this moment since the walls of my room are closer, and everything I see through the window is further). Moreover, (b) some distances are instantiated twice: one might be seeing *red* at (ϕ, θ, d) and *blue* at (ϕ', θ', d). On these grounds, distance is beginning to seem more and more analogous to colour, shape, or motion. Clark is tempted by the following:

> **Uniqueness of place*: Visual location p occurs at most once.

In fact, this is plausibly false, as is shown by our example of a reflection colocated with a tree seen through the reflecting window. There do not seem to be any structural facts about location as opposed to direction. So there is no obstacle to saying that distance is a part of the empirical content of vision. This seems to imply that, *pace* Clark, distance is a quale. It is not clear why one should object to this.

On this assumption, visual location is a mixture of a formal element (direction) and a quale of distance. Even so, the quale of distance is unique in that it is *relative* to a specific feature: we don't see distance *per se* but the distance *of some descriptive feature*. So the complementarity of place and feature noted earlier still has force. This is what remains of Clark's verdict that there is a difference between how descriptive features and locations are presented. Here is what he says about this:

We need two different kinds of place-holders in any schema describing the contents of sensory experience. It cannot be collapsed to univariate form. We cannot capture those contents by substituting different qualities Q in a schema of the form
    appearance of qualities Q.
Instead we need two place-holders:
    appearance *of* qualities Q *at* region R.
Here Q and R are place-holders to be filled in by qualitative and spatial dimensions respectively. The two play different roles, which cannot be interchanged. (2000, 60)

The task undertaken in the following section is to give an account of how 'region R' is presented.

Before we get to that, however, a remark about realism. I called the above argument 'Kantian'. Now, Kant famously thought that his argument about space and time implied that space and time have no reality independent of perceiving minds. To hold that space is 'formal', is, according to him, to imply that it is 'solely from the human standpoint that we can speak of space, of extended things, etc'. I have been resisting this form of argument in the case of colour. The similarity space of colour is constructed by the human colour-vision system—by our receptivity to colour, in short—yet, as we have argued in Chapter 8, section IV, the colour properties are physically specifiable and also subject to standards of correctness. Exactly the same holds for space. That the human visual system constructs a representational system for space, and that the visual apprehension of space inherits characteristics from this construction, does not imply that what we visually apprehend is merely subjective. Indeed, there is, in the case of the visual representation of space, a greater fidelity to the characteristics of external space than there is in the representation of colour. The structure of spatial coordinates is influenced by the optical laws of projection through lenses, which maintain certain elements of external structure, and distance is estimated with good accuracy by a variety of means, some optical (binocularity), others not. The spatial form of conscious vision is, as we have noted elsewhere, perspectival in nature. This reflects a rearrangement of raw spatial information for the organism's purposes. Despite such rearrangement and special purpose processing, the visual representation of space corresponds more closely, both in dimensionality and in resolution, to the structure of objective physical space than the spatial representations of other modalities—though in the case of echo-locating bats, auditory space takes over this role. Thus, it is appropriate to hold that spatial coordinates used by the human visual system map on to and represent real space in something like the sense of Chapter 8, section IV (though the criterion of *physical* specifiability may need to be modified to accommodate space). The point to take from the above discussion is just that because of the peculiar structuring role it plays in vision, it displays certain peculiarities that one would not expect of other sense modalities. There is not, in audition or olfaction, a connected spatial plenum as there is in vision.

II. Seeing Objects

What is the function of visual locations relative to descriptive features? What is the purpose of the indexing they provide? Clark approaches the question through something he calls the Many Properties problem, which he attributes to Frank Jackson (1977, 65). How do you tell the difference between:

Scene 1: red square next to green triangle
Scene 2: red triangle next to green square?

The mere occurrence of *red, green, square*, and *triangle* will not do the job, since both scenes incorporate all and only occurrences of these qualities. What we need is that different pairs of these qualities must be bound together—*red* with *square* in Scene 1, *red* with *triangle* in Scene 2. Clark proposes that binding occurs by features being jointly *predicated* of some subject. 'Feature overlap demands predication not merely conjunction', he says (2000, 68). And he proposes that 'place-times' function as subjects for visual feature predication. As far as visual representation is concerned, we have referential elements to pick out places, descriptive elements to characterize the places thus picked out, Clark suggests. This is the difference between visual elements that characterize 'region *R*' and those that intimate occurrences of 'quality *Q*'. In short, *red* and *square* are predicated of the same place in Scene 1, while *red* and *triangle* are predicated of the same place in Scene 2. In Feature Integration Theory (Chapter 2, section IV, and Chapter 3, section IV), all sense-features are indexed by locations. Clark converts this to the claim that features are *predicated* of locations.

I have recounted Clark's argument at length because it is extremely important and far-reaching. But it does not go quite far enough. Many, perhaps most, visual states go beyond merely locating descriptive features in a three-dimensional spatial matrix. This can be demonstrated by a further application of the Many Properties problem. Consider the famous *phi* phenomenon demonstrated by the psychologist, Max Wertheimer, in 1912, and other cinematographic phenomena investigated by A. Körte in 1915. (For descriptions of these phenomena, I rely on Dan Dennett, 1991, 114, and Albert Bregman, 1990, 21–3.)

You are sitting in a darkened room: a blue light comes on, and then goes off; after an interval, another blue light comes on, somewhat displaced in position from the first light. Let the interval between these occurrences be long, and the second light will be perceived as different from the first one. Let the interval be short, and the first light will be perceived as moving to the second location; thus, the second flash will appear to have emanated from the same individual thing as the first one. As far as synchronic properties are concerned (i.e. excluding movement), there is no *descriptive* difference between the two visual presentations: aside from the temporal interval between the two appearances of *blue*, there is no difference in the synchronic features seen at the two moments. However, one is perceived as containing two blue lights, and the other as containing a single blue light moving from one position to another.

Körte, for his part, extended and elaborated these observations into an early theory of motion perception. He considered four lamps arranged as follows:

O   O   O   O

There is a greater gap between the two pairs of lamps than between the two in each pair. One would expect a uniformly moving particle to take longer to span the gap between the pairs. Körte found that if the temporal interval between the second lighting and the third is not lengthened proportionate to the distance, you will see two different particles moving—two distinct *phi*-phenomena, one on the left and one on the right. If, however, you increase the time between the second and third flash, you will see a single particle moving across the four positions. More recently, Zenon Pylyshyn and his co-workers, have demonstrated that criss-cross movements of light spots are tracked on the basis of spatio-temporal continuity and the minimization of total movement, even when (as above) there are several possible interpretations of the light-place sequences (see Pylyshyn 2001 for an extensive review and discussion).

These presentations demonstrate that the visual system is sensitive to motion. It is able to discriminate individual spatially extended sequences of unrelated events from the trajectories of a single particle. This evidence was later supplemented by the discovery of a 'motion-blind' patient, who had suffered a lesion in a particular part of the brain—Zihl et al. 1983. This patient saw all motion as a series of stills. No *phi* for her. This evidence suggests that the visual system contains a separate module dedicated to the detection of motion.

Returning now to our original simple *phi*-phenomenon, the two presentations—blue lights with different time intervals between flashes—are equivalent with respect to features and locations. That is both presentations consist of one blue flash at one location, followed by a later flash at a second location. Consider the following *feature-location* assumptions made by the visual motion-processing system:

> *Interval Long.* If Blue-here at time $t1$ and Blue-there at time ($t1 + 150$ *msec*), then Blue-here does not belong to the same object as Blue-there.
> *Interval Short.* If Blue-here at time $t2$ and Blue-there at time $t2 + 50$ *msec*, then Blue-here belongs to same object as Blue-there.

What would the references of 'Blue-here' and 'Blue-there' be? What are the stimuli assigned to the sensory class *blue* in these presentations? They cannot simply be *locations*. Both presentations deal with the same two locations: it is therefore not possible to make sense of the difference between the two presentations, and of the identity claim in *Interval Short*, in terms of locations. The stimuli must then be presented as *material objects*. Thus, the visual system's operating assumptions can be put like this:

> *Interval Long.* If Object 1 appears to be located here at time $t1$ and Object 2 to be located there at time $t1 + 150$ *msec*, then Object 1 is not the same as Object 2.

> *Interval Short.* If Object 1 appears to be located here at time *t1* and Object 2 to be located there at time *t1 + 50 msec*, then Object 1 is the same as Object 2—this object has moved from here to there.

Clark solved the Many Properties problem by proposing that vision attributes qualities to regions of space. His solution does not work here, for motion cannot be attributed to places. Places do not move, nor do place-times.

Why *material* objects? Let us consider a version of the *phi*-phenomenon generated by Paul Kolers and Michael von Grünau in response to a query from Nelson Goodman. What would happen if the first light was blue, as in the above presentation, and the second one red? Here is Dennett's description of the new *Interval Short* phenomenon:

> Two different colored spots were lit for 150 msec (with a 50 msec interval); the first spot seemed to begin moving and then change color abruptly *in the middle of its illusory passage* toward the second location. (1991, 114)

This demonstrates that the bearers of visual features are capable not only of movement but of qualitative *change*. These objects are capable of manifesting one quality in one location at one time, and an incompatible quality in another location at another time. Now, as Aristotle very long ago remarked:

> It seems most distinctive of substance that what is numerically one and the same is able to receive contraries. In no other case could one bring forward anything, numerically one, which is able to receive contraries. For example, a colour which is numerically one and the same will not be black and white, nor will numerically one and the same action be bad and good; and similarly with everything else that is not substance. A substance, however, numerically one and the same, is able to receive contraries. For example, a man—one and the same—becomes pale at one time and dark at another, and young and old, and bad and good. Nothing like this is to be seen in any other case. (*Categories* 5, 4a10–22)

In the colour-*phi*-phenomenon we see a single object move from place to place and take on contrary qualities. This shows that the things we see are what Aristotle calls 'individual substances'. (Vision fails to respect Aristotle's theory of *secondary* substances, or substance types, however, for if a picture of a rabbit is flashed at location one, and a picture of a duck at location 2, one sees what appears to be a rabbit moving from the first to the second location while changing to a duck in mid-trajectory. As we shall see in a moment, Aristotelian ontology reasserts itself in post-visual processing.)

The conclusion that vision attributes features to material objects is reinforced by a recent experiment by Blaser, Pylyshyn, and Holcombe (2000). These researchers demonstrated the converse of the *phi*-phenomenon, namely that the visual system is capable of tracking several objects superimposed on one another *in the same location*. The display consisted of two (or more) superimposed patterns varying independently of one another. For instance, a typical display consisted of a red disc with parallel dark stripes running in one direction and a bright bar with a different orientation. The pattern of stripes would change smoothly, independently of changes in the bright bar. For instance, the whole pattern of stripes might rotate smoothly or change in thickness and separation, at the same time as the bar changed in brightness. Observers saw these patterns as distinct objects in the same location, and were able to track them independently. It was found that 'when observers attempt to attend to a particular feature of one of the [objects] . . . they actually by default attend to the object as a whole; consequently, processing is enhanced for all of its features' (197). In other words, if they were tracking the rotation of one pattern, they were more likely to notice a shift in the colour of this pattern than any change in the other. If they were tracking both objects simultaneously, then, because their attention is divided between the two, their performance with regard to noticing secondary shifts and changes is diminished (cf. Baylis and Driver, 1993). These results show that these observers were attending to features by attending to the objects to which these features were attributed, and not by attending to the features directly (see Scholl 2001 for a disussion of object-oriented attention). This explains how a reflection can be seen in the same place as a thing seen through the reflecting window. It implies, by the way, that in such a case, the same visual location is seen *twice*: once in each of two objects.

These visual apprehensions of features in objects are the product of data-processing that occurs relatively late in the visual process—in 'middle vision', as it is sometimes said. This is significant: for as we saw, Clark's proposal that features are attributed to regions of space is influenced by Treisman's Feature Integration Theory, which is a process of *early* vision. Now, the later a process is in vision, the more profoundly it affects conscious vision. Thus, conscious vision is organized more around objects than around places. This organization feeds, apparently, into the early stages of the use of *sortals*. For as Susan Carey and Fei Xu (2001) have shown, what Aristotle calls 'secondary substances', i.e. fundamental classifiers of individual substances such as *rabbit, bird, person*, etc., are intimately tied up with how we perceive the continuity of objects. Carey and Xu argue that this use of classifiers traces to a system that is independent of the primitive motion-detecting module responsible for *phi*-phenomena in visual processing: it is, they say, 'fully conceptual, drawing on kind information for decisions about individuation and numerical identity' (181). Their conclusions show that vision is committed, so to speak, to an ontology of material objects at several different levels. The simple objects of motion processing provide base continuity conditions for the more richly structured objects of our intuitive ontology.

Let us define a material object as a spatio-temporally confined and continuous entity that can move while taking its features with it. Films and lights as well as three-dimensional objects with mass count as material objects by this definition. Spots of light cast by a moving light, or images projected in a 'motion' picture do not count as material objects: but as the *phi*-phenomenon demonstrates, vision encodes them as such. Since spatio-temporal continuity is a defining criterion of material objects, we may replace Clark's theory that features are attributed to locations with one that makes the subject material objects.

We saw in the last section that regions of space are visually represented by means of a combination of a *formal* component of direction, together with an *informative* component of depth. We have now concluded that the primary objects of vision are material objects: all features are attributed to these. Since depth is informative, a feature, it too must be attributed to material object—depth is simply the distance this seen object is from the viewer. Two further conclusions can be drawn from this. First, regions of space are seen only as occupied by a material object at a certain distance: we do not *see* regions unless we see a material object there, though unseen locations still form a part of the total visual representation. We are so to speak visually aware of objects in a complete scene; however, we do not see all parts of this scene since in some such parts, there is nothing to be seen. Second (and more controversial), one sees a material object in every direction, in some directions perhaps only an illusory material object like the sky, but a material object in every direction nonetheless.

To summarize, then. Perceptions of change and motion demand an identity that underlies change. Locations do not provide such an identity. Hence the proper representation of visual states demands reference to *objects*, which can continue through time. The scenes mentioned earlier can be analysed as follows:

> Scene 1: One material object that is red and square next to another that is green and triangular.
> Scene 2: One material object that is red and triangular next to another that is green and square.

Objects solve both the static and the dynamic form of the Many Properties problem. The *phi*-phenomenon and the tracking of multiple objects in the same place demonstrates that feature binding occurs on material objects, not just locations (cf. Campbell 2002: 'Visual attention can be allocated to objects rather than to locations', 34–5; see the evidence and discussion in the pages following).

III. The Peculiarities of Visual Location

One might think that sensory reference to material objects occurs in all sensory modalities. Not so. I shall now argue that vision is unique in this respect.

Audition too demands attribution to something other than places, but only vision demands material objects.

Visual states are in *object-attribute* form. The following, for instance, expresses the content of a typical visual state: *That disc is blue and shiny* (or, more accurately, *that thing is round, flat, blue, and shiny*). Since objects like discs are seen as located in space, the attribution of a colour to an object has spatial form. However, this visual state does not merely intimate the co-locatability of roundness and blueness, their presence in the same place: it intimates, in addition, that both inhere in an individual object with temporal reidentification conditions that go beyond descriptive similarity. Mere co-location gives me no reason whatsoever to think that the shininess and the blue will stay together. This visual state, however, leads me to expect that they will, that each will move when its bearer does, and that *this* disc, with these visual features, might be different from another disc with the same features, though the two discs might swap places. Though the co-location leads me to expect feature-continuance, it is also compatible with being later informed about change, e.g. with the disc becoming, a moment later, an ellipse, or becoming red, while retaining its numerical identity. Because they carry these additional expectations, states in object-attribute form do something more than merely describe. They also identify the objects to which they attribute descriptive features. The feature containment of the object-attribute form is logically more demanding than that of simple feature location, because it assigns features to objects with spatio-temporal continuity, and not merely to places at moments. (The results of Blaser et al. 2000, discussed in the previous section, confirm the above claims.)

Historically, many philosophers have treated of feature location, and even of the object-attribute form, as if they were universally present in all sense modalities, not just the visual. Some have suggested that one could not experience *any* perceptual feature without locating it somewhere, or indeed (some say) without attributing it to an object. This, one might suppose, was part of what Aristotle had in mind when he insisted that '*All the other things* are either said of the primary substances as subjects or in them as subjects' (*Categories* 2b8)—for what he seems to mean is that *all* descriptive features, including sensory features, *must* be attributed to material objects. Kant too thought that feature-location was the same in different sense-modalities: he meant to include all sense-modalities when he claimed that space underlies *all* outer intuitions, that it is, as he put it, 'the condition of the possibility of appearances' (*Critique of Pure Reason*, A24). Kant is assuming that all modalities share a single spatial matrix, or at least that there is a common space that contains spaces proprietary to the different modalities—'touch space', 'sight space' and so on (as Russell 1914 called them)—and that this common space provides a matrix for the location of all sense-features, regardless of modality. Aristotle and Kant are committed to the thought that the *same* form of feature placement is involved whenever a descriptive feature is presented in perception, possibly even that perceptual description was always in object-attribute form, regardless of which sense modality is involved. They did *not* think vision was a distinctive form of presentation in this respect. And even empiricists like Russell, who keep the modality-specific spaces separate, never suggested that visual representations of space might be structurally different from auditory ones, or that the basic form of feature-containment might be different in different modalities.

This kind of treatment fails to do full justice to the peculiar character of *visual* experience. Think of olfaction. I am aware of an acidic odour. *Where* is that odour? Perhaps, as Kant thought, it needs to be *some*where—*here*, where I am. But it is not precisely located in external space as a colour appears to be—it is diffuse, not contained. Smells do not have a definite size, as instances of colour do. They have, at best, a *primitive*—that is, an undifferentiating—feature-location structure—every smell of which I am aware is simply here. Of course, one is able to trace the source of an odour by moving objects to one's nose and sniffing them, or by moving oneself with respect to them—when I want to know what smells bad in the refrigerator, I sniff each thing in turn; when I want to know where the bad smell in my kitchen comes from, I walk around sniffing. To locate smells, one needs to be active. When one moves, one makes use of chemical gradients, sensing how olfactory concentrations vary with position. Since this involves movement, tracing the source of a smell is necessarily extended in time. At an instant, or without movement, one's olfactory perception does not contain the idea of direction or distance. Further, it does not come in object-attribute form. This is connected to the fact that odours linger: the salad has been eaten but the bouquet of the dressing stays a while—without differentiating location. Smells are not sensed as inhering in an object; synchronically, they are not even sensed as located in a particular direction; they are never experienced as at a definite distance away.

In Chapter 4, section I. 4 we encountered the following Feature Exclusion Principle:

> A fully determinate feature excludes other features *of the same type*. If *FD* and *FD** are distinct fully determinate features of the same type, there is some range of individuals, *x*, such that *x* cannot be both *FD* and *FD**.

The kind of individual that figures in this principle—the range of objects, *x*, to which it is appropriate to attribute features in a particular exclusion range—depends on the feature-placing structure of features in that exclusion range. When I see *green* and *blue* simultaneously, they cannot be in the same part of the same object, though they can be in the same place provided that they are in different objects. Smells, however, co-locate with unrestrained promiscuity. In the kitchen where a salad-dressing is being made, I smell olive oil and garlic. Where are these odours? Simply *here*. They coexist in a place without combining. This means, that the range of individuals invoked for olfactory features in the above principle cannot be objects or places. There would be no incompatibilities if such individuals were invoked. The individuals have to be smells themselves. No one smell can be both garlicky and olive-oily—these are two smells, not one—though both smells can be traced to a single object. More importantly, the co-locatability of all smells means that you cannot simultaneously be aware of *two* instances of the same garlicky smell. There may, of course, be two things in your vicinity that smell garlicky. But both simply contribute to the same garlicky smell in your area. You can't distinguish two smells for the two objects. You would have been able to do this if it were possible to place smells in distinct locations or distinct objects.

Smells do not come in object-attribute form. Of course, physical objects may be identifiable as the *source* of odours. But this is different from saying that they are subjects for the smells as predicates. The salad-dressing on the kitchen counter is the source of the odours of olive-oil and garlic. But the smells are not there on the kitchen counter; they are diffused throughout the room. Neither the room nor the salad-dressing is the bearer of the odour. As the feature-exclusion principle implies, what we smell are *smells*; only secondarily is the olfactory state directed towards the salad-dressing: the odour of olive oil *comes from* the dressing. This is enough to cast doubt on, or at least significantly to modify, how we understand, Kant's claim that 'intuition' relates us to objects. Smells are, of course, 'objects', if that term is used in a more accommodating sense than Kant intended. That is, it should not escape one's notice that smells are external objects distinct from olfactory sensations: they have existence outside our own minds, they are public entities to which more than one person has access. In this sense, they count as stimuli, and thus olfaction conforms to the Sensory Classification Thesis. But they are not individual substances in Aristotle's sense, reidentifiable objects that move around in space: they are not the receptacles of sensory attributes. This should lead us to question Aristotle's idea that 'all the other things' stand in a predicative relationship to 'primary substances'. *Pace* Aristotle in the *Categories*, a smell is neither a primary substance nor *in* a primary substance.

Now think about sounds. Notice first that sounds too do not stand in an *attributive* relationship to objects. If I see *green* in an object, then I am seeing a green (or partially green) object—*green* is here predicated of, attributed to, the object. But when I hear middle C coming from a violin I do not thereby hear a middle C violin; it makes no sense to characterize the violin that way. True, objects are characterizable by the sound they make—there are squeaky violins, baritone singers, alto saxophones—but the inferential path from auditory experience to such dispositional characterizations is quite indirect.

Why is this? Perhaps because our ears use sounds *emitted* by objects, rather than sounds *reflected* by them. By contrast, our eyes primarily take information from light reflected by objects, not from light emitted by them. The sounds emitted by objects vary a lot with what they are doing or what is happening to them. The timbre and range of a voice is a good clue to identity and we do indeed characterize people or voices by the timbre of the sounds they emit—baritone singers and alto saxophones, as we remarked a moment ago. But the volume and pitch of a sound somebody emits is obviously not a constant, and cannot be used to characterize the person. We can, and in general material objects can, emit different tones at different times. What we hear then are entities independent of the identity of their producers, and we hear sounds, not people—at least in the first instance.

Audition conveys a lot of spatial structure, much more than olfaction—all the same, auditory experience does not have, primarily, a feature-*placing* structure, rather it has a feature-*direction* structure, and though it is true that there is some sense of distance in sounds as well, this is not as precise as the directional aspect. (Distance in audition seems to be connected with the degradation of auditory signals: the more 'noise' there is in a sound, the further away it will seem to be. In the bat, audition conveys an extremely precise sense of distance, but this depends on the bat's own production of auditory probes. Unlike ourselves, the bat is able to gather and use information about acoustic reflectance. It is at least possible that bats hear certain sounds in object-attribute form.) Sounds come from a particular direction. They may even be heard as emanating from objects: I may hear a *violin* making a musical sound, or a *person* speaking—though this kind of object-specificity does seem to depend to a great extent on visual identification. (This is why the ventriloquist's dummy is so compelling an illusion.) However that might be, sounds are not generally presented (as visual features are) as *in* a place. Audition is too two-dimensional for that.

Moreover, sounds combine even when they come from different places. Though it may be clear from the quality and direction of the sounds that the violins are playing C and the violas G, it is also the case that the two together sound a fifth. (It is not invariably the case that these will combine: whether the violins and violas will merge or stay separate depends on other musical cues. In the simplest case, they might be playing a tune in unison, at different pitches. In this case, they will be heard as one unit. In a more complicated case, they may constitute two different voices in a fugue: here, they will be heard as separate, but their joint production of chords will still contribute to the musical experience.) This phenomenon of *simultaneous*, or *spectral*, integration marks a radical difference between sounds and colours or odours. The complexions of two persons standing next to each other never combine into a single whole; nor do their perfumes—but their voices might. On the other hand, smells are always co-located (though not merged): sounds may be co-located or not. Spectral integration is a producer-independent auditory experience, and this shows why sounds do not enter into an attributive relation with their producers. Since musical sounds are, so to speak, free both to be heard independently, and to combine, they are perceived as existing separately from their producers.

This said, audition does have objects that are distinct from sounds. These objects are usually voices, or more generally 'auditory streams', as Albert Bregman (1990) has called them in a pioneering study. Tones heard in succession associate with each other by *sequential* integration to form temporally extended objects. These objects are subjects for properties, and pose their own version of the Many Properties problem which we discussed earlier in the visual domain. Bregman puts the point as follows:

> Suppose that there are two acoustic sources of sound, one high and near and the other low and far. It is only because nearness and highness are grouped as properties of one stream and farness and lowness as properties of the other that we can experience the uniqueness of the individual sounds rather than a mush of four properties. (11)

The principles that govern sequential integration are analogous to Gestalt principles of association, but Bregman argues that the objects thus formed are perceived as unitary wholes because they behave in ways that approximate ecological truths. For example, vision manifests a 'principle of exclusive allocation': no sensory element is attributed to more than one object at a time. For example, an edge will be seen as an edge of at most one object: this accounts for figure-ground reversals, which depend on an edge being associated with different parts of a drawing successively. Bregman argues that this reflects an ecological constraint, namely the 'very low likelihood (except in jigsaw puzzles) that the touching edges of two objects will have the same shape' (13). In exactly the same way, since it is unlikely that one sound will terminate exactly when another begins, sudden discontinuities in sound patterns are attributed to at most one stream. Bregman gives an example of a sequence of notes like the following (where height represents pitch, though Y is a variable):

$$B$$
$$A$$
$$X \quad X \quad X \quad Y \quad \quad Y \quad X \quad X \quad X$$

It turns out that if the Ys get associated with the Xs by means of contextual cues such as proximity or similarity of timbre, then A and B are heard as separate events. But if the Ys get associated with A and B, YABY is heard as a single unit, and the relationship between A and B is more difficult to hear. This is strictly analogous, Bregman plausibly claims, with perceptual switches due to the exclusive allocation of edges in visual figure-ground reversals: the Ys cannot be allocated both to the Xs and to the AB sequence. This phenomenon gives credence to the idea that audition reifies sounds and auditory streams in the same way as vision does material objects.

As remarked before, it is not uncommon for philosophers to assimilate the form of all the sense-modalities to the object-attribute structure of vision. For example, Sydney Shoemaker (1990, 97) says that secondary qualities are experienced 'as belonging to objects in our external environment—the *apple* is experienced as red, the *rose* as fragrant, the *lemon* as sour'. We have just found that the second and third clauses of his assertion need to be qualified: there are substantial differences amongst the sense modalities with regard to how they localize and attribute their descriptive percepts. True, secondary qualities are always experienced as occurring in the external environment (tastes in an slightly odd but still recognizable sense of 'external', i.e. in the mouth), but they do not always implicate material objects. In other words, it is right for Shoemaker to insist that secondary qualities are *not* experienced as occurrences within the perceiver, as changes in *her* inner conscious state. But this does not imply that they are attributed to external movable and reidentifiable objects as the only alternative to self-ascription: we have seen that in audition and olfaction, secondary qualities are attributed, in the first instance, to modality-specific environmental events or conditions, i.e. to sounds and smells, and only by inference to the objects that are responsible for these.

In much the same way, John Campbell (2002) makes a slight, but discernible, misstep concerning the objects of audition. He claims that in order to identify a helicopter as the source of a particular noise, you should be able to identify the heard helicopter with the seen helicopter.

Otherwise, your auditory demonstrative would not be referring to a helicopter at all, but to something different, namely, a sound . . . . So when your auditory system is organizing the auditory information from that helicopter into a single whole, it is using a principle of integration that depends on vision; it depends on the knowledge you have, on the basis of vision, of what such an object is. (63–4)

It is certainly true that vision primes your identification of sound as coming from the helicopter. What is not true is that your auditory system attaches that sound, by predication, to a visual representation of the helicopter. As Bregman shows, auditory objects are sequentially integrated series of sounds. It is true, of course, that the helicopter will emit just such an auditory stream. It may also be true that the sounds it emits come to be sequentially integrated by a mechanism, the function of which is precisely to identify and integrate sounds that emanate from a single object. The point is that this mechanism operates without reference to a visual category. For example, I might hear two annoying sounds from the garden next door without seeing their source—a loud high-pitched hedge trimmer and an equally loud low-pitched lawnmower. I distinguish these as two separate *auditory* objects: two auditory streams, not two material objects. Similarly, when I am at a choral concert, I can hear the tenor and baritone parts separately, even though I may not be able visually to verify which singers are emitting which. As we just said, it is a part of the evolutionary function of this kind of auditory segregation that it helps me count the sources of sound and correlate them with objects identified visually. Nevertheless, the auditory stream is the primary object created by sequential integration. Auditory demonstratives do not refer to material objects.

Shoemaker and Campbell *are*, however, right about vision. That is, vision *does* refer to material objects. We will need to investigate how this comes to be.

IV. On Sensory Idiosyncrasy

In Chapter 13, we will investigate how visual objects, as opposed to visual features, are presented to us in experience. In order to do this, we will be taking note of certain neurophysiological mechanisms of vision. This will strike some readers as superfluous. As philosophers, we are interested in *psychological* and *phenomenological* descriptions of sensory experience, they will say. While few doubt that these descriptions are ultimately grounded in physiology, this grounding seems to many like an accident. Vision could just as easily have been realized on a silicon medium, it has been argued. This shows that the actual realization of vision in flesh is irrelevant or inessential to visual phenomena. Why should we pay attention to an inessential aspect of the phenomena we seek to understand? Let's call this line of thought the Functionalist Paradigm.

The Functionalist Paradigm is confounded by the idiosyncrasies of individual sensory systems revealed by our investigation above. Consider the following facts.

> Vision places features in material objects. There is no such intermediate category as ecological 'sights' (or internal visual sense data) which vision pastes together as material objects.

> Visual features are tightly contained in material objects and in the places where material objects reside. They do not combine across material objects and across places.

By contrast:

> The direct objects of audition are *sounds*. We are frequently able to determine whence and from which material objects these sounds come, but the sounds and their characteristics are not *attributed* to these sources as predicates are to subjects.

Moreover, audition displays two distinct modes of combining sounds:

> Sounds from distinct locations may be 'simultaneously integrated' into chords: these do not always come from any particular place, since the component notes may emanate from different directions.

> Sounds may also be 'sequentially integrated' into auditory streams. These streams are, as we saw, subjects for auditory features like *near* or *far, high* or *low*, but they are, in other respects, very different from material objects.

The ontology of visual representations is thus radically different from that of auditory representations.

Such peculiarities of sensory systems can be explained only by reference to physical reality: the nature of the sensory input, the character of the receptors, and the organization of the data-processing system downstream from these receptors. Consider first the influence of the different kinds of receptors present in the visual and auditory systems. The retina receives an image cast by a lens; there is no such thing as an acoustic lens; sound does not form an image in this way. The auditory receptor is the basilar membrane. This is, in effect, a spectrometer: each part of this membrane responds to sound of a particular frequency. Thus the membrane is a linearly arranged spectrogram: a graph of amplitudes for each frequency. There are no spatial parameters recorded at this stage, hence all sound-locations—directions, distance, etc.—are processed later. One immediate consequence is that spatial representation is *not* part of the *form* of auditory representation: that is, there is no counterpart in audition of the formal requirement for visual scenes that every direction is represented once and only once. Here already we see how the form of representation is constrained by the physical character of the receptor—a physiological fact.

The Functionalist may not feel much threatened by this simple example—perhaps it is easily accommodated—nonetheless, it carves out a role, however small, for physics and physiology within psychology and phenomenology. The effects of physiology on the post-receptoral processing of the auditory image is much harder for the Functionalist to dismiss. As it turns out, the physiology of the auditory data-stream is strikingly similar to that of the visual stream. In the first place, the auditory cortex incorporates several 'tonotopic' maps of auditory features; that is, it preserves the spectrographic organization of the basilar membrane, just as the primary visual cortex preserves the two-dimensional spatial organization of the retina. This application of one and the same neurophysiological architecture to a radically different data-stream accounts for many of the differences between vision and audition. In audition, a number of computations have to be organized by frequency, whereas in the visual stream, computations are organized by place. We saw earlier, for example, that there are precise analogues in audition of

Gestalt grouping operations in vision, but these grouping operations are done by differences and similarities of frequency, not place. As Bregman (1990) says of groupings like the one discussed above:

In [vision] the grouping is predicable from the Gestalt psychologists' proximity principle, which states roughly that the closer the visual elements in a set are to one another, the more strongly we tend to group them perceptually. The Gestalt psychologists thought of this grouping as if the perceptual elements ... were attracting one another like miniature planets in space with the result that they ended to form clusters in our experience. If the analogy to audition is a valid one, this suggests that the spatial dimension of distance in vision has two analogies in audition. One is separation in time, and the other is separation in frequency. Both, according to this analogy are distances, and Gestalt principles that involve distance should be valid for them. (18–19)

That these Gestalt principles operate on frequency is not just enabled, but more importantly, compelled by the spectral organization of information on the basilar membrane and auditory cortex. In each modality, elements that are adjacent or near to one another in the primary cortical representational area have a certain 'attraction' on one another. However, adjacency has a quite different representational significance in each. Adjacent elements in audition are close together in frequency, adjacency in vision signifies closeness with regard to direction of origin. It seems therefore that the brain is taking advantage of a *physiological* relation—adjacency—in the procedures it uses to analyse incoming data. Physiology is thus a determinant of the phenomenology of perception.

Bregman himself essays a Functionalist explanation of auditory Gestalt principles. He insists that ecology explains why visual and auditory grouping are so different:

The way to get at [differences between vision and audition] is to consider the differences in the way in which information about the properties of the world that we care about are carried in sound and in light. The fact that certain Gestalt principles actually are shared between the senses could be thought of as existing because they are appropriate methods for scene analysis in both domains. (ibid., 36)

It is certainly true that as Bregman says, the methods used by each sense modality are going to be *appropriate*—that goes almost without saying. The question is: why do they use the same methods of grouping proximal elements, even though visual proximity reflects proximity of direction and auditory proximity is proximity of pitch? It is hard to resist the conclusion that there is a 'preadapted'—i.e. antecedently available—mechanism that has been taken over by each system and adapted by evolution to serve the divergent ends of the two systems. Without denying, then, that ecology is important, it is clear that physiology is important too. The methods used by each system are dictated by what the preadapted neurophysiology allows and admits.

Now, some Functionalists think that this conclusion is contra-indicated by the 'multi-realizability' of sensory processes. A visual or auditory process can be duplicated in silicon: indeed, technological progress has already been made towards the manufacture and use of a silicon prosthesis for the primary visual cortex. Clearly then it does not depend on its actual realization in nerves and cortical organization. But this argument confuses the *proximal* explanation of process by more or less contemporaneous physical events with the *historical* explanation of process by evolutionary antecedents. The correct point to make here is that auditory and visual processes can take place without the appropriate neurophysiological substrate. In this sense, neurophysiology is not necessary for vision, even for the idiosyncratic form that vision takes in different species. But it is a completely wrong-headed point to take from this the completely different moral that the neurophysiology of the brain was irrelevant to the historical evolution of idiosyncratic sensory process. (Larry Shapiro 2000 arrives at a similar conclusion, though by a different process of argument.) Vision and audition take the form they take in us because of ancestral neurophysiological facts. Some of those ancestral facts persist in the present day. One will not understand the oddities of human sensory mechanisms if one ignores them. It is true that when one analyses visual data-processing in algorithmic terms, one need not invoke the nature of the substrate, except in order to account for certain performance parameters — processing time and the like. But if one wants to understand *why* visual processing is the way it is—why we see the things we see in the way we see them—the biological facts are central.

13

Visual Reference

In Chapter 12, we argued that objects, not locations, were the primary targets of visual feature-attribution. Vision places features in material objects, not in locations. In this chapter, we investigate *how* vision deals with objects.

I. Motion-Guiding Vision

Think of an incident like this:

> *Ex. 1* You are walking on a quiet trail in a park. Suddenly, a cyclist passes you on the left. As she passes, she catches your attention, and you turn your head and eyes to see her better.

Philosophical intuition, and possibly introspection, might lead you to describe this incident in the following way: as a *consequence* of seeing something passing, you redirected your gaze to look at it. When you look at the passing figure you get other information. For instance, you might find that it is a woman wearing a yellow sweater. Accordingly, you might be inclined to reconstruct this visual incident in the following way: your attention was drawn by the sight of a woman wearing yellow, and that, consequently, you redirected your gaze. On reflection, you might weaken this claim. You might concede that pre-attentively you were not really aware of a *woman*. So you might think that you ought not to describe the initial incident in object-attribute form, and be more non-committal about the actual features of which you were aware before you turned your head. This would be wise, since peripheral vision offers us very little informational content. So the best might be to make a quite cautious statement: your attention was drawn by your awareness of a sudden movement to your left. This made you turn to look, and *after* you did, you saw a woman wearing a yellow sweater.

Put in this way, *Ex. 1* seems similar in structure to the following:

> *Ex. 2* You are walking on a quiet trail in a park. You hear somebody call your name. You turn around to look. It is your friend from work.

In actual fact, the two incidents do not have the same structure. In *Ex 2*, the sound of your name *does* prompt you to turn around to look. But in incidents like *Ex 1*, no such descriptive feature draws your attention; probably, you were not aware of anything at all before your attention was caught. For as natural as it seems to philosophical intuition that visual awareness of *something* must have been responsible for your turning your head, this distorts the structure of vision. As numerous recent studies of the extra-conscious uses of vision show (see Milner and Goodale 1995 and Weiskrantz 1998 for reviews), the processes that provide you with conscious awareness of visual features— colour, sudden motion, etc.—is in fact independent of and parallel to the one that controls gaze redirection.[1] Thus, gaze-redirection is independent of all the sense-features discussed in Chapter 1, i.e. of those that are present in visual awareness and conscious visual memory. The inclination to diagnose *Ex. 1* as parallel to *Ex. 2* is wrong not because it overestimates *how much* information you get through peripheral vision; it is wrong because that information is more or less insulated from gaze-redirection (though as I shall argue, they do have an effect on visual consciousness in an unexpected way.)

Now think of another case: reaching out to touch something or to pick it up.

> *Ex. 3* You are visiting somebody in her office. She offers you coffee: 'Take the blue cup,' she says. You scan the table for the blue cup—there are several cups sitting there—and having identified it, you reach out and pick it up with thumb and two fingers around the handle and hold it out to be filled with coffee. You deliberately choose that grip—you don't wrap your whole palm around the cup, since this risks your being splashed when the coffee is poured.

Philosophical intuition might lead you to think that throughout this process, you were guided by the blue shape in your visual field. For the standard empiricist view of perception maintains that you will have constructed and tracked a three-dimensional representation of an object out of the information conveyed by such sensations as that of blueness and shape. This representation enables you to move your hands to pick up the cup. Putting detail aside, the causal relations implied by this account are almost universally accepted by philosophers (Andy Clark 2001 and Campbell 2002, 55–6, are exceptions).

Though the role of conscious visual experience in *Ex. 3* is much greater than it is in *Ex. 1*, this philosophical intuition too underestimates the role that unconscious visual processes play. Before we get to that, however, let us examine what is *right* about the intuition. Remember from Chapter 1, section I, that there are visual features—*descriptive* sense-features, as we shall call them

---

[1] I do not want to exaggerate the independence of these two processes: there are elaborate cross-connections between the two streams just mentioned. But they are independent enough that the redirection of gaze will occur even in the absence of the representational stream—as in patients with 'blindsight'.

throughout this chapter—that characterize stimuli grouped together by the visual system for epistemic purposes. In Chapter 9, we suggested that these features provide the perceiver with relatively stable, object-centred information about stimuli, which she can hold for a period of time, in order to weigh its implications in the light of other incoming information and past experience. In order to play this role, descriptive features are presented in conscious states of visual awareness; they can also be recalled in conscious memory states which possess some of the same qualitative character as the aforementioned states of visual awareness. All the traditional empiricist sense-features fall into this category—*blue, round, moving*, and so on. Now, in *Ex. 3*, the *initial identification* of the object is driven by descriptive sense-features. 'Take the blue cup', your host says, and you identify which one she means by scanning for *blue* coinstantiated with a cup-shape. Moreover, the kind of grip you use to pick the cup up is guided by your conscious apprehension of its descriptive sense-features. You see that it has a handle; past experience tells you that you should grip the *handle* while hot coffee is being poured. Employing conscious volition, you reach for the handle with a 'precision grip'. So conscious processes of vision and intention play an important role in this action.

However, once the object has been identified and the type of grip chosen—once the action has, as it were, been launched—the guidance of the hand is taken over by a system that is independent of the one that provides experiential information about shape, size, and colour. For it has been known since the early 1980s that one's ability to handle objects in one's immediate vicinity, like one's ability to redirect one's gaze to a passing object, is also governed by visual states that contain no information concerning the *descriptive* features these objects possess. To be sure, these guidance systems are put into play by conscious volition, as we have just seen, and further, they are constantly corrected and redeployed by information from the descriptive sense-feature system. If you suddenly change your mind and go for green cup instead, conscious vision will come back into play. Nevertheless, the trajectory of the hand itself, and even many last-minute adjustments to it, are carried out without reference to the consciously available sense-features provided by the descriptive system. The visual system that guides the hand is much quicker to react and much more coercive than the epistemic system. It does not hold its information in abeyance waiting for a context-sensitive decision; it simply guides bodily motion in predetermined—sometimes innate, sometimes learned, but almost never novel—ways. There is, in short, a repertoire of actions that conscious volition is able to deploy for its own purposes, and these actions are neither volitionally controlled nor under conscious visual guidance. Action is hierarchically organized, as Charles Sherrington already realized (Gallistel 1980), and we now know that the more subordinate levels of bodily action are served by a visual system that operates somewhat independently of conscious descriptive vision.

Ex. 3 has the structure suggested by Andy Clark's (2001) *Hypothesis of Experience Based Selection,* which states that 'Conscious visual experience presents the world to a subject in a form appropriate for the reason-and-memory based *selection* of actions' (512; my emphasis). Clark is careful to emphasize that once the target and the form of action have been 'selected', as he puts it, its bodily execution is under the guidance of visual information that is not consciously available. Along somewhat different lines, John Campbell (2002) insists that while conscious attention to a thing is what enables you to select (from all the information available to you at a given moment) information about *that* thing, and to use this information to arrive at beliefs regarding its descriptive features, he is very much aware of the fact that there are 'underlying information processing systems' at the service of these actions which operate in the background, without consciousness or intentional intervention. Campbell, in effect, applies the Hypothesis of Experience Based Selection to the epistemic action of scrutinizing an object.

Not all bodily motion is initiated in an experience-based manner: *Ex. 1* is an example of non-consciously initiated behaviour. However, as was suggested in Chapter 10, section II, conscious sensory experience is a way of putting information at the disposition of the perceiver without commanding action: correspondingly here, action-*selection* is responsive to and guided by conscious experience, while automatic action is neither initiated nor guided by conscious sensation. Note that in *Ex. 3*, after action-selection has occurred, the bodily motion takes place more or less automatically, and is therefore under non-conscious visual guidance.

These functions are independent, it seems, because they take place in distinct data-processing streams in the brain (Schneider 1969; Ungerleider and Mishkin 1983; Milner and Goodale 1995). The processing of sense-features (*yellow, blue, cylindrical,* etc.) occurs in a succession of neurological formations that runs from the primary visual cortex, located at the back of the head in the occipital lobe of the brain, to a part located just behind the ears, in the lower temporal lobe. This physiological pathway is often called the *ventral stream* in virtue of the fact that it proceeds downwards to the infero-temporal region. (Think of the brain as in the shape of a fish: the ventral area is below.) This ventral data-stream accounts for much (though not necessarily all) of what we have been calling *descriptive vision,* the visual capacity for sensory classification.

The processing required for bodily motion occurs in other data-streams, particularly (1) a pathway that flows from the eyes through certain mid-brain (i.e. non-cortical) structures including the superior colliculus (SC), and (2) a cortical stream that diverges from the ventral stream some way downstream of the primary visual cortex and running upwards to the parietal lobe at the top of the head. The latter pathway is entitled the *dorsal stream,* in contrast to the ventral stream, where descriptive processing occurs. *Ex. 1,* in which your eyes moved involuntarily to a salient stimulus before you were able to attribute any features to it probably involves the superior colliculus, which registers changes in the scene and directs attention to the locus of such changes. In *Ex 3*, the initial identification of the target was descriptive: it involved descriptive vision, or the 'ventral stream'. Once the cup was identified and became a target of volitionally initiated manipulation, its coordinates were passed to the dorsal stream which then processed information for bodily motion and orientation. The dorsal stream operates without access to information about descriptive features of this target: once the cup had been identified as the target of manipulation, bodily action on it was guided independently of the blue sensum.

Let us call the action-relevant vision that emerges from these sources *motion-guiding*. (Like 'descriptive vision', 'motion-guiding vision' is a term that takes the functional implications of the above account on board without making a specific commitment to what areas of the brain are involved.) Motion-guiding vision may be pre-attentive and merely orienting as in *Ex 1*, or post-attentive and motion-controlling as in *Ex 3*—as we have seen, different visual systems are involved in these events in different combinations. In both cases, there is at least a phase of the action during which vision operates independently of the descriptive features that are the primary stuff of visual awareness and conscious recall. Motion-guiding vision is characterized (a) by its eponymous function of orienting the body when it is performing motor functions, and (b) by its independence from the feature-processing, i.e. classificatory, parts of vision. The output of motion-guiding vision does not, moreover, have any lasting effect on the system. The link between motion-guiding vision and bodily motion is direct; it is not routed through consciousness. The epistemic parts of the brain are apprised neither of its computations nor of the kind of memory and learning—procedural memory—of which it avails itself.

When one or other of the motion-guiding data-streams are physically damaged, patients show diminished physical action-related abilities.[2] Depending on which area is damaged, their ability to reach out for or handle objects might be impaired, or they might not be able properly to orient their bodies towards visual stimuli, and so on. However, if, in such cases, the ventral stream is spared, their descriptive vision is left more or less intact. In these cases, a subject might retain the ability to describe objects she sees even while displaying a significantly impaired ability to handle these objects. For example, she might be able to *describe* with only a little less than normal accuracy the orientation and distance of a slot into which she is asked to post

---

[2] A good account, with bibliographical information, of the phenomena described in this paragraph and the next can be found in Milner and Goodale (1995), Weiskrantz (1997), and Goodale (2001).

a letter, but still be unable to *perform* this action correctly without painful trial and error—her hand might miss the slot altogether on the first attempt, or hit it at the wrong angle; she might have to readjust by a relatively difficult process of comparing the angles of the letter and the slot and computing a correction.

On the other hand, when the opposite deficit occurs, that is, when the various motion-guiding data-streams are left intact but the ventral stream is damaged, patients lose aspects of descriptive vision, but retain some ability to navigate and move about in the world. Such a patient might be able to pick up an object, though he might be almost completely incapable of describing its shape. Again, the patient might lose the ability to see a particular *kind* of feature: he might become completely colour-blind, or be unable to recognize faces. In an early demonstration of the two different kinds of vision, Gerald Schneider (1969) demonstrated that rats who are able to navigate their environments more or less satisfactorily were nevertheless unable to recognize food as food.

These selective impairments are evidence of visual specialization. In particular, they show that the visual control of motor behaviour occurs, at least to some extent, independently of descriptive vision. The visual processing that accounts for your ability to catch a ball arises at least in part from sources independent of those that underlie your ability to identify it as blue, or as a ball. Now, some investigators are still somewhat sceptical about the observations on brain-damaged patients (Gazzaniga, Fendrich, and Wessinger 1994). In many such cases, the brain areas involved are not cleanly ablated or completely damaged, and they retain some residual capacity. Thus, the conclusions drawn from the evidence are, to some degree, extrapolative, and not absolutely forced by the evidence. Some have sought to diminish the extent and importance of the conclusions drawn above. Instead of attributing the conjunction of spared and retained ability to specialization, some are inclined to say that both are attributable to the fact that a fraction of the brain is intact, while some is damaged. For instance, one might suppose that what happens when losing the ability to catch a ball is that some learning is forgotten as a consequence of the insult to a part of the brain. (The opposite disability is harder to account for: action without awareness.) However, this sort of response is gradually losing credibility as physiological and psychological evidence for multiple visual data-processing streams accumulates.

The evidence supporting specialization is, moreover, supplemented by psychological observations involving normally sighted humans. Some of these consist in handicapping descriptive vision in various ways, for example, by subjecting it to cognitive illusions, such as the size-contrast effects familiar from the Ebbinghaus illusion or the Müller–Lyer diagram (Aglioti, DeSousa, and Goodale 1995; Goodale and Haffenden 1998). (We shall return to these illusions in a moment.) These illusions are produced by descriptive vision, and it has been found that motion-guiding vision is largely (though not always entirely) unaffected by such temporary handicaps. Another strategy is to explore dissociations of descriptive and visual-motor ability in normally sighted subjects. In one experiment, subjects were told that a small light would suddenly appear in the periphery of their visual fields, and instructed to reach for it when it did. While they were reaching for the light, it was displaced. The light was moved during an eye-saccade: since they were looking in a different direction, the subjects did not see it move. When they looked again, the light was at a new position. Subjects failed to notice the shift, *but were able to reach for the shifting light smoothly* (Goodale, Pélisson, and Prablanc 1986). It seems clear that information regarding the shift was available to the hand, as it were, through dorsal stream processing (which is less dependent on the target being fixated on the fovea), but failed to register in whatever part of the brain is responsible for reporting such happenings to conscious visual awareness. Thus, it supports the idea that what seems introspectively to be a smoothly integrated ability to notice and report visual stimuli and to act appropriately on the information revealed by these stimuli actually arises from a fragmented process with several independent components.

Such experiments argue for the partition of cognitive function amongst the various streams: descriptive and motion-guiding vision are somewhat independent of one another, even though there is cross-communication. This specialization seems to go with a distinction in terms of the form of representation that emerges from each stream. Motion-guiding vision is involved in controlling our limbs, and to subserve this function, it seems to locate objects in space in *agent-centred* terms.[3] It is directly concerned with bodily orientation with respect to environmental objects, reach, grasping, and the physical manipulation of objects. It therefore represents objects in terms of their distances and angles relativized to parts of the body such as the head, the eye, or the hand. These representations of spatial relationships change as we move: whenever our hands or our heads change position or attitude, these representations have to be updated. They have no lasting significance for two reasons. First, the hand does not need to remember where it was a moment ago; how it gets to its target depends wholly on where it is *now*. Secondly, agent-centred spatial information has no epistemic significance. For precisely

---

[3] This hypothesis is due to Melvyn Goodale and David Milner (1992); until recently, it was more standard to suppose that the dorsal stream computes spatial relations as such—it is often called the 'where' channel, contrasting with the 'what' channel constituted by the ventral stream (see Ungerleider and Mishkin 1982 and Ungerleider and Haxby 1994). The Goodale–Milner view has gained strength in the last few years. One of its great advantages is that it allows for ventral-stream representations of spatial information. However, it is not clear how, for the purposes of cross-talk, the object-centred coordinates of the dorsal stream get converted into the agent-centred coordinates of the ventral stream and vice versa.

the reason that it relates objects to the perceiver, it does not provide information about these objects in themselves, and are unsuitable for being filed away in object representation files. For these reasons, they are not stored in the memory system that is connected to descriptive vision and epistemic facilities, i.e. memory that facilitates conscious recall (Goodale and Haffenden 1995; Goodale 2001). Consequently, motion-guiding vision cannot be used for the purposes of comparing two objects, whether these are seen at the same or at different times.

Descriptive vision, on the other hand, is connected with *scene-centred* representations of the world: it makes us aware of qualities that objects possess independently of perceivers—this includes relations of one object to another. The spatial relations that enter into ventral-stream transactions are perspectively influenced but still object-centred: they organize seen objects into a three-dimensional representational array in which each is related to the others in ways that roughly instantiate the laws of Euclidean geometry. These spatial relations are presented in a way that does not make them a matter of reach or availability to the grasp of our fingers or hands. Ventral-stream representations do not change radically when we shift our own positions or move our limbs, because they inform us about the interrelations of seen objects, not merely the relations in which they stand to us. Even when we walk around a pair of objects, and left becomes right and right left, or walk towards them and far becomes near, the continuity is maintained, and no incoherence results. We know instinctively which object file should receive information about which object. These spatial representations are suitable for storage in the memory of conscious recall, and for the use of general terms.

II. Seeing Objects Non-Descriptively

Motion-guiding vision is a collection of somewhat independent visual data-streams that make it possible for us to perform actions like picking up a fork, posting a letter, avoiding obstacles, and catching a ball. Most scientists say that it does not contribute to sensory consciousness. This is not exactly correct. What is true is that it does not provide us with a certain kind of datum: that is, it does not classify visual stimuli, or give us the means by which to compare or differentiate visual stimuli. Consequently, motion-guiding vision does not provide us with the kind of conscious visual datum that we get from descriptive vision. However, motion-guiding vision furnishes us with the capacity to come into contact with and physically manipulate physical objects. The attention-securing events described in section I above constitute a kind of demonstrative reference to visual stimuli—a connection between the visual system and a stimulus that supports physical manipulation or interaction, and does not depend on the attribution of descriptive visual features to it. The result of this connection established by motion-guiding vision is, as we shall find in the following section, that these objects acquire a feeling of *presence*. Predictably enough, this feeling of presence is, as it were, inarticulate: that is, it supplements, but does not provide, awareness of the objects' features. Nevertheless, it makes a difference to the quality of one's visual awareness of an object.

John Campbell (2002, ch. 3) gives a good account of this kind of connection between visual system and stimulus. He suggests that visual attention is a largely non-descriptive facility for singling out objects for physical manipulation and visual description, and strongly resists the traditional idea that conscious visual processing of descriptive data is required for reference. One part of his apparatus, however, is potentially a source of misunderstanding concerning the role of descriptive elements in visual reference to objects. For he thinks that Gestalt principles of grouping are part of what allows us to use perceptual demonstratives.

The Gestalt organization of the visual field, when you are consciously attending to the object, must also play a role, since different objects can be close together, and there must be a way in which the subject can decide to verify visually a proposition about one rather than another of those objects, and it must be possible for the subject to decide to act on one rather than another of those objects. (89)

This argument is undoubtedly correct. In order to single out a spatially extended object like a door-handle or mail-box slot, I must group its elements together and distinguish them from those of other objects that visually abut it. Something like Gestalt organization is necessary to accomplish this. Thus, in order to make a decision to act on some object in your visual field, for example the blue cup in *Ex. 3*, you must have grouped its elements together into a coherent shape.

It might be thought that the same point must apply to visually guided motion. (I do not mean to suggest that Campbell thinks this himself.) You might think that in order to grasp and manipulate an extended object, I *must* group its elements together into a single coherent whole. Suppose that I am about to open a door. I identify the handle and reach out to turn it, forming my hand to conform to the shape of the handle, and making contact with it smoothly. My shaping my grip to match the handle seems to presuppose that motion-guiding vision possesses and employs information about the gross contour of the object. I want now to argue that this is wrong. There is no need to build Gestalt grouping into the kind of visual contact with an external stimulus that supports physical interaction. Motion-guiding vision does not demand even this much descriptive information. It is, as one might say, purely deictic.

To see how motion-guiding vision can do without shape information, let us consider first more simple ways of acting on a distant object, and consider how these simpler ways can be elaborated to yield something like the sophisticated dexterity of humans. Consider a bird spearing a fish. We may suppose that, parallel to *Ex 3* above, this bodily action is executed in three stages:

1. Descriptive identification of target. The bird identifies a certain object as a fish. (It does not lunge at rocks.) At this stage, all of its capacities for visual perception are called into play. Not just Gestalt organization, but object features are needed here. Recall that it is the *blue cup* that you reach for in *Ex. 3*. You needed to identify it as such in order to match object with invitation.

2. Formulation of action-plan. This stage is at least partially non-perceptual: it does build on the previous stage because the action that is planned has specific reference to the object there identified, but is subject to various contingencies of context. You don't hold the cup in your palm, but in your fingers, since the latter is easier for the person pouring coffee. The bird, similarly, has to get into appropriate position to spear the fish.

3. Lunging at target. Once the bird has 'decided' to go for a particular fish, motion-guiding vision takes over and guides the beak to the target. Note that since the beak is closed, and the tip of the beak is effectively a one-dimensional point, no shape information or Gestalt organization is required for this action. Reference is made to a single point on the body of the fish, and that is all that is needed.

In this sequence, motion-guiding vision comes into play only at stage 3; it requires no descriptive data such as that which feeds into Gestalt organization.

Now imagine a slightly more complicated task. The bird wants to eat the fish it has just caught. Now, it is dealing with a three-dimensional target, not a mere point. The bird opens its mouth; the aperture of the mouth can be assumed to covary with target size, though it will likely be larger; the head is 'launched' towards the fish. Now comes the analogue of stage 3: motion-guiding vision takes over and executes the closing of the beak around the fish. Here, you might think, it needs to estimate the size of the target, since it must close its beak around the fish with appropriate force. This is just what we need to deny because we are trying to show that the motion-guiding system is purely *deictic*, i.e. makes reference to an object relative to the perceiver's own body *without intermediary descriptive information*. Giving this system shape-information means that something entirely new has to be added to it relative to what is needed for the spearing function: Gestalt organization and size-estimation would have to be added to and integrated with motion-guiding vision in order to make *biting* possible. But without size-estimation, how are we to account for the accuracy of grasp?

Fortunately, there is an alternative to size-estimation. Instead of assuming that the whole beak aperture needs to match the target at the point when the mouth closes around the fish, we can suppose that in the final stages of

Lunging, each part of the open beak, the top part and the bottom part, are *separately* guided to different spots on the surface of the fish. Like spearing, this does not require size-estimation; it simply requires *two* guidance mechanisms similar in informational and computational structure to that which we imagined to be involved in the simpler case of spearing. Each carries a *part* of the beak to a point.

This, one would think, is analogous to how human grip control develops. Humans are capable of many different kinds of grip. It appears that, as with the bird, descriptive information that might be used for a rough estimate of grip type and size is transferable from the *Descriptive identification* phase. Estimates of distance necessary for *reaching* for an object, information concerning the nature of the object, and the action to be performed on it all inform the action-plan. This information too is available in the first phase of the execution-schema above. By contrast, hand and finger flexion occur relatively late in the performance of reaching-and-manipulating tasks; the neurons that control these movements only come into play after the grip has been chosen. In a precision grip, the kind of grip used when we pick up a grain of rice, the fingers close around the target well after the *Lunging* phase has been launched, when motion-guiding vision is in control. No whole-object size or shape information is needed for this. Once the hand gets near the object, each finger can be individually guided to a different spot on the surface of the object.

Evolutionary considerations support this conjecture. Finger-control is a recent add-on. Going down the phylogenetic tree, it is only in apes that we find individual control of fingers. Human digital dexterity is unparalleled among contemporary species, and developed only 1.8 million years ago in *pananthropus robustus* (Jeannerod 1998, 32). This late development would not have been feasible in evolutionary terms if it demanded a complete reorganization of motion-guiding vision, which is very ancient. The conjecture of individual finger guidance makes such re-engineering unnecessary.

Of course, the suggestion being made here is speculative. It seems reasonably well-established, however, that grip type, size, and force are determined early in a reach-and-manipulate task, and that hand and finger flexion occur in the later stages. Since these later stages are under the guidance of motion-guiding vision later, it seems plausible to suppose that whole-shape information is used only in the first two stages of action outlined above. There is some empirical evidence in support of the conjecture. For there are preliminary indications that while descriptive vision estimates shapes 'holistically', motion-guiding vision is sensitive to the action-relevant dimension only (Ganel and Goodale 2003)—when one picks up an ellipsoid by one axis, motion-guiding vision does not seem to have information about the size of other axes. This is exactly what one would expect if the hypothesis on offer were correct. For the fingers to close around an object under individual guidance, no information is needed concerning the object-dimensions in directions other than those in which the fingers operate.

The conclusion that I wish to draw from this discussion is that there is in motion-guiding vision a wholly or largely non-descriptive reference to parts of material objects, a *deictic* element akin to ostension in language. Campbell (2003) posits a similar connection, and locates it in *conscious attention to an object*. His suggestion can be made compatible with mine if what he calls 'conscious attention' includes not only the identification of an object in the first two stages of physical action, but also the connection in phase 3 which makes physical manipulation possible. It is, in any case, the latter which is non-descriptive and deictic in character.

Motion-guiding vision gives me access to the cup of coffee that I lift to my lips. It locates the cup relative to my hand and my mouth independently of the visual system that gives me information about its more permanent visual qualities. I will now argue that motion-guiding vision is responsible for the inarticulate feeling of presence that we feel when we are visually conscious of three-dimensional objects. Visual scientists usually hold that motion-guiding vision contributes nothing to visual consciousness—that 'vision is more than seeing' as Goodale (2001) puts it. Without contesting that vision is indeed more than seeing, I want to insist that there is more to conscious vision, 'seeing', than descriptive vision provides.

III. Vision and the Feeling of Presence[4]

What would seeing—conscious vision—be like if we *lacked* motion-guiding vision? We have a partial answer in the following observation: we would not see things as an arm's length away, hurtling towards ourselves, or 'head-turning' (as the passing cyclist in *Ex. 1* was). We would, of course, continue to see things as three feet away or as moving in a trajectory that will soon intersect with our own. But these descriptive attributes would possess little ergonomic significance (aside from epistemic significance). I might classify an object as 'Three feet away, which is roughly as far as I can reach', but though this kind of description would help me *think* about and *verbally describe* spatial relations in my immediate vicinity, it is not in the limb-centred form that would help me control my bodily parts while reaching out to the thing. Conversely, there would be no exact phenomenological equivalent of 'hurtling towards one'. One often sees something as describing a trajectory that will soon intersect with one's own.

---

[4] The following discussion of pictorial seeing derives from a talk, 'How Real Do Pictures Look?' given at a number of universities. Numerous people made helpful points while discussing these papers: I particularly remember Alastair Macleod, Colin Macleod, and Steven Stich. I am grateful to Vincent Bergeron and Dustin Stokes for probing and insistent questions which forced fundamental changes, and to Dom Lopes for excellent advice at an early stage of my thinking about these matters.

Imagine seeing that but experiencing no urgent impulse to duck. That is what it would be like to lack motion-guiding vision.

There is more. For as I shall now argue, our visual states present us with an *assembled* message, a message that has a descriptive element as well as a referential one. Motion-guiding vision is responsible for the latter. This referential element of visual states constitutes a kind of direct connection between perceiver and distal stimulus, and creates a feeling of reality of presence. Consider a singular proposition: 'John is tall'. This proposition can be entertained without being asserted. Similarly, a visual scene can be imagined or dreamed. In normal visual perception, however, the scene is not simply imaged, but seems to present the perceiver's own surroundings as so. I will refer to this as a 'feeling of presence'. The feeling of presence is similar to assertion: attached to a visual scene, the feeling of presence asserts it, so to speak—it makes one feel that the scene being described is present.

Now, the way that a scene gets 'asserted' by vision is different from how a proposition gets asserted in linguistic communication. I'll say what I take to be the difference first without any argument.

We normally think of asserting a proposition as an operation performed on the whole content. This operation can be represented as follows:

ASSERTED: John is tall.

The 'assertion' operation acts on the whole proposition, 'John is tall', distinguishing it from the same proposition merely entertained. I want to argue that in perception, a similar effect is achieved by a deictic sign or demonstrative.

Consider:

[THAT] is tall.

A deictic such as the above is *not* normally enough to mark off an asserted proposition. It is perfectly possible to ostend an object and entertain the thought that it is different in some way than it actually is. I think of my daughter. She is often late. I wish that she would arrive for dinner at the pre-arranged time. In so wishing, I am, as it were, peeling a descriptive predicate off a particular person—i.e. I am peeling the actual lateness off her—*while still thinking about **her***. (This is what makes it different from wishing merely that I had a punctual daughter.) Thus:

$[x = \text{Sheila}]$: I wish x were punctual.

Clearly, the deictic does not ensure assertion in this case: I am not asserting that my daughter is punctual; on the contrary, I *wish* that she were.

In perception, by contrast, the deictic operator that purports to put a perceiver directly in contact with a distal object *cannot normally be exercised except in visual states that are produced by actually looking at something.*

It is impossible to exercise such a deictic operation in mere visual imagining—
or so it will be argued. I look at my sofa: it is black. Thus:

$[x = \text{That}]$: x is black.

Now, I can try to peel the descriptive feature, *black*, off the sofa. Thus, I can
try to entertain a visual image of the sofa in blue. However, as I shall be arguing, this new state of visual imagining would not contain the deictic element.
Only visual states produced by actually *looking* contain deixis; visual imaging
does not. So in trying to peel the visual feature off the sofa, I lose the deictic
element produced by looking at it. The visual image I entertain would not
therefore be about *that* sofa, but only about a sofa that looks the same in
other respects. I can *think* about this particular sofa being blue, much as
I think of my daughter (she herself) being punctual. But I cannot visually
imagine this very sofa looking other than it does; visual images do not link
(with a few exceptions to be noted later) to particular objects. (This might
sound counter-intuitive: remember that the argument supporting this claim
is still to come.)

  Visual states produced by *looking* have an implied assertion operator—they
convey to us an act of sensory classification performed by the visual system
on an object that is present. By contrast, visual states produced by visual
imaging have no such operator. However, states produced by looking can be
descriptively the same as states of visual imagining; that is, they may present
the same visual features in the same places. Clearly, then, the assertion
operator in visual states produced by looking—the feeling of presence—is
not to be traced to any descriptive difference. The proposal being made here
is that the assertion operator is to be traced to the deictic element in visual
states produced by looking. This deictic element explains why looking at
the sofa gives me the feeling (correct or mistaken) of dealing with something
present which looks *so*, while visual imagining does not. *This*, I claim, is the
element of 'vivacity' by which Hume differentiated impressions from mere
ideas. (I am grateful to Ori Simchen for helpful discussion of the above.)

  Crucially, my claim is that visual deixis is provided by motion-guiding vision,
while the visual features attributed to ostended objects is provided by descriptive vision. It is in this sense that I claim that visual states are *assembled*.

IV. What is it Like to View an Object Non-Referentially?

Let us embark now on an argument to support the claims just made. The
argument depends on the existence of a kind of seeing—*seeing in pictures*
(cf. Wollheim 1973)—which, in unimpaired humans, forces motion-guiding
vision and descriptive vision apart. A consideration of this kind of seeing
will help us understand the sensuous force of visual deixis where merely intro-
specting the content of everyday visual states does not.

Pictorial vision is 'dual', or 'twofold' as Dominic Lopes (1996) puts it. When we look at a picture, we see

(a) The picture itself. Generally, it is a surface on which coloured dyes have been applied by a painter or by some photochemical or electronic process, or on which coloured light is projected. Vision enables us to describe this surface, its size and position, its texture and colour, and so on. This surface belongs to a manipulable object: it is at a certain distance from ourselves, and we can move towards it, or reach out to touch it. Thus, with respect to looking at the picture itself—the 'picture-as-object,'—both descriptive and motion-guiding vision are engaged, just as it is with any other three-dimensional visual object.

When we look at a picture, we also see

(b) The thing it depicts. We see this thing, as I shall say, *in the picture* (as contrasted both with seeing the picture itself, as an object, and also with seeing the thing in reality). That is, we are, with regard to the object in the picture, in something like the same visual state as we would be if we were looking at the thing itself.

Now, it is clear that seeing in pictures is *not* a straightforwardly sensory phenomenon with regard to the entire range of things that are depicted. Monet depicts the straw hats worn by a distant boater with just a squiggle of white. More than likely, he has not caused in the viewer *just* the visual qualia that would have been created by a boater in a straw hat at that distance. More likely, he has created visual qualia that the viewer is able to interpret as a depiction of a straw hat, given a certain amount of background knowledge. I want to concentrate here on the very simple sense-features that can be seen *in* a picture just as a matter of seeing, and with no background knowledge. In particular, I would like to concentrate on simple spatial qualities and relations such as occlusion, distance, orientation, shape, and comparative size. In recent studies, Jan Koenderink and Andrea van Doorn (2003) superimposed on pictures of a nude female torso (a subject chosen for its undulating surface) a manipulable gauge figure under the control of an observer. They asked observers to adjust this gauge figure so that 'clings to the pictorial surface'. These subjects found it easy to 'establish a fit in picto-rial space'; the experimenters were then able to read depicted tilt and slant off the adjusted gauge figure. There was, of course, no tilt or slant in the surface of the picture itself: it is the depicted nude torso whose surface displays a mix of angles. Thus, it can be argued, indeed it seems quite clear, that with respect to these simple spatial qualities, a picture *can* put you in visual states recognizably like those caused by the real thing. (I am grateful to Dustin Stokes for making me restrict my claim about seeing in pictures to simple descriptive features.)

Seeing in pictures engages descriptive vision. This is why we can learn about a thing by looking at an accurate pictorial depiction. From the famous self-portrait of Rembrandt in the National Gallery of Art in Washington, DC, we learn that he had, in middle age, a fleshy anxious face, big eyes and nose, wispy moustache, double chin, thick neck. (At least we learn that the person Rembrandt imagined had these features.) These features of Rembrandt are not just *inferred* from features of the self-portrait, or assembled in the way that they could have been from a verbal description such as the one offered above. There is, in the experience of looking at the picture, *some* component that resembles the experience we would have had if we had looked at Rembrandt directly—the claim is that certain spatial properties and relations are presented this way. From this component we learn about his appearance in much the same way looking at the picture as we would have looking at *him*. In particular, the three-dimensional features of the face are portrayed by creating visual cues in the two-dimensional surface of the picture that mimic three dimensionality. This is the phenomenon I am referring to when I say that we see these spatial qualities *in* the picture.

Now, if seeing three-dimensional qualities in a picture is so much like seeing them in real life, how do we know that the picture is actually two-dimensional, not three-dimensional? In standard cases, we are not fooled by a picture: we know that what we see in the picture is not actually there. This means that the experience of seeing an object in a picture, even the experience of the spatial qualities we are talking about, must be saliently different from that of seeing it in real life. What is this difference? What in the phenomenology of vision corresponds to the two kinds of seeing involved when we look at a picture? This question is usually discussed in terms of descriptive vision alone—psychologists ask what descriptive features enable us both to see the thing in the picture and to see it as merely depicted.

This standard answer goes something like this. Pictorial vision is twofold because, in addition to the visual cues naturally provided by the picture itself—the texture of the canvas, the reflections off the photograph, etc.—the marks made on its surface give us visual cues similar to those the depicted object would have given us if it had been present. These additional cues account for the second thing we see, the thing in the picture. Now, the two things that we see when we look at a picture are visually very different from one another, and so the descriptive cues they provide are in conflict. Most saliently, the picture of Rembrandt is flat, and Rembrandt himself is three dimensional. Descriptive vision detects both the flatness cues given us by the picture, and the depth cues created by the artist in order to depict the man.[5]

---

[5] Lopes (1996, ch. 2) and Miller (1999) have relevant discussions. Miller shows that the effect of some illusions, such as the Ponzo illusion, is reduced when they are inserted into a pictorial context.

These contradictory cues seem to be segregated; they lead to two different visual representations that exist side-by-side, though they cannot be attended to simultaneously. Sometimes, the visual cues that emanate from the two representations interfere with one another. For instance, in another famous painting by Rembrandt, the man depicted in 'The Artist in His Studio' looks very short, this despite the fact that the picture is drawn in classic perspective. Painters usually compensate for two-foldness when they want their subject to look the right size and in this particular picture, Rembrandt, for whatever reason, has not done this. Similarly, lines that converge to a perspectival vanishing point look one length qua lines on the surface of the picture, another length viewed three dimensionally, and this may cause distorted relations of size. (This is the Ponzo illusion.) At other times, there is no cross-interference, but the fact that things can be seen in two different ways, as representers and things represented, is in itself unusual. This simultaneous possibility of distinct visual representations in the act of looking at a picture is a distinctive feature of pictorial seeing. Or to put it in another way: it is distinctive of pictures among objects of vision that they provide cues that lead to two different representations. Because of this, the thing depicted cannot, it seems, be seen in exactly the same way as it is in real life.

This is the standard account of the duality of pictorial seeing, though as Dominic Lopes (1996, ch. 2) argues, the difference it points to is not absolute. In the case of *trompe-l'oeil* pictures, pictures in which flatness cues are masked or diminished at certain angles by extremely salient depth cues, the three-dimensional effect can be startling. If the duality of pictorial seeing derived entirely from the two kinds of descriptive cue that pictures offer us, and if one of these kinds of seeing (i.e. seeing the picture itself) is suppressed in an exercise of *trompe-l'oeil*, then the latter ought to approach real-life seeing. But this is not what happens. The three-dimensional effect of *trompe-l'oeil* technique may be startling (and this is what it makes it a '*trompe*'), but in many situations we continue to see them as pictures. There is something more here that needs to be explained. (I'll return to *trompe-l'oeil* later.)

What about motion-guiding vision? The picture-as-object engages motion-guiding vision, and consequently we are able to grasp it, adjust it, move it. By contrast, the thing depicted does *not* engage this visual system. This difference, I shall argue, is crucial to the phenomenology of seeing objects in pictures. More importantly for our present purposes, it reveals a crucial feature of real-life seeing.

That the depicted thing fails to engage motion-guiding vision is suggested by some interesting recent experiments making use of the kinds of visual illusions that artists use to convey the impression of depth. These illusions involve configurations of lines that also occur in projections of three-dimensional scenes: while viewing the latter, these configurations lead to accurate estimates of depth. The two-dimensional counterparts create 'illusions' of orientation,

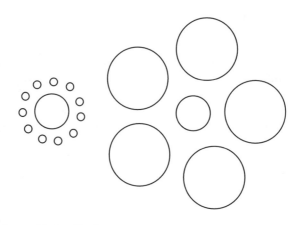

FIG. 13 Titchener Circles Illusion.

size, and depth. (The precise explanation of these illusions is controversial. It is often said that estimates of nearness and depth interact with apparent size to produce a composite impression of actual size at a distance, but this is almost certainly too simple with respect to the flat figure: see Gillam 1998.) The Titchener circles illusion consists of two equal-size circles, one surrounded by an annulus of larger circles, the other by one of smaller circles (Fig. 13). The circle surrounded by smaller circles looks bigger; in order to make the two circles look equal, this circle needs to be reduced in size. The experiment consisted in recreating the Titchener circles illusion with flat poker-chip type discs positioned in front of a normally sighted observer. All observers *saw* the central discs in the illusory way, but in reaching for them (see Fig. 14), their grip was scaled according to the actual size of the disc (Aglioti, DeSousa, and Goodale 1995).

These illusions correspond to pictorial devices that artists use to convey the impression of depth. If one were going to depict two equal-size objects one further away than the other, one might do so by scaling the two objects in relation to surrounding objects—the scaling instanced in the illusion is characteristic of *unequal* objects. In the psychological experiment, the perceptual impression of disc size is correlated to how observers would perceive it in a picture. The fact that grip size was correlated to the actual size of the discs, rather than their illusory size, shows that the visual system guiding the hand did not respond to the size-contrast illusion. According to Melvyn Goodale and Keith Humphrey (1998), these results are replicable with other illusions used to convey depth and size in pictures (e.g. the Müller-Lyer and Ponzo illusions). Motion-guiding vision is impervious to the very visual effects that help us to see depicted objects, i.e. objects in pictures.

What happens when size-contrast illusions are embedded in the depiction of a three-dimensional scene? It depends on how the observer is looking

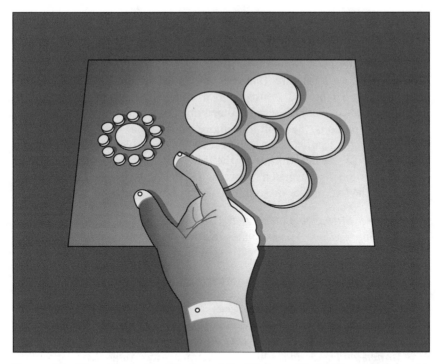

FIG. 14 The Three-dimensional Version of the Titchener Circles Illusion (the hand is not fooled).

Source: Adapted from Aglioti et al. (1995) with the authors' permission.

at the picture. If she is looking at the picture itself, then the situation is no different from the above. Attending to the surface of the picture alone, an embedded size-contrast illusion will have much the same effect as in the simple flat display. When the observer is attending to the *depicted* scene, however, things are different. In this context, the very relations that in the non-pictorial case contributed to a size-contrast illusion, now contribute to the perception of depth within the depicted scene. Thus, these relations change their meaning. However, when one reaches to the picture in order to touch the figures, motion-guiding vision reacts to the lines themselves, not to what they depict. That is, it will reach or grasp in ways appropriate to that part of the drawing which represents the object, but not in ways appropriate to the depicted object. When, for instance, a ball is represented as a coloured ovoid itself, a normal viewer will instinctively be able to make reaching and grasping motions appropriate to that ovoid itself, but not those appropriate to the ball depicted. Even if instructed: 'Pick up the *ball*' she will not be able to do the right sort of thing. At the same time, she will be able to describe the depicted ball accurately. (The hand can *learn* to use descriptive vision for physical manipulation by trial and error: this is illustrated by the acquired ability of microsurgeons who operate on internal organs using images projected on a television monitor, by mimes, and by technicians who handle dangerous materials remotely with robotic arms.)

Consider now a picture that employs some size-contrast illusion to engender the perspectival sense of two equal-sized spheres A and B at different distances from the viewer. When one looks at the figures themselves, i.e. not as depictions, they will look more nearly equal than they really are. However, when one attends to the objects *in the picture*, one forms an impression of relative size appropriate to the things that are depicted. Thus, there is a dissociation or mismatch between the deliverances of the two visual systems in the two modes of seeing. This can be schematized as follows:

Observer attends to picture itself
Descriptive vision: Mis-estimates relative size of elements A and B.
Motion-guiding vision: Correctly estimates relative size of A and B.

The two systems contradict one another with respect to A and B.

Observer attends to depicted scene
Descriptive vision: Correctly estimates relative size *and three-dimensional spatial relations* amongst objects *depicted by A and B.*
Motion-guiding vision: Offers no estimate regarding depicted objects but correctly estimates relative size of the figures on the surface of the picture (as before).

The two systems do not contradict one another since they are here engaged with different tasks. With respect to the depicted scene, then, the information concerning the depicted object is simply *unaccompanied* by any parallel message from motion-guiding vision. In pictures, you see depth through only one system; whereas in real life you get information about depth from both.

Return then to the example of Rembrandt's self-portrait. The thing depicted, Rembrandt, cannot be touched or moved by virtue of the seeing afforded us by this picture of him: more relevantly, we cannot move our hands *as if* we were dealing with this depicted object. The picture itself engages feature-attributing as well as motion-guiding vision. The thing it depicts, when we see it in the picture, engages only feature-attributing vision. We see its descriptive features though we lack motion-guiding vision of it. My claim amounts to this: when normally sighted individuals see things in pictures they replicate some aspects of the real-life vision of patients afflicted with *optic ataxia*, a condition in which, because of lesions to the parietal lobe (i.e. to the dorsal stream), objects are seen as they normally are in conscious vision, but cannot be handled appropriately. (I am grateful to Vincent Bergeron for forcing me to clarify my line of thought here.)

Let's summarize the argument up to this point. Pictures evoke in us an awareness of the same descriptive visual features of objects as real-life scenes—features that we use for epistemic purposes. From a feature-attribution point of view, many things that can be seen in real life can also be seen in a picture, and *in the same way*: When we look at a picture, this kind of input accounts for why we construct a three-dimensional representation of the depicted object side-by-side with one of the picture itself. What then is the phenomenological difference between a 'hyper-realist' picture and real life? The standard story appeals to the flatness cues that pictures provide. However, the engagement of motion-guiding vision is another important difference. We have just seen that though we are able accurately to report on the visual features of depicted objects, we are unable to make appropriate bodily motions with respect to them. This difference entails that we do not have agent-centred experiences of depicted things. When we see a thing in a picture, we cannot visually locate it in ways that guide bodily motion with respect to it.

Motion-guiding vision sends its output directly to parts of the body. Psychologists often conclude that this output never reaches consciousness. I have been arguing that this is not correct. It is true that descriptive vision gives us experiential qualia concerning descriptive features, and motion-guiding vision does not do this. Nevertheless, the absence of motor affordances affects how we experience a scene with which motor-guiding vision is uninvolved. Now, what holds of pictures holds equally of visually imagined scenes. Visual imagination consists of an activation of the ventral stream: this is how we recreate in ourselves the experience of sense-features when we are not looking at anything. Visual images are not, therefore, accompanied by motion-guiding information. As I shall argue in the following section, this entails that deixis does not occur with respect to depicted scenes. It also does not occur within mental images. Visual deixis is, as we argued in the previous section, crucial to the feeling of presence in our visual experience of real things. Motion-guiding vision is implicated in the feeling of presence.

V. Locating Pictured Objects

Motion-guiding vision places an object of sight into a set of spatial relations used for the control of the perceiver's own limbs. Consequently, it locates the object relative to the viewer herself, automatically updating the location of the object in these terms as she or her limbs move. Motion-guiding vision computes locational information in a characteristic *form*, but the actual information it presents overlaps with that which descriptive vision provides. This is particularly true of spatial information. Looking at myself in the mirror while picking something up, I can see my hand moving towards another object. This is information about my own body, but it is presented in object-centred coordinates, just as information about somebody else's body would be.

My hand, however, is being guided by information that is presented in a different form. As noted earlier, it is not easy to use information in the form available from the mirror to guide my hand—you can verify this by trying to follow instructions concerning an unfamiliar task while obstructing the direct visual path to your hand, and using the mirror image instead.

I possess descriptive vision concerning my own limbs. I can look at them, examine them, even notice them. But the channel that provides me with information in this form is not the one that directly provides guidance to my limbs as I move them. Suppose that I am trimming my finger-nails. I notice that the nail of my left index-finger is too long, and decide to clip it. So far, I have been using information provided to me by descriptive vision, and in the form characteristic of that system. What I have seen so far is precisely comparable to my noticing that *your* nail is too long. As I begin to move my other hand to clip the over-long nail, motion-guiding vision takes over. The hand is guided by information about where the target is relative to itself; as it moves towards the target, the information continues to place it at the 'origin' of the system—at point zero—with the target taking on continually changing coordinates in this system of coordinates. Motion-guiding vision treats my active hand as privileged in this case, since it computes spatial coordinates relative to it, but the target hand has no such privilege. For the purposes of executing this action, motion-guiding vision treats it much as if it were somebody else's.

In the classical paradigm, sensation affords us conscious awareness of the retinal image. This image is, in a sense, egocentric: the perceiver is, as it were, in a fixed position relative to the scene thus presented. So one might think that motion-guiding vision is providing the limbs with a visual image very much as the classical empiricists imagined it to be. This would not be quite correct. The analogy leaves out the movement of the eye itself. The eye scans the scene, and as it does so, the image of one and the same object will move about on the retina; for instance, as my eye rotates in its socket, the image of the keyboard in front of me will move from the right to the left of both retinae. So if my hands are to be reliably guided, the movement of the eye has to be discounted: the image has to be stabilized in this manner at least. The authors of the classical paradigm did not recognize this; presumably, they did not know of the constant unconscious movement of the eyes. Also the classical paradigm assumed that visual sensation provides the perceiver with a two-dimensional image, whereas the ventral stream, at least (though not the superior colliculus) operates with three-dimensional representations. But in one way, the information that motion-guiding vision provides to the limbs *is* as described by the classical paradigm. As far as motion-guiding vision is concerned, the perceiver is always at the origin of the coordinate system, always in the zero-position.

Now, descriptive vision affords you with object-centred representations. When you walk around two objects, their left–right orientation reverses, but they do not seem to move: as you move around them, and look at them from the other side, you receive information about their relative position that does not have to be laboriously decoded—as mirror image information often does. It can be smoothly filed away in the correct object files without the need for translation into some other form. This shows that the 'left–right' aspect of visual awareness is a relatively superficial characteristic. When you look at something in real life you receive two 'files' of spatial information about it, one of these files contains information about its location relative to you: thus, you are able to cross-index descriptive information with information presented in egocentric coordinates and locate things relative to you.

The point about pictures is that since the spatial and temporal relations depicted in them come only in object-centred form, they are generally disconnected from one's own—that is, a picture gives you no information of location relative to yourself. Suppose you are looking at a picture of two men shaking hands. *Where* are they? As far as what you can tell by seeing in the picture, the question has no answer. The space *within* the picture is connected, as any good three-dimensional space should be: since the two men are shaking hands, they are spatially connected to one another in quite determinate ways. But their spatial relations are visually represented in object-centred, not viewer-centred coordinates. As a consequence, you, the viewer, are not, so to speak, in the picture. Where are the men *in relation to you*? Of course, you know where the *picture* is. It's right in front of you, where it can be grabbed or pushed; at least, it is clearly spatially related to things that can be so handled. That's how it is with the picture itself: you can pick it up, adjust the way it hangs on the wall, brush a speck of dust off it, clean it—clearly you know where it is relative to you. I can't, without practice and training, do any of these things with depicted things: indeed, it is difficult even to *pretend* to do so, or at least not convincingly to an observer. Without the hard-gained skill of an accomplished mime, one cannot smoothly reach out to the self-portrait and grab the depicted nose (in pretence), making the correct movements of your hands. Descriptive vision offers you an epistemic, but not a motor, affordance.

The availability of agent-centred spatial relations creates a *feeling* of presence in real-life seeing which is missing when we see things in pictures. Of course, this feeling can be mistaken. Holographic images can engage motion-guiding vision: they can provide you with an deictic element, and consequently an 'asserted' visual image, though the deixis refers to nothing and the assertion is false. But then seeing a hologram is not (phenomenologically) like seeing in a picture—it is more like seeing in real life. What I am suggesting is that the feeling of presence in real-life seeing is a product of seeing objects as *ready to hand* (to misappropriate a phrase of Heidegger's). The feeling is not inferred from visual sensation; it is not acquired by a reasoned judgement about the reality of certain objects of sight. Moreover, it is not the consequence solely of descriptive differences between the pictured object and the real thing. It is, at least in part, a phenomenological consequence of motion-guiding vision, vision mediated by the dorsal stream. Mark this distinction: phenomenological but not descriptive. There is something in perceptual experience that relates the perceiver to a particular object. This something is not, however, a feature that this object shares with others. Rather it is the feeling that one is, as Alva Noë and Kevin O'Regan (2002) put it, 'perceptually coupled' to the object. This feeling cannot be duplicated in imagination: it is not stored in memory. Mere visual images do not incorporate the feeling of presence.

Of course, you may sometimes be subject to the illusion that the pictured space connects to your own. *Schippol 1994* is a large photograph by Andreas Gursky: it depicts the Amsterdam airfield with its taxiways, runways, etc., as seen from within the terminal through the huge glass pane of a concourse. Now, the oddity of this photograph is that every bit of it is in sharp focus. The bottom edge of the photograph depicts the floor of terminal concourse: standing close to the photograph you can look down at this, and then shift your gaze up at the green open spaces of the airfield outside, still in focus. Thus you replicate the act of scanning as it would occur if you were there in that concourse at Schippol. Though there is some phenomenological oddity in being able to accomplish this without simultaneously changing the focus or binocular disparity of your eyes, Gursky's photograph (or rather the large format print) creates the illusion of being there at the airport, in a way that a normally focused small-sized photograph could not have done. (Call up the photograph on the Internet and the effect is absent.) This is one of the things *trompe-l'oeil* technique has to do: elide the disconnection between the space in which the viewer stands and the space of the depicted objects.

In the normal case of looking at a picture, there is a disconnection. Your space stops just where the space of depicted objects begins. The picture is *there*, right in front of you, but the men it depicts are not. Agent-centred spatial coordinates are needed to make the connection between the two spaces, and seeing in pictures, which depends on descriptive vision, cannot provide them. The space in the picture lacks, if you will, a *here*. Think again of the picture of the two men shaking hands. How far away from you do they look? I am not sure that one can answer this question. Unlike the photograph by Andreas Gursky, which creates a fake reference point right by your feet, there is no connecting point to your own location.

Now, many observers *claim* (in response to such questions put by myself) that objects in a picture look a determinate distance away. I am inclined to think this response reflects a misunderstanding of my poorly put questions, a confusion between the picture and the things it depicts, but suppose for a moment that there is an answer. Suppose that a depicted man in a particular picture looks from various visual cues to be 10 feet away from you. Now, close your eyes and move three steps closer. Open your eyes. How close does he now look? No closer than before. (I have observed that size cues play no part in people's responses to my questions: the things depicted subtend a very different angle than they would if they were really at the reported distance.) And if you had kept your eyes open while approaching the picture, you would have no impression of moving towards the man (as opposed to towards the picture). Again, look at a man in the foreground of the picture. Let's suppose that he looks 10 feet away from you. Now look at something in the background. It looks (let us imagine) to be 40 feet away from the man—it is on the other side of a road from him. (Spatial relations within a picture are often quite easy to decode.) It follows that the background things must look 50 feet away from you. But do they? Cover up the man in the foreground, or delete him. Now how far do the buildings look? There is no reason to think that they will look 50 feet away now. These phenomena show that even if one has some kind of vague feeling of egocentrically expressed distance with regard to objects in pictures—and once again, I am highly sceptical that this is really so except in instances like the Gursky picture—this feeling is imprecise, evanescent, and highly disconnected.

What one sees in a picture is also temporally dislocated. *When* did two men in the picture shake hands? At the same time as each other. But when was that? The picture does not tell us. If we were seeing it non-pictorially, the answer would be obvious: 'now.' However, as with space, the time within a picture is internally connected, but not to the observer.

This relates to a point about episodic memory—the kind of memory in which you recall sensory images from the past as past. There is a difference, often noted by philosophers, between remembering a scene by 'reviving a perception' of it (as Locke put it) and merely by recalling a verbal description or image. There are certain memories of which you the remembering subject are a part. You may remember how you heard of the events of 11 September 2001. You remember seeing a headline, or an interrupted TV show, or somebody breathlessly giving you the news. You not only remember the news; you remember your own involvement: how you felt, where you were, etc. This is an example of episodic memory. By contrast, semantic memory does not involve you. You remember your friend's birthday, but you don't necessarily remember the incident of having that information imparted to you. This kind of memory is called 'semantic'. The point to be noted is that subjective involvement and temporal reference are essential parts of episodic memory: such memory presents some incident as involving the subject and as having occurred in the past: it has an 'A-series' aspect (as McTaggart called it), a relation to the now. On the other hand, your memory of your friend's birthday has no such temporal reference. What you remember is a fact, not an incident of which you were a part.

Note that this is not a matter of what or how much information the memory contains. A verbal memory can contain as much information as an episodic one, or even more. Nor is it a matter of the episodic memory being like a sensory image, while the verbal one is 'propositional'. An eidetically *imagined* scene can be 'pictorial' in form and presentation, but still not contain any relative-to-the-now temporal information. So can a certain sort of remembered scene: an expert art-historian or curator might be able to remember what the Mona Lisa looks like, and to recover information about the picture from this memory. For instance, looking at a field guide to trees in Italy, he might be able to inspect his image of the Mona Lisa and identify the trees in the background. This may be accomplished without reference to *seeing* it; in such a case, the image might be temporally neutral. In episodic memory, however, you remember yourself looking at the scene (Wheeler et al. 1997; cf. Martin 2001), or you see yourself in it. John Sutton (2003) says that in such a memory 'temporal orientation is by particular times rather than simply by rhythms and phases.' This is an important point: the temporal information available in episodic memory is not merely relational (as temporal information about objects in a picture is). Actually, it understates the point to say simply that episodic memory relates events to 'particular times': it is a matter of the memory containing relative-to-the-now indexing of times, not merely a reference to them. It is not all in B-series form, i.e. merely in terms of a temporal sequence in which the now cannot be located. (Such indexing might be relatively sparse: it may only reveal that the scene occurred before now, and be silent about when, or when relative to other memories.)

Like a picture, a merely imagined scene will be temporally coherent internally, even though disconnected from the now; an episodic memory, by contrast, presents itself as connected to the present. It does not merely contain reference to particular times or temporal ranges, but is essentially in the past, essentially before the now. This is precisely the kind of point I am trying to make about spatial relations within a picture: because motion-guiding vision is not involved, there is no place depicted objects are relative to oneself. In real life vision, on the other hand, there is a here and a now—an indexed aspect with regard both to time and space. The hypothesis advanced here is that motion-guiding vision is responsible for this. No theory is offered concerning the temporal aspect of episodic memory: the phenomenology is merely noted. It is important, however, to distinguish, as in the case of vision, the eidetic or descriptive content of the memory from the feeling of the now in the case of vision or of the past in the case of episodic memory. Otherwise, it becomes a mystery how a *recalled* image, i.e. one that is the *same* as the original, can change with respect to contained tense—see Martin (2001) for a discussion of this. For exactly the same reason, the feeling of the past in episodic memory cannot be a matter of recalling the feeling of the present in the original perception. If this were so, it would be a mystery how a feeling of the present could become, upon recall, a feeling of the past. The memory theorist needs to hang the A-series temporality of memory on something other than its eidetic aspect, and also on something other than its phenomenal feeling of presence.

These points closely parallel one made in a much quoted passage from Frege.

> If someone wants to say the same today as he expressed yesterday using the word 'today', he must replace this word with 'yesterday'. Although the thought is the same its verbal expression must be different so that the sense, which would otherwise be affected by the differing times of utterance, is readjusted.

A perceptual state and an episodic memory of that perceptual state are presentations of the same thing—they have as David Kaplan (1989) puts it, the same *content*. But they have different ways of presenting this content—they have different *characters*. One aspect of this difference is precisely the same as the difference between 'It is raining today', and 'It was raining yesterday' spoken on the following day (in the same place). The theory offered above offers a mechanism for the spatio-temporal indicator in perception—from a philosopher's point of view, it proves the possibility of this kind of indication of the present. Since episodic memory has a different character, the same theory will not suffice to explain the temporal indicator in such memory. The possibility of such indication stands in need of explication and proof.

VI. Seeing Individuals

In section I above, we saw that a (normally sighted) person might be able to reach for an object, but not see where it is: subjects were able to reach for something that had shifted during an eye-saccade though they did not consciously notice the change of location. This indicates that subjects are able to establish a sensorimotor connection with an object, to become 'perceptually coupled' with it as Noë and O'Regan say (2002, 571), without being *conscious* of its location. So the kind of contact that we have with objects in real-life vision (i.e. in contrast with pictorial vision) seems to be independent of object-centred representations of location with which we are presented in visual consciousness. The feeling of presence that accompanies seeing real objects, which I have been connecting with the ability to reach out and touch or manipulate these objects, seems to be, as far as conscious visual experience is concerned, a *pure* demonstrative, a cognitive relationship between perceiver and object, devoid of all descriptive content.

I have been arguing that motion-guiding vision places us in the space and the time which the object of vision also inhabits. This does not tell the whole story about how we see space and time. Clearly, *descriptive* vision has a great deal to do with processing the spatio-temporal relations that one ordinarily sees. This is demonstrated in the above discussion of pictures, since it is descriptive vision that gives us information about spatial relations *within* pictures. These spatial relations, however, are presented in object-centred coordinates, which means that they are subject to transformations that adjust for one's changing perspective as one moves. As one moves towards and around things, they do not look altered in position, absolutely or relative to each other; the sequence of images one receives is so encoded that the differences amongst them are integrated into a single unchanging reality with differences of perspective. This temporal stability is a mark of the object-centred spatio-temporal framework provided by descriptive vision. It is a different kind of framework than the agent-centred one provided by motion-guiding vision. What matters to agent-centred vision is where something is in relation to yourself. It does not retain prior positions: your next movement with respect to an object is determined by where you and it are now, not on your trajectory up until now.

Now, the lack of a direct perceptual link between perceiver and an object in a picture has interesting consequences for the possibility of using a demonstrative in order to refer to the latter. Put aside familiar objects and faces for a moment. Suppose that you are looking at a painted portrait. Can one refer to the subject as 'that man'? It doesn't seem so because there may be no such man: the depicted object might be a figment of the painter's imagination. Demonstratives demand a direct link between gesture and object, a link unmediated by belief. But as has been argued there is a formal disconnection between the gesturer's spatial coordinates and those of the object she ostends: 'that object' cannot mean the same thing here as when one ostends an object seen as in real life, because the location information is not available to the gesturer in egocentric terms. When I look at an object in a painting, the visual experience itself offers me no assurance that there even is such an object, and no information about its location relative to myself. So the normal mechanisms of demonstration simply do not work in this case. As a corollary, one might think that the normal mechanisms of *reference* are inoperative too. So it seems natural to say that what one sees in a picture is a description, with no demonstrative attached. When I *imagine* a place or a face, there is no particular person I see, but when I have an episodic memory or visual perception, there must be.

M. G. F. Martin (2001) makes this point well:

When I see or taste an apple, there is a particular object, and indeed a specific event involving that object, which I come to perceive. Two episodes of seeing might present objects indistinguishable in their qualities, in the same relative locations to the viewer, and yet be experiences of different objects and different events. When we turn to imagery, however, the particularity and specificity drops away. If asked to visualize a green apple, you may well succeed in bringing to mind an image of an apple. But, in many contexts, it is simply inappropriate to press the question which apple you have imagined. In visualizing an apple, there need be no particular apple which is imagined. (275)

Is it the same with the picture of the man? I am suggesting that it is, indeed, that (with an exception to be noted immediately) you *cannot* visualize a particular object, or see one in a picture. Martin (who explicitly notes the parallel with pictures) does not go so far. He insists: 'One can, if one wants, imagine the very green apple now nestling in A. A. Gill's pocket.' I doubt this: you can imagine a green apple, and imagine *that* it is the one now nestling in A. A. Gill's pocket (whether or not there is indeed such an apple), but imagining *that* something is a particular entity is different from visualizing a particular entity. There is no difference between the apple you imagine in A. A. Gill's pocket and a qualitatively similar one, no difference that makes one and not the other the apple you imagined. There is, however, a difference between the apple you see and a qualitatively similar one. That difference is not, of course, qualitative. It is relational. The difference is that motion-guiding vision perceptually couples you to the one and not to the other. As a result, the apple you see is the one that is endowed with a feeling of presence.

The *complete* denial of particularity in pictures is too extreme. Can I not pick up a picture and say: 'This man is my father'? Yes I can, but because of a different kind of visual mechanism. Vision offers us immediate knowledge of faces; this knowledge is for the identification and reidentification of other members of our own species for stable social and sexual relations. When I identify somebody as the same person as so-and-so, I use descriptive information, of course. However, consider what happens when I get this information right, but the person is not the same as so-and so. For instance, suppose I misidentify my friend's twin as my friend. In such a case, the sensory system has worked correctly, but the human activity it is supposed to subserve—social relations—is disrupted. Though it operates on purely descriptive information, face recognition is *for* certain social relations, but in this case it does not play its role correctly. When I point to a picture and say, 'This is my father', I am relying on face-recognition. It is quite different when I look at a green apple, or imagine it. Perception has no mechanisms that aid in the reidentification of green apples; they are a fungible asset, as far as human evolution goes. So in the absence of motion-guiding vision, which 'perceptually couples' me to a particular green apple, I couldn't see such a thing. In short, there is nothing in my experience of a pictured (or imagined) green apple that makes it an experience of a particular green apple.

The knowledge of a face is *identity-regarding*: it tells us who somebody is, and connects them with individuals encountered before. This allows me to connect pictures with people seen in the past. I may not know where a person seen in a photograph is now, but I can connect their identity with people I remember seeing. This is enough to legitimate the demonstrative used with a picture. In the normal case, my gesture ostends the man I point to; when I point to the picture, however, and say 'This man is my father', the gesture takes in a man I saw in the past, connected to the face in the picture by the identity-regarding relationship of facial recognition. Thus interpreted, the picture might give me wholly new information about the man in the picture. It shows him riding a bicycle wearing the blazer and cap of the Madras Bicycle Club. (There is no such club, I hasten to say.) Vision has told me something I did not know about a specific person. To somebody who had never been visually acquainted with my father, the picture simply depicts a man in MBC gear. To me, it tells me something about a man not wholly identified by the picture itself.

This said, it seems a natural extension that I could use *your* face-recognition capacity to ensure reference too. Suppose I ask you to go to the airport to meet a friend, and give you a photograph to help you recognize the person. I say: 'This is Mary, the woman I want you to meet.' I refer to Mary through identity-regarding features depicted in the photograph, and my memory of Mary. Your visual system can't yet refer to Mary. So far your perceptual state is equivalent to what John Perry (2001) has called a 'detached belief'—a belief that in your present state of mind has no attributive force. The picture is valuable because it will enable you to recognize Mary as soon as you lay eyes on her, courtesy of the demonstrative and my introduction.[6] When you finally lay eyes on Mary, it will be as if I was there and performed the introduction in the flesh. The photograph of my father led me backwards in time, courtesy of the identity-regarding relation of face recognition; the photograph of Mary leads you forward in time to the reference.

Similarly, it is clear that one can track something as it moves. This is what the *phi*-phenomenon proves. Motion too is an identity-regarding feature. So this is possible: A. A. Gill shows me an apple in his hand; I form a visual image of the apple he shows me flying out of his hand and landing on the table. The apple I visually imagine on the table is indeed A. A. Gill's. Notice, however, that this requires the use of motion as an identity-regarding feature.

VII. Features and Their Locations

This casts some light on the nature of visual representation of space. The space in which we see objects is charted by a combination of motion-guiding and descriptive devices. In the first instance, motion-guiding vision gives you, directly, reference to certain objects, or rather to points on their surfaces. We may assume that motion-guiding vision is not able to engage distant

---

[6] There may be an external fact of the matter about which individual is represented in a picture. This painting is not just of a man, it is of Rembrandt, because that is who was sitting for it; this photograph is not just of a green apple; it is of the green apple in A. A. Gill's pocket, because I happened to be pointing my camera at that very apple. So one might say that one is looking at Rembrandt in the painting, at that apple in the photograph. I do not wish to deny this: my point is that there is nothing in the *experience* of either picture that makes it a particular individual, unless it portrays an identity-regarding descriptive feature.

objects: our distance cues are not very accurate beyond a certain range. Our grasp of spatial relations in a distant mountain range is likely very little different from that of objects in a picture. Thus, this might be called 'near-space' or *N*. (The term is intended to cover *only* the points and locations of which motion-guiding vision provides information, although descriptive vision provides information about points equally close in.)

The representation of near-space is unstructured, merely a set of egocentric coordinates for (small) material objects near by: it carries no information about how these points are related to one another, and in particular no systematic scheme of spatial description, like Cartesian coordinates, in which these are presented. *N* is also disconnected and discontinuous. It is restricted to discrete objects near by, and encodes body-centred locations for these. There is no guarantee that if two points are represented in near-space, every (or any) intermediate point will also be represented.

Descriptive vision, on the other hand, gives you (a) object-centred characterizations of space, (b) spatial relations that locate objects relative to one another, including objects that happen to exist in near-space, and (c) certain identity-regarding features, such as faces and motions, that make object-identification possible. Let's call this scheme of coordinates and relations 'descriptive space'. *D* is more structured than *N*: while one may not be able to *see* every point in it, one does see that there is nothing in between certain disconnected objects. Objects that can be manipulated are encoded by *both* kinds of vision, more distant objects are related to the ones in near-space by spatial relations provided primarily by descriptive vision.

Nearby objects have what one might think of as ergonomic potential. They are seen both as things one is able to manipulate with appropriately oriented motions of one's limbs, and also as things that stand to one another in spatial relations that do not change as one's own position changes. It is not clear exactly how this cross-indexing works: presumably, it is *object*-oriented. Possibly, places identified separately by the two systems will be identified with one another when we get visual feedback from acting on something. My attention may be caught by a passing object, and I might turn my head to look at it; I get a descriptive fix on the object only when my gaze fixes on something that seems to have been the cause of the distraction. It seems clear, on the other hand, that there cannot be direct translation of near-space coordinates into descriptive coordinates and vice versa: the computational task seems too complicated.

Distant objects, objects outside near-space, are presented in purely object-centred terms. However, since these distant objects are related to nearby ones by descriptive spatial relations, they too can have ergonomic potential, indirectly. That is, though one cannot use motion-guiding vision to reach for or orient one's body with respect to an object 30 feet away, one can relate it to one's own position by descriptive cues relative to nearby things, and thus one can estimate how to get to it by walking or running. One can form a route in advance that will take you to this object. Such a route may involve circumnavigating an obstacle that one can see. As one approaches this one updates one's own position with respect to this obstacle. When one actually gets to it, motion-guiding vision enables one to steer around it. To summarize, visual space contains a *here* and an ergonomically structured *near-space* as well as a set of object-centred relations *R* which connect objects both to one another and to those in your near-space. Further, there has to be a cross-reference between *R* and near-space, which allows us to cross-identify points.

As standardly characterized in philosophical discussions, a visual datum includes reference to space and time— 'Green there (now)'. The spatial reference is sometimes taken as alluding to an inner visual field, sometimes to an external location in three-dimensional space (Clark 2000, ch. 3). In Chapter 12, we saw that features are attributed in the first instance to material objects, reconstructed out of visual cues located around small parts of their surfaces, the latter being directly referred to by motion-guiding vision. This invalidates one aspect of the traditional theory: visual representations are not two-dimensional. Also, the traditional theory supposes that the time of the visual experience is the same as that of the scene represented in it. This is not true in general: imaginings and memories are counter-examples. Visual representations that are the result of actually looking at something are in fact related to the now—at least when they are not of objects in pictures—but as we have seen this is a contribution of motion-guiding vision. Through motion-guiding vision we latch on to particular objects, not just because their features happen to individuate them, but directly and independently of their features. Descriptive vision also helps us latch on to particular objects, through identity-regarding relations such as those of face recognition and motion.

In the more standard presentation, features have an independent status; material objects are constructed out of them. In the alternative version presented here, material objects come first; features are attributed to them after they are identified. This brings us back to the Sensory Classification Thesis of Chapter 1. The claim made there was that sensory systems assign *distal* stimuli to classes. The perspective offered in Part V on the nature of visual (and other sensory) objects, and on how we identify these, vindicates this postion. After motion-guiding vision identifies a material object as something to attend to, descriptive vision assigns it to descriptive classes.

Conclusion

The model of perception presented in this book is not completely surprising in all of its aspects, but does present a comprehensive alternative to traditional theories of perception. The latter are not firmly in the saddle in contemporary philosophical endeavours; in the absence of comprehensive alternatives, however, they provide the default position where there is no apparent reason to believe otherwise. For this reason, the idea that sensation is a point-by-point transformation of receptor states, mostly out of favour with philosophers, still turns up in unexpected forms in unexpected contexts.

The paradigm of perception presented here has two parts, one has to do with sense-features, the other with the external objects that constitute the objects of sensory states: material objects in the case of human vision and bat audition, other sorts of objects in other cases.

Let's talk about objects first, the distal stimuli about which sensory states give us information. There are two kinds of visual system that engage with external stimuli, descriptive vision and motion-guiding vision. (The picture may be less complicated in some other sensory systems.) Descriptive vision is a system or collection of systems that provides us with information that gets incorporated into our consciously available record of the external world. It recognizes material objects by means of three processes:

First, it carves objects out of the retinal array, drawing lines between these objects and allocating these lines or 'edges' to individual objects.

Second, it allocates the sense-features it finds in the retinal image to objects created in the first step above.

Third, it makes visual scrutiny of these objects possible by means of a facility known as attention (cf. Campbell 2002). Attention typically considers one object at a time; thus, even where a single colour or similar motion is assigned to adjacent objects, this can only be known by attending to the objects separately and comparing them. A single act of visual scrutiny comprehending two objects simultaneously is impossible.

On the other hand, there is motion-guiding vision. This system or collection of systems guides bodily motion below the level of conscious volition; it is engaged by specific objects in the vicinity, and helps the limbs act upon these. Conscious volition specifies an action at an abstract level. The exact movement of the limbs, the muscular control necessary to achieve this, etc., are neither known nor consciously controlled. Motion-guiding vision steps into this gap, and assists the body to move appropriately. It was argued in Chapter 13 that when motion-guiding vision combines with descriptive vision, it gives a feeling of presence to the sense-features detected by the latter system.

Descriptive sensory systems have a mode of operation that is more or less independent of motion-guiding vision. Their job is the construction of an explicit and consciously recallable record of objects in the world. To this end, they function as automatic sorting machines that assign stimuli to distinct sensory classes—this is what was called the Sensory Classification Thesis.

Sensory classification can act automatically or in a non-coercive fashion (Chapter 10); further, it can guide deliberate action or it can serve an epistemic role. The thesis advanced in this book is that descriptive vision is, for the most part, non-coercive and epistemic. It is non-coercive in the sense that it posts its classificatory determinations for further scrutiny and decision by other systems, and for the most part it does not force any particular reaction to its results. ('For the most part' because some of the determinations of descriptive vision have automatic and coerced epistemic consequences in the form of priming, habituation, and conditioning—see Chapter 10, sections I and II.) Descriptive vision 'posts' the results of classification by means of states of sensory consciousness. When a perceiver is in such a state, she is aware of the results of sensory classification, but is not compelled to act in any particular way in accordance with it.

In this book, the sensory process is presented as culminating in a proposition-like state, a state which expresses the answer to a yes-no question, or a state which extracts numerical information from sensory input. This contradicts what one might call the 'pictorial' paradigm of perception, which imagines visual sensation to be much like a moving picture of the world, and other forms of sensation in analogous ways. It is not clear that this pictorial paradigm makes sense. A picture of x is something which, when viewed, puts us into a visual state that is similar in relevant ways to that which we enjoy when we view x itself. In the light of this explication, what does it mean to say that visual sensation is a picture? We never look at visual sensation: it simply is not an object of sight. Thus, we cannot be put into any visual state by looking at visual sensation.

In this book, each sensation is treated as a sign or symbol of a feature that is being attributed to an object. When motion-guiding vision engages an object, and we attend to that object, the system's determinations of that object's sense-features become available to us. Sensory qualia are not in any sense *pictures* of these sense-features; they merely signal the presence of certain sense-features.

This conception of sensation allows us a rich account of sensory specialization across biological kinds. In the view of sensation as a picture, it is a puzzle how two organisms can see different things when they look at the same scene. After all, they are both entertaining naturally produced pictures of the same scene, and there cannot be much variation between these. From the Sensory Classification perspective inter-organism differences make perfect sense. Organisms of different kinds need different information about the world. Consequently, they have evolved sensory systems with different informational functions.

List of Definitions and Named Theses

Definitions

Only explanations of terms used in a technical sense are included under this heading. More substantive and controvertible definitions, for example, the definition of *colour*, are included under the heading 'Theses', below.

Analogue and digital (See Chapter 3, sections I to III)

Dretske's definitions

A signal carries the information that *s* is *F* in *digital* form if and only if it contains no information about *s* other than that which is nested in *s* being *F*.

A signal carries the information that *s* is *F* in *analogue* form if and only if it carries additional information about *s* that is not nested in *s* being *F*.

Goodman's definition

A notational scheme is *analogue* if it is syntactically dense, that is, if the scheme provides for infinitely many characters so ordered that between each two there is a third.

Colour Look (Chapter 11, section II.1)

Stimulus *x* presents observer *O* with colour-look $\mathscr{L}$ at *t* if and only if *x* occupies region $\mathscr{L}$ in *O*'s colour similarity-space at *t*.

Component-Incompatibility (see also Feature-Incompatibility) (Chapter 4, section I.4)

Sense-features *F* and *G* are *component*-incompatible if they cannot be components of the same colour.

Determinable (Chapter 4, section I.2–3)

Determinables are sensory classes the perceptual grasp of which involves grasping certain relations of intensification that can be used to generate their subclasses.

Exclusion Range (Chapter 4, section I.4)

A (complete) *exclusion range* is a determinable *E* such that
    (1) *E* includes at least one fully determinate feature *F*, and
    (2) If any member of *E* excludes another fully determinate feature *F'*, then *E* includes *F'*, and
    (3) Any determinable that includes a member of *E* is itself a member of *E*.

Feature-Incompatibility (see also *Component-Incompatibility*) (Chapter 4, section I.4)

Sense-features *F* and *G* are *feature* -incompatible if no full determinate that falls under *F* also falls under *G*. (Notice that any two fully determinate features will be feature-incompatible with one another.)

Full determinates (Chapter 4, section 1.3)

Full determinates are classes that admit of no more than a just-noticeable difference between any two members with regard to the relations of intensification by which they are generated from the determinables that include them. Full determinates are the *infimae species* of sensory classification.

Generative Hierarchy (Chapter 4, section 1.3)

A tree-like structure that arrays determinate features under their determinables.

Hardin's Catalogue (Chapter 7, section I)

A list of mismatches between the similarity spaces of perceived colour and of its physical counterparts.

Response Condition

The *response condition* of a cell C is a proposition p such that C *normally* responds positively (i.e. evinces a firing rate higher than its resting state) when p is true within C's receptive field.

Richness Argument: See Chapter 3, section VII.

Sensation and perception: See Chapter 3, section I.

Similarity Space

A spatial arrangement of sense-features from a single exclusion range, with the distance between two features proportionate to their dissimilarity.

Subclass

X is a subclass of Y relative to classification scheme S if there is a feature F significant in S such that X consists of all and only those members of Y that possess F. Here F is the defining property of X within Y.

Theses

In the following list, theses contested by the author are marked with an asterisk (*)

Classificatory Equivalence Thesis (Chapter 1, section II.4)

Two stimuli present the same appearance in some respect if and only if they have been assigned to the same sensory class.

Codependency Thesis for Phonemes (Chapter 9, section I)

We perceive phonemes because humans produce them. We produce phonemes because humans perceive them.

Coevolution Thesis

Perceptual systems coevolve with effector systems. Their function is to provide effector systems with information specific to the performance of the behaviours produced by the effector systems, much as it is the function of effector systems to use the information available to them to do things that are advantageous to the organism they serve.

Colour Relativism (Chapter 11, section II.1)

Stimulus *x* **is** *Col* (where *Col* is a colour term) to observer *O* in circumstances *C* if and only if *x* **looks** *Col* to observer *O* in circumstances *C*. (Note here that the expression 'looks *Col*' alludes to a colour-look by means of the same colour term as is used on the left side of 'if and only if'.)

Colourist Intuition (Chapter 7, section III)

The difference between black and white and colour vision is the substitution of certain experiences for others—reds, greens, etc., in places where previously there was only black and white and grey.

Counterfactual Principle of Colour Attribution (Chapter 11, section II.1)

'*x* is *Col*' is true if and only if *x* would look *Col* to a standard observer in standard conditions.

Dispositional Principle of Colour Attribution (Chapter 11, section II.1)

'*x* is *Col*' is true if and only if *x* has the disposition to look *Col* to a standard observer in standard conditions.

Disunity of Colour Thesis (Chapter 6)

I. There is no *ecologically characterized* class of properties such that colour vision *must* consist (in whatsoever kind of organism it may occur) in the capture of some or all of the members of this class.

II. There is no *subjectively characterized* class of experiences such that colour vision *must* consist (in whatsoever kind of organism it may occur) in having some or all of the experiences.

Error Theory of Colour Perception (Chapter 8, section II.3)

(a) Colour sensation assigns (what it takes to be) distal objects to certain classes, and

(b) Colour sensation conveys to the perceiver the message that these classes correspond to some system-independent property, and

(c) This message is false.

Feature Exclusion Principle (Chapter 4, section I.4)

A fully determinate feature excludes other features *of the same type*. If *FD* and *FD** are distinct fully determinate features of the same type, there is some range of individuals, *x*, such that *x* cannot be both *FD* and *FD**.

Functional Definition of Colour (Chapter 6, section III)

A colour classification is one that is generated from the processing of differences of wavelength reaching the eye, and available to normal colour observers only by such processing.

**Functional Definition of Colour Vision, first pass (F*)* (Chapter 6, section III)

Colour vision is the perceptual discrimination capacity underlying differential responses to light differing in wavelength only.

Functional Definition of Colour Vision (Chapter 6, section III)

Colour vision is the visual discrimination capacity that relies on wavelength discriminating sensors to ground differential *learned* (or conditioned) responses to light differing in wavelength only.

Fundamental Principle of Colour Attribution (Chapter 11, section II.2)

'*x* is *Col*' is true if and only if *x* really is the colour something visually appears to be when it presents the *Col*-look.

**David Lewis's Definition of Colour* (Chapter 6, section II.)

> *D1. Red* is the surface property which typically causes experience of red in people who have such things before the eyes.
> *D2. Experience of red* is the inner state of people which is the typical effect of having red things before the eyes.

A *colour* is any first component of a corresponding pair. A *colour experience* is any second component

Look Exportation (Chapter 11, section II.2)

Col is the colour-property something visually appears to have when it looks *Col*.

Meta-response (Trace) Schema (Chapter 6, section III. Strengthens the *Perceptual Grasp* schema by characterizing effects of perception on subsequent conditioning, learning, etc.)

For some class of features *R* and some class of behaviours *S*, if organism *O* is rewarded when it responds to a stimulus that has feature **r**, which is a member of *R*, with behaviour **b**, which is in *S*, then the probability that *O* will respond to a future **r**-thing with **b** rises.

Nominalism, Constrained (Chapter 1, section I.3; cp. *Nominalism, Extreme*)

Sensory classification is constrained by the environmental activities of an organism, and is *wrong* if it does not aid these activities.

***Nominalism, Extreme* (Chapter 1, section I.3; cp. *Nominalism, Constrained*)**

There is nothing common to the members of a sensory class other than that they belong to this class, having been assigned to it by the system on some consistent basis.

***Passive Fidelity Principle* (Chapter 2, section II)**

The sensory process preserves the receptoral image; sensory consciousness corresponds to the latter except where it has decayed in the process of transmission.

***Perceptual Grasp* (Chapter 3, section VI: the *Meta-Response Schema* is supposed to capture situations when an organism *represents* the feature in question.)**

An organism perceptually grasps a sense-feature F if and only if there is some (learned or innate) behaviour pattern B that it executes in the presence of things that are F, but not in the presence of things that differ from the former only insofar as they are not F.

***Phenomenological Constraint on Colour (Strong)* (Chapter 5, section III)**

If an organism does not experience red, green, yellow, and blue, it does not experience colour at all.

***Phenomenological Constraint on Colour (Weak)* (Chapter 5, section III)**

If an organism does not possess colour experiences that result from multiple pigments and opponent processing, it does not experience colour at all.

***Phonetic Codependency Thesis* (Chapter 9, section I)**

We perceive phonemes because humans produce them. We produce phonemes because humans perceive them.

***Pluralistic Realism Thesis* (Chapter 8, section IV)**

In general, organisms from different biological taxa may represent different distal features, and all of these features may be real in the action-relative sense.

***Posteriority of Appearance Thesis* (Chapter 1, section II.4)**

Appearance follows sensory classification as the record thereof. It is not the basis or ground for sensory classification.

***Punctuated Equilibrium Assumption* (Chapter 8, section IV)**

Most species are in evolutionary equilibrium *most* of the time. Thus, for most species now there is no mismatch between sensory capacities and specialized sensorily guided activities.

***Realism, Action-Relative* (See Chapter 8, section IV)**

Sense experience E (or neural state N) represents distal feature F in the action-relative sense for a member of species S if

(a) *F* is the physically specifiable response condition of *E* (or *N*), and
(b) misclassifying things as *F* disrupts some innately or developmentally specified use to which *E* (or *N*) is put by members of species *S*.

Realism, Correspondence (Chapter 5, section IV)

A positive answer to either of the following questions.

Does the classificatory basis for sensory classes reflect some system-independent property of distal stimuli?
Does the experienced similarity of stimuli correspond to some similarity relation that can be specified in a system-independent way?

**Revelation* (after Johnston 1997/1992, 138; see Chapter 11, section I.2. *Transparency* is an attempt to capture what is plausible about this principle.)

The *intrinsic nature* of canary yellow is *fully revealed* by a standard visual experience as of a canary yellow thing (and the same goes, *mutatis mutandis*, for the other colours).

**Same-Cause, Same-Effect Principle* (Chapter 2, section II)

There are similarities and dissimilarities present in the retinal images of various situations that are sufficient to account for similarities and dissimilarities in an organism's response to those situations

Sense experience (Chapter 10, section IV; see also *Sensory State*)

A sense experience is
(a) a signal issued according to a convention developed during an evolutionary game of pure coordination,
(b) in order to inform an effector system of the guidance for action provided by a perceptual state,
(c) in such a way as not to coerce action in the way that drives or feelings do: sensory experience is not intrinsically, i.e. outside the context of the system, causally apt for ensuring a particular epistemic action, and hence it should be possible for such experiences to have been deployed as signals of different sensory determinations.

Sensory Content, Primary (Chapter 9, section IV)

The primary content of a sensory state is that the situation is right for a certain action or actions, these actions having been associated with this state by evolution. These actions may include epistemic actions.

Sensory Content, Secondary (Chapter 9, section IV)

The secondary content of a sensory state is the physically specifiable environmental situation in which it is functionally correct to perform the associated action.

Sensory Classification Thesis (Chapter 1, section I.1.)

I

(a) Sensory systems classify and categorize; they sort and assign distal stimuli (i.e. external sensed objects) to classes.

(b) Ideally—i.e. when they are functioning as they should, and in circumstances to which they are well-adapted—they do so on some consistent basis.

(c) The results of this activity have a lasting (but not necessarily permanent) effect on the perceiver in the form of conscious memories and changed dispositions with regard to the associative triggering of conscious experiences.

II

A *sense-feature* is a property a stimulus appears to have by virtue of an act of sensory classification. For example, the *colours* are the properties that distal stimuli appear to have when colour vision assigns them to classes in accordance with its own classification scheme. *Red* is the property characteristic of one such class: it is the property a thing appears to have when colour vision assigns it to this class.

Sensory State (Chapter 10, section IV; see also *Sense Experience*)

A sensory state is

(a) a classificatory state (in the sense of Chapter 1),

(b) formed by a process of sub-personal automatic data-processing on neural records (transductions) of ambient energy patterns,

(c) which evolved for the purpose of guiding epistemic actions.

Sensory Equivalence, Three Principles of (see Chapter 9, section III)

(1) *Resemblance* x and y sensorily appear (on a particular occasion) to resemble each other if there is some epistemic action E, such that the sensory experience of x and the sensory experience of y (on that occasion) suggest that x and y be treated similarly with respect to E.

(2) *Non-resemblance* x and y sensorily appear (on a particular occasion) *not* to resemble each other if there is some epistemic action E, such that the sensory experience of x and the sensory experience of y (on that occasion) suggest that x and y *not* be treated similarly with respect to E.

(3) *Indiscriminability* x and y are indiscriminable (on a particular occasion) relative to a particular sensory modality or submodality if the sensory experience of x and the sensory experience of y in that modality (on that occasion) suggest that for *all* epistemic actions associated with that modality or submodality, x and y should be treated exactly the same.

Sensory Ordering Thesis (Chapter 1, section I.5; Chapter 4, introduction)

Sensory systems create *ordered* relations of similarity and dissimilarity among stimuli, relations which grade the degree of similarity that one sensed object bears to another. (The Sensory Ordering Thesis is a more widely applicable version of condition I (a) of the Sensory Classification Thesis above, and may be supplemented with suitably modified versions of the remaining clauses of that Thesis.)

***Sensory Process, Three Stages of* (Chapter 1, section II.2; Afterword to Part II)**

A. Stimuli: material objects and the packets of energy that they send to our sensory receptors.

B. Sensory classes: the groups that the system makes of the stimuli, and sense-features, the properties that stimuli in a given sensory class share in virtue of belonging to that class.

C. Sensations: events in sensory consciousness with a particular subjective 'feel'. These events are like labels that the system attaches to stimuli in order that we may know that they have been assigned to a particular class.

***Sensory Signalling Thesis* (Chapter 1, section II.1; Chapter 10, section III)**

A sensory experience is a signal issued in accordance with an internal convention. It means that the sensory system has assigned a stimulus to a certain category—the same category as when other tokens of the same signal are issued.

***Similarity of Effect* (Chapter 5, section I)**

x and *y* will appear similar only to the degree that they have physically similar effects on sensory receptors (thus causing these receptors to have physically similar outputs).

***Similarity of Functional Relevance* (Chapter 5, section IV)**

If *x* and *y* are similar from the point of view of an organism's way of life, then the organism *may* gain an evolutionary advantage if its sensory systems co-classifies them, and thus makes them appear similar to one another.

***Similarity of Process* (Chapter 5, section IV)**

Two stimuli appear to be similar because the sensory process they occasion results in physically similar output.

***Species-Relative Realism* (Chapter 8, section IV)**

Sense experience *E* (or neural state *N*) represents feature *F* for a member of species *S* if
    (a) *F* is the physically specifiable response condition of *E* (*N*), and
    (b) misclassifying things as *F* disrupts some innately or developmentally specified use to which *E* (*N*) is put by the members of species *S*.

***Transparency* (Chapter 11, section I.2)**

A visual experiences as of a canary-yellow thing is:
    (a) sufficient for knowing how to classify canary-yellow things for the purposes of inductive inference (etc.), and
    (b) sufficient together with experiences as of lime-green things to know how to differentiate canary-yellow things from lime-green things.

***Universalism (with regard to sensation)* (Chapter 9)**

Since sensation consists in a more or less faithful projection of the state of the sensory receptors, it is the same across species, except for imperfections.

Literature Consulted

The following is a necessarily incomplete attempt to list (relevant) works consulted during the course of writing this book. Not all are cited within the main text; some were relevant to my research, but not in so specific a way as to facilitate citation. A few were not consulted but only indirectly cited, i.e. through their citation in other works.

Where page references are to a reprinted version, items are listed as (x/y), x stands for the year of the cited reprint, and y for the original publication. Classic historical works are not listed below. They are cited in the text by title and the standard reference apparatus used by scholars.

Aglioti, S., DeSousa, J. F. X., and Goodale, M. A. (1995). 'Size contrasts deceive the eye but not the hand', *Current Biology* 5: 679–85.
Akins, Kathleen (1993). 'What is it Like to Be Boring and Myopic?', in B. Dahlbom (ed.), *Daniel Dennett and His Critics*. Oxford: Blackwell, 1993: 124–60.
—— (1996). 'Of Sensory Systems and the "Aboutness" of Mental States', *Journal of Philosophy* 93: 337–72.
Albers, Josef (1975/1963). *Interaction of Color*. Revised edn., New Haven: Yale University Press.
Allman, John Morgan (1999). *Evolving Brains*. New York: HPHLP, Scientific American Library.
Almog, Joseph, Perry, John, and Wettstein, Howard (eds.) (1989). *Themes from Kaplan*. New York: Oxford University Press.
Arbib, Michael (1987). 'Levels of modeling of mechanisms of visually guided behaviour', *Behavioral and Brain Sciences* 10: 407–36.
—— (ed.) (1995). *The Handbook of Brain Theory and Neural Networks*. Cambridge, Mass.: Bradford Books, MIT Press.
Ariew, A. (1996). 'Innateness and Canalization', *Philosophy of Science* 63 (Proceedings): S19–S27.
Ariew, André, Cummins, Robert, and Perlman, Mark (eds.) (2002). *Functions*. Oxford: Oxford University Press.
Armstrong, David (1967). *A Materialist Theory of Mind*. London: Routledge & Kegan Paul.
—— (1978). *A Theory of Universals*. Cambridge: Cambridge University Press.
—— (1989). *Universals: An Opinionated Introduction*. Boulder, Colo.: Westview.
Atran, Scott (1990). *Cognitive Foundations of Natural History: Towards an Anthropology of Science*. Cambridge: Cambridge University Press.
Austin, J. L. (1962). *Sense and Sensibilia*. Oxford: Clarendon Press.
Averill, Edward Wilson (1985). 'Color and the Anthropocentric Problem', *Journal of Philosophy* LXXXII: 281–304.
Ayer, A. J. (1953). *The Foundations of Empirical Knowledge*. London: Macmillan.
Ayers, Michael (2002). 'Is Perceptual Content Ever Conceptual?', *Philosophical Books* 43: 5–17.
Barlow, Horace B. (1972). 'Single units and sensation: a neuron doctrine for perceptual psychology?', *Perception* 1: 371–94.

—— (1996). 'Banishing the Homunculus', in D. C. Knill and W. Richards (eds.), *Perception as Bayesian Inference*: 425–50.

—— (1999). 'Feature Detectors', in Wilson and Keil: 311–14.

Baylis, Gordon, and Driver, Jon (1993). 'Visual Attention and Objects: Evidence for Hierarchical Coding of Location', *Journal of Experimental Psychology: Human Perception and Performance* 19: 451–70.

Berlin, Brent, and Kay, Paul (1969). *Basic Color Terms: Their Universality and Evolution*. Berkeley: University of California Press.

Bermúdez, José Luis (1995). 'Nonconceptual Content: From Perceptual Experience to Subpersonal Computational States', *Mind and Language* 10: 333–69.

—— (2000). 'Naturalized Sense Data', *Philosophy and Phenomenological Research* 61: 353–74.

Blachowicz, James (1997). 'Analog Representation Beyond Mental Imagery', *Journal of Philosophy* 94: 55–84.

Blaser, Erik, Pylyshyn, Zenon W., and Holcombe, Alex O. (2000). 'Tracking an Object through Feature Space', *Nature* 408: 196–99.

Block, Ned (1995). 'On a confusion about a function of consciousness', *Behavioral and Brain Sciences* 18: 227–47.

—— (1998). 'How Not to Find the Neural Correlate of Consciousness', in O'Hear: 23–34.

Boghossian, Paul, and Velleman, David (1997/1989). 'Colour as a Secondary Property', *Mind* 98: 81–103. Reprinted in Byrne and Hilbert (1997a): 81–103.

—— (1997/1991). 'Physicalist Theories of Color', *Philosophical Review* 97. Reprinted in Byrne and Hilbert (1997a): 105–36.

Bouwsma, O. K. (1942). 'Moore's Theory of Sense-Data', In P. A. Schilpp (ed.), *The Philosophy of G. E. Moore: Library of Living Philosophers*, vol. 4. Chicago: Northwestern University Press.

Braddon-Mitchell, David, and Jackson, Frank (1997). 'The Teleological Theory of Content', *Australasian Journal of Philosophy* 75: 474–89.

Bradley, Peter A. (unpublished). 'On Being a Color'.

Bradley, Peter A., and Tye, Michael (2001). 'Of Colors, Kestrels, Caterpillars, and Leaves', *Journal of Philosophy* 98: 469–87.

Bregman, Albert S. (1990). *Auditory Scene Analysis: The Perceptual Organization of Sound*. Cambridge, Mass.: Bradford Books, MIT Press.

Brewer, Bill (2002a). Summary of *Perception and Reason*, *Philosophical Books* 43: 1–4.

—— (2002b). 'Reply to Ayers', *Philosophical Books* 43: 18–22.

Brindley, G. S. (1960). *Physiology of the Retina and Visual Pathway*. London: Arnold.

Brooks, Rodney (1991). 'Intelligence Without Reason', In *Proceedings of the 12th International Joint Conference on Artificial Intelligence*. Morgan Kaufman.

Burnyeat, M. F. (1982). 'Idealism and Greek Philosophy: What Descartes Saw and Berkeley Missed', *Philosophical Review* 90: 3–40.

Byrne, Alex (2001a). 'Do Colours Look Like Dispositions? Reply to Langsam and Others', *Philosophical Quarterly* 51: 238–45.

—— (2001b). 'Intentionalism Defended', *Philosophical Review* 110: 199–240.

—— (2003). 'Color and Similarity', *Philosophy and Phenomenological Research* 66: 641–65.

Byrne, Alex and Hilbert, David R. (1997a) (eds.). *Readings on Color*, vol. 1: *The Philosophy of Color*. Cambridge, Mass.: Bradford Books, MIT Press.

—— (1997b) (eds.). *Readings on Color*, vol. 2: *The Science of Color*. Cambridge, Mass.: Bradford Books, MIT Press.

—— (1997c). 'Colors and Reflectances', in Byrne and Hilbert (1997a): 263–88.

—— (2003). 'Color Realism and Color Science', *Behavioural and Brain Sciences* 26: 3–21.

Callan, D. E., Jones, J. A., Munhall, K., Callan, A. M., Kroos, C., and Vatikiotis-Bateson, E. (2003). 'Neural Processes Underlying Perceptual Enhancement by Visual Speech Gesture', *Cognitive Neuroscience and Neuropsychology* 14: 2213–18.

Campbell, John (1997/1993). 'A Simple View of Colour', in Byrne and Hilbert (1997a): 177–90. Reprinted from J. Haldane and C. Wright (eds.), *Reality, Representation, and Projection*. Oxford: Clarendon Press, 1993.

—— (2002). *Reference and Consciousness*. Oxford: Oxford Cognitive Science Series, Clarendon Press.

Campbell, Keith (1969). 'Colours', in R. Brown and C. D. Rollins (eds.), *Contemporary Philosophy in Australia*. London: Allen & Unwin.

Carey, Susan, and Xu, Fei (2001). 'Infants' Knowledge of Objects: Beyond Object Files and Object Tracking', *Cognition* 80: 179–213.

Carnap, Rudolf (1928). *Der Logische Aufbau der Welt*. Berlin: Weltkreis. Translated by Rolf A. George (1967) in *The Logical Structure of the World & Pseudoproblems in Philosophy*. Berkeley and Los Angeles, University of California Press.

Cervantes-Pérez, Francisco (1995). 'Visuomotor Coordination in Frogs and Toads', in Arbib (1995).

Chalmers, David (1996). *The Conscious Mind*. Oxford: Oxford University Press.

Chatterjee, Soumya, and Callaway, Edward M. (2003). 'Parallel Colour-Opponent Pathways to Primary Visual Cortex', *Nature* 426: 668–71.

Chisholm, Roderick M. (1957). *Perceiving: A Philosophical Study*. Ithaca NY: Cornell University Press.

Churchland, Patricia S., Ramachandran, V. S., and Sejnowski, T. J. (1994). 'A Critique of Pure Vision', in C. Koch and J. Davis (eds.), *Large-Scale Neuronal Theories of the Brain*. Cambridge, Mass.: Bradford Books, MIT Press.

Churchland, Paul M. (1988). *Matter and Consciousness*. Revised edn., Cambridge, Mass.: Bradford Books, MIT Press.

—— (1995). *The Engine of Reason, the Seat of the Soul*. Cambridge, Mass.: Bradford Books, MIT Press.

Clark, Andy (1997). *Being There: Putting Brain, Body, and World Together Again*. Cambridge, Mass.: Bradford Books, MIT Press.

—— (2001). 'Visual Experience and Motor Action: Are the Bonds Too Tight?', *Philosophical Review* 110: 495–519.

Clark, Austen (1993). *Sensory Qualities*. Oxford: Clarendon Press.

—— (2000). *A Theory of Sentience*. Oxford: Oxford University Press.

Cohen, Jonathan (2000). 'Color Properties and Color Perception: A Functionalist Account', PhD thesis, Rutgers University, New Brunswick, NJ.

—— (2003a). 'On the Structural Properties of the Colours', *Australasian Journal of Philosophy* 81: 78–95.

—— (2003*b*). 'Color: A Functionalist Proposal', *Philosophical Studies* 113: 1–42.

—— (2003*c*). 'Perceptual Variation, Realism, and Relativization, or: How I Learned to Stop Worrying and Love Variations in Color Vision', *Behavioural and Brain Sciences* 26: 23–4.

Cohen, Jonathan, and Meskin, Aaron (forthcoming). 'On the Epistemic Value of Photographs', *Journal of Aesthetics and Art Criticism*.

Cowey, A., and Stoerig, P. (1995). 'Blindsight in Monkeys', *Nature* 373: 247–9.

Crick, F., and Koch, C. (1995). 'Are We Aware of Neural Activity in Primary Visual Cortex?', *Nature* 375: 121–3.

Cronly-Dillon J. R., and Gregory, R. L. (1991) (eds.), *Evolution of the Eye and Visual System*. Basingstoke and London: Macmillan.

Currie, Gregory (1995). *Image and Mind: Film, Philosophy, and Cognitive Science*. Cambridge: Cambridge University Press.

Davis, Steven (ed.) (2000). *Color Perception: Philosophical, Psychological, Artistic, and Computational Perspectives*. New York and Oxford: Oxford University Press.

Dawkins, Richard I. (1976). *The Selfish Gene*. New York: Oxford University Press.

Dedrick, Don (1996*a*). 'Can Colour Be Reduced to Anything?', *Philosophy of Science* 63 (Proceedings): S134–S142.

—— (1996*b*). 'Color Language Universality and Evolution: On the Explanation for Basic Color Terms', *Philosophical Psychology* 9: 497–524.

Delattre, P. C., Liberman, A. M., and Cooper, F. S. (1955). 'Acoustic Loci and Transitional Cues for Consonants', *Journal of the Acoustical Society of America* 27: 769–73.

Dennett, Daniel C. (1987*a*). *The Intentional Stance*. Cambridge, Mass.: Bradford Books, MIT Press.

—— (1987*b*). 'Eliminate the Middletoad! (Invited Peer Commentary on Ewert)', *Behavioral and Brain Sciences* 10: 372–3.

—— (1991). *Consciousness Explained*. New York: Touchstone Books, Simon & Schuster.

—— (1995). *Darwin's Dangerous Idea: Evolution and the Meanings of Life*. New York: Touchstone Books, Simon & Schuster.

De Valois, Karen (ed.) (2000). *Seeing*. San Diego: Academic Press.

De Valois, R. L., Cottaris, N. P., Elfar, S. D., Mahon, L. E., and Wilson, J. A. (2000). 'Some Transformations of Color Information from Lateral Geniculate Nucleus to Striate Cortex', *Proceedings of the National Academy of Science USA* 97: 4997–5002.

Dominy, N. J., and Lucas, P. W. (2001). 'Ecological Importance of Trichromatic Vision in Primates', *Nature* 410: 363–6.

Dretske, Fred (1981). *Knowledge and the Flow of Information*. Cambridge, Mass.: Bradford Books, MIT Press.

—— (1984). 'Seeing Through Pictures (Abstract of a comment on Walton [1984])', *Noûs* 18: 73–4.

—— (1993). 'Conscious Experience', *Mind* 102: 263–81.

—— (1995). *Naturalizing the Mind*. Cambridge, Mass.: Bradford Books, MIT Press.

Eilan, Naomi (1998). 'Perceptual Intentionality, Attention and Consciousness', in O'Hear (1998: 181–202).

Elster, Jon (1984). *Ulysses and the Sirens: Studies in Rationality and Irrationality*. 2nd edn., Cambridge: Cambridge University Press.

Enns, J., and Rensink, R. A. (1991). 'Preattentive Recovery of Three-dimensional Orientation from Line Drawings', *Psychological Review* 98: 335–51.

Evans, Gareth (1982). *The Varieties of Reference*. Oxford: Clarendon Press.

Ewert, Jörg-Peter (1987). 'Neuroethology of Releasing Mechanisms: Prey-catching in Toads', *Behavioral and Brain Sciences* 10: 337–68.

Firth, Roderick (1949). 'Sense-Data and the Percept Theory. Part I', *Mind* 57: 434–65.

—— (1950). 'Sense-Data and the Percept Theory. Part II', *Mind* 58: 35–56.

Flanagan, Owen (1984). *The Science of the Mind*. Cambridge, Mass.: Bradford Books, MIT Press.

Fodor, Jerry A. (1982). *The Modularity of Mind*. Cambridge, Mass.: Bradford Books, MIT Press.

—— (1998). *Concepts: Where Cognitive Science Went Wrong*. Oxford: Clarendon Press.

Gallistel, C. R. (1980). *The Organization of Action: A New Synthesis*. Cambridge, Mass.: Bradford Books, MIT Press.

—— (1990). *The Organization of Learning*. Cambridge, Mass.: Bradford Books, MIT Press.

Ganel, Tzvi, and Goodale, Melvyn A (2003). 'Visual Control of Action but Not Perception Requires Analytical Processing of Object Shape', *Nature* 426: 664–7.

Gärdenfors, Peter (2000). *Conceptual Spaces: The Geometry of Thought*. Cambridge, Mass.: Bradford Books, MIT Press.

Gazzaniga, M. S., Fendrich, R., and Wessinger, C. M. (1994). 'Blindsight reconsidered', *Current Directions in Psychological Science* 3: 93–6.

Gibson, Eleanor, Adolph, Karen, and Eppler, Marion (1999). 'Affordances', in Wilson and Keil: 4–6.

Gibson, J. J. (1950). *The Perception of the Visual World*. Boston: Houghton Mifflin.

—— (1979). *The Ecological Approach to Visual Perception*. Boston: Houghton Mifflin.

Gigerenzer, Gerd (1991). 'How to Make Cognitive Illusions Disappear: Beyond Heuristics and Biases', *European Review of Social Psychology* 2: 83–115.

Gigerenzer, Gerd, Todd, Peter M., and the ABC Research Group (1999). *Simple Heuristics That Make Us Smart*. New York: Oxford University Press.

Gillam, Barbara (1998). 'Illusions at Century's End', in Hochberg: 95–136.

Goldsmith, Timothy (1990). 'Optimization, Constraint, and History in the Evolution of the Eyes', *Quarterly Review of Biology* 56: 281–322.

Goodale, Melvyn A. (1987). 'The Compleat Visual System: from Input to Output. (Invited peer commentary on Ewert)', *Behavioral and Brain Sciences* 10: 379–80.

—— (2001). 'Why Vision Is More than Seeing', in MacIntosh: 187–214.

Goodale, M. A., and Haffenden, A. (1998). 'Frames of Reference for Perception and Action in the Human Visual System', *Neuroscience and Biobehavioral Reviews*: 161–72.

Goodale, M. A., and Humphrey, G. K. (1998). 'The Objects of Action and Perception', *Cognition* 67: 181–207.

Goodale, M. A., and Milner, A. D. (1992). 'Separate Visual Pathways for Perception and Action', *Trends in Neurosciences* 15: 20–5.

Goodale, M. A., Pélisson, D., and Prablanc, C. (1986). 'Large Adjustments in Visually Guided Reaching Do Not Depend on Vision of the Hand or Perception of Target Displacement', *Nature* 349: 154–6.

Goodman, Nelson (1972/1970). 'Seven Strictures on Similarity', in Goodman, *Problems and Projects*, Indianapolis: Bobbs-Merrill: 437–47. Reprinted from L. Foster and J. W. Swanson, *Experience and Theory*. Boston: University of Massachusetts Press.

—— (1976). *Languages of Art*. 2nd edn., Indianapolis: Hackett; 1st edn., Indianapolis: Bobbs Merrill.

—— (1977/1951). *The Structure of Appearance*. 3rd edn., Boston: Reidel; 1st edn., Indianapolis: Bobbs-Merrill.

Gould, Stephen Jay (2002). *The Structure of Evolutionary Theory*. Cambridge: Belknap Press of Harvard University Press.

Gregory, Richard L. (1970). *The Intelligent Eye*. London: Weidenfeld & Nicolson.

Gregory, R. L., and Cronly-Dillon, J. (eds.) (1991). *Vision and Visual Dysfunction*. Vol. 2: *Evolution of the Eye and Visual System*. London: Macmillan.

Grice, H. P. (1957). 'Meaning', *Philosophical Review*.

—— (1961). 'The Causal Theory of Perception', *Proceedings of the Aristotelian Society*, supplementary vol. 35.

Griffiths, Paul (1997). *What the Emotions Are*. Chicago: University of Chicago Press.

Hanson, Norwood Russell (1958). *Patterns of Discovery: An Inquiry into the Conceptual Foundations of Science*. Cambridge: Cambridge University Press.

Hardin, C. L. (1984). 'A New Look at Color', *American Philosophical Quarterly* 21: 125–33.

—— (1988). *Color for Philosophers: Unweaving the Rainbow*. Indianapolis: Hackett.

—— (1992). 'The Virtues of Illusion', *Philosophical Studies* 68: 371–82.

—— (2003). 'A Spectral Reflectance Doth Not a Color Make', *Journal of Philosophy* 100: 191–200.

Hardin, C. L., and Maffi, Luisa (1997) (eds.). *Color Categories in Thought and Language*. Cambridge: Cambridge University Press.

Harman, Gilbert (1990). 'The Intrinsic Quality of Experience', *Philosophical Perspectives* 4: 31–52.

—— (1996). 'Explaining Objective Colors in Terms of Subjective Reactions', *Philosophical Issues* 7 (1996). Reprinted in Byrne and Hilbert (1997). Page references to the latter.

Harnad, Stephen (1987). 'Category Induction and Representation', in Harnad (ed.), *Categorical Perception*. Cambridge: Cambridge University Press: 535–65.

Harvey, Jean (2000). 'Colour-Dispositionalism and its Recent Critics', *Philosophy and Phenomenological Research* 61: 137–55.

Hatfield, Gary (1990). *The Natural and the Normative: Theories of Spatial Perception from Kant to Helmholtz*. Cambridge, Mass.: Bradford Books, MIT Press.

Haugeland, John (1982). 'Analog and Analog', in J. Biro and R. Shahan (eds.), *Mind, Brain, and Function*. Norman OK: Oklahoma University Press: 213–25.

Hayek, F. A. (1952). *The Sensory Order: An Inquiry into the Foundations of Theoretical Psychology*. Chicago: University of Chicago Press.

Heck, Richard G., Jr. (2000). 'Nonconceptual Content and the "Space of Reasons" ', *Philosophical Review* 109: 483–523.

Helmuth, Laura (2003). 'Brain Model Puts Most Sophisticated Regions Front and Center', *Science* 302: 1133.

Herrnstein, Richard J., and Boring, Edwin G. (1965). *A Source Book in the History of Psychology*. Cambridge, Mass.: Harvard University Press.

Hilbert, David R. (1987). *Color and Color Perception*. Stanford: Centre for the Study of Language and Information, CSLI Lecture Notes 9.

—— (1992). 'What is Color Vision?', *Philosophical Studies* 68: 351–70

Hill, Christopher S. (1991). *Sensations: A Defence of Type Materialism*. Cambridge: Cambridge University Press.

Hochberg, Julian (1998). *Perception and Cognition at Century's End*. San Diego: Academic Press.

Hubel, David H. (1988). *Eye, Brain, and Vision*. New York: Scientific American Library.

Huffman, Donald D. (1998). *Visual Intelligence*. New York: W. W. Norton.

Hughes, Howard C. (1999). *Sensory Exotica: A World Beyond Human Experience*. Cambridge, Mass.: Bradford Books, MIT Press.

Humphrey, Nicholas (1992). *A History of the Mind: Evolution and the Birth of Consciousness*. New York: Simon & Schuster.

—— (1995). 'Blocking out the Distinction Between Sensation and Perception: Superblindsight and the Case of Helen', *Behavioral and Brain Sciences* 18: 257–8.

Hurvich, Leo M. (1981). *Color Vision*. Sunderland, Mass.: Sinauer.

Husserl, Edmund (1931/1913). *Ideas: General Introduction to Pure Phenomenology* (tr. W. R. Boyce Gibson). New York: Macmillan.

Huxley, Aldous (1936). *The Doors of Perception*. London: Chatto & Windus.

Imaizumi, Takato, Tran, Hlen G., Swartz, Trevor E., Briggs, Winslow R., and Kay, Steve. A. (2003). 'FKF1 is Essential for Photoperiodic-Specific Light Signalling in *Arabidopsis*', *Nature* 426: 302–6.

Ingle, D. J. (1987). 'Ewert's Model: Some Discoveries and Some Difficulties', *Behavioral and Brain Sciences* 10: 383–5.

—— (1991). 'Functions of Subcortical Visual Systems in Vertebrates and the Evolution of Higher Visual Mechanisms', in Gregory and Cronly-Dillon: 152–64.

Jackson, Frank (1977). *Perception*. Cambridge: Cambridge University Press.

—— (2000). 'Philosophizing about Colour', in Davis (2000): 152–62.

Jackson, Frank, and Pargetter, Robert (1987). 'An Objectivist's Guide to Subjectivism about Colour', *Revue Internationale de Philosophie* 41: 127–41.

Jacobs, Gerald H. (1981). *Comparative Color Vision*. New York: Academic Press.

Jameson, Dorothea, and Hurwich, Leo M. (1989). 'Essay Concerning Color Constancy', *Annual Review of Psychology* 40: 1–22. Also reprinted in Byrne and Hilbert (1997b).

Jameson, Kimberly (forthcoming). 'Culture and Cognition: What is Universal about the Representation of Colour Experience?', *Journal of Culture and Cognition*.

Jameson, Kimberly, and Alvarado, Nancy (2003). 'The Relational Correspondence between Category Exemplars and Names', *Philosophical Psychology* 16: 25–49.

Jeannerod, Marc (1997). *The Cognitive Neuroscience of Action*. Oxford: Blackwell.

Johnson, W. E. (1964/1921). *Logic Part I: Propositions and Relations*. New York: Dover Books. Republished from the 1921 edn. Cambridge: Cambridge University Press.

Johnston, Mark (1997/1992). 'How to Speak of the Colours', in Byrne and Hilbert (1997a): 137–76. Reprinted with a postscript from *Philosophical Studies* 68: 221–63.

Kahneman, Daniel, Treisman, Anne, and Gibbs, Brian J. (1992). 'The Reviewing of Object Files: Object-Specific Integration of Information', *Cognitive Psychology* 24: 175–219.

Kaplan, David (1989*a*). 'Demonstratives: An Essay on the Semantics, Logic, Metaphysics, and Epistemology of Demonstratives and Other Indexicals', in Almog et al.: 491–563.

—— (1989*b*). 'Afterthoughts', in Almog et al.: 565–614.

Katz, Jerrold J. (1964). 'Analyticity and Contradiction in Natural Language', in J. A. Fodor and J. J. Katz (eds.), *The Structure of Language*. Englewood Cliffs, NJ: Prentice-Hall: 519–43.

Katzir, Gadi (1993). 'Visual Mechanisms of Prey Capture in Water Birds', in Zeigler and Bischoff: 301–15.

Kay, Paul (1999). 'Color Categorization', in Wilson and Keil: 143–5.

Kay, Paul, and McDaniel, Chad K. (1997/1978). 'The Linguistic Significance of the Meanings of Basic Color Terms', *Language* 54: 610–46. Reprinted in Byrne and Hilbert (1997*b*).

Keeley, Brian L. (2002). 'Making Sense of the Senses: Individuating Modalities in Humans and Other Animals', *Journal of Philosophy* 99: 5–28.

Koch, C., and Braun, J. (1995). 'Towards the Neuronal Correlate of Visual Awareness', *Current Opinion in Neurobiology* 6: 158–64.

Koechlin, Etienne, Ody, Chrystèle, and Kouneiher, Frederique (2003). 'The Architecture of Cognitive Control in the Human Prefrontal Cortex', *Science* 302: 1181–5.

Koenderink, Jan J., and van Doorn, Andrea (2003). 'Pictorial Space', in H. Hecht, R. Schwartz, M. Atherton (eds.), *Looking Into Pictures: An Interdisciplinary Approach to Pictorial Space*: 239–403.

Kording, Konrad P., and Wolpert, Daniel M. (2004). 'Bayesian Integration in Sensorimotor Learning', *Nature* 427: 244–7.

Kubovy, Michael, and van Valkenberg, David (2001). 'Auditory and Visual Objects', *Cognition* 80: 97–126.

Laming, Donald (1997). *The Measurement of Sensation*. Oxford: Oxford Psychology Series 30, Oxford University Press.

Land, Edwin (1977). 'The Retinex Theory of Color Vision', *Scientific American* 237 6: 108–28.

Land, E. H., and McCann, J. J. (1971). 'Lightness and Retinex Theory', *Journal of the Optical Society of America* 61: 1–11.

Langsam, Harold (2000). 'Why Colours *Do* Look Like Dispositions', *Philosophical Quarterly* 50: 68–75.

Lerdahl, Fred (2001). *Tonal Pitch Space*. Oxford: Oxford University Press.

Lettwin, J. Y., Maturana, H. R., McCulloch, W. S., and Pitts, W. H. (1959). 'What the Frog's Eye Tells the Frog's Brain', *Proceedings of the Institute of Radio Engineers* 47: 1940–51.

Levine, Joseph (1983). 'Materialism and Qualia: The Explanatory Gap', *Pacific Philosophical Quarterly* 64: 354–61.

Lewis, David (1999/1966). 'Percepts and Color Mosaics in Visual Experience', in Lewis (1999*a*): 359–72. Reprinted from *The Philosophical Review* 75: 357–68.

—— (1966). 'An Argument for the Identity Theory', *Journal of Philosophy* 63: 17–25.

Lewis, David (1969). *Convention: A Philosophical Study*. Cambridge, Mass.: Harvard University Press.

—— (1999/1971). 'Analog and Digital', in Lewis (1999*a*): 159–65. Reprinted from *Noûs* 5: 321–7.

—— (1972). 'Psychophysical and Theoretical Identifications', *Australasian Journal of Philosophy*: 249–58.

—— (1999/1983). 'New Work for a Theory of Universals', in Lewis (1999*a*): 8–55. Reprinted from the *Australasian Journal of Philosophy* 61: 343–77.

—— (1997). 'Naming the Colors', *Australasian Journal of Philosophy* 75: 325–42.

—— (1999*a*). *Papers in Metaphysics and Epistemology*. Cambridge: Cambridge University Press.

—— (1999*b*). *Papers in Philosophical Logic*. Cambridge: Cambridge University Press.

Lewontin, Richard (1985/1980). 'Adaptation', in Lewins and Lewontin, *The Dialectical Biologist*. Cambridge, Mass.: Harvard UP. Reprinted from *The Encyclopedia Einaudi*, Milan.

Liberman, A. M., Cooper, F. S., Shankweiler, D. P., and Studdert-Kennedy M. (1991/1967). 'Perception of the Speech Code', *Psychological Review* 74: 431–61. Reproduced in Miller, Kent, and Attal (1991): 75–105.

Liberman, A. M., and Mattingly, I. G. (1991/1985). 'The Motor Theory of Speech Perception Revised', *Cognition* 21: 1–36. Reproduced in Miller, Kent, and Attal (1991): 107–42.

Lopes, Dominic M. (1996). *Understanding Pictures*. Oxford: Clarendon Press.

—— (1997). 'Art Media and the Sense Modalities: Tactile Pictures', *Philosophical Quarterly* 47: 425–40.

Lotto, R. Beau, and Purves, Dale A. (2002). 'Rationale for the Structure of Color Space', *Trends in Neurosciences* 25: 84–8.

McCullogh, Warren S., and Pitts, Walter (1943). 'A Logical Calculus of the Ideas Immanent in Nervous Activity', *Bulletin of Mathematical Biophysics* 5: 115–33.

McGilvray, James A. (1983). 'To Color', *Synthese* 54: 37–70.

—— (1994). 'Constant Colors in the Head', *Synthese* 100: 197–239.

McGinn, Colin (1996). 'Another Look at Color', *Journal of Philosophy* 93: 537–53.

McGurk H., and MacDonald, J. (1976). 'Hearing Lips and Seeing Voices', *Nature* 264: 746–8.

McLaughlin, Brian (2003*a*). 'Color, Experience, and Color Experience', in Quentin Smith (ed.), *New Essays on Consciousness*. Oxford: Oxford University Press.

—— (2003*b*). 'The Place of Color in Nature', in R. Mausfeld and D. Heyer (eds.), *Colour Perception: Mind and the physical world*. Oxford: Oxford University Press: 475–502.

McLelland, James L., and Elman, Jeffrey L. (1986). 'The TRACE Model of Speech Perception', *Cognitive Psychology* 18: 1–86. Reproduced in Miller, Kent, and Attal (1991): 175–260.

Macdonald G. F. (ed.) (1979). *Perception and Identity: Essays Presented to A. J. Ayer, with His Replies*. London: Macmillan.

MacIntosh, Jill (ed.) (2001). *Naturalism, Evolution, and Intentionality, Canadian Journal of Philosophy*, supplementary volume 27.

Mackie, J. L. (1976). *Problems from Locke*. Oxford: Clarendon Press.

Marcel, Anthony J. (1983*a*). 'Conscious and Unconscious Perception: Experiments on Visual Masking and Word Recognition', *Cognitive Psychology* 15: 197–237.

—— (1983*b*). 'Conscious and Unconscious Perception: An Approach to the Relations between Phenomenal Experience and Perceptual Processes', *Cognitive Psychology* 15: 238–300.

—— (1988). 'Phenomenal Experience and Functionalism', in Marcel and Bisiach: 121–58.

—— (1998). 'Blindsight and Shape Perception: Deficit of Visual Consciousness or of Visual Function', *Brain* 121: 1565–88.

Marcel A. J., and Bisiach, E. (eds.) (1988). *Consciousness in Contemporary Science.* Oxford: Clarendon Press.

Marr, David (1982). *Vision.* New York: W. H. Freeman.

Martin, M. G. F. (2001). 'Out of the Past: Episodic Recall as Retained Acquaintance', in C. Hoerl and T. McCormack (eds.), *Time and Memory: Issues in Philosophy and Psychology.* Oxford: Clarendon Press: 257–84.

Masland, Richard H (2001). 'Neuronal Diversity in the Retina', *Current Opinion in Neurobiology* 11: 431–36.

—— (2003). 'Vision: the Retina's Fancy Tricks', *Nature* 423: 387–8.

Matthen, Mohan (1988). 'Biological Functions and Perceptual Content', *Journal of Philosophy.* LXXV: 5–27.

—— (1992). 'Colour Vision: Content and Experience', *Behavioural and Brain Sciences.* 15: 46–7.

—— (1997). 'Teleology and the Product Analogy', *Australasian Journal of Philosophy* 75: 21–37.

—— (1998). 'Biological Universals and the Nature of Fear', *Journal of Philosophy* XCV: 105–32.

—— (1999). 'The Disunity of Color', *Philosophical Review* 108: 47–84.

—— (2001*a*). 'Human Rationality and the Unique Origin Constraint', in Ariew et al.: 341–72.

—— (2001*b*). 'Our Knowledge of Colour', in MacIntosh: 215–46.

—— (2003). 'Color Nominalism, Pluralistic Realism, and Color Science', *Behavioural and Brain Sciences:* 39–40.

Maund, Barry (1995). *Colours: Their Nature and Representation.* Cambridge: Cambridge University Press.

Maynard Smith, John (1982). *Evolution and the Theory of Games.* Cambridge: Cambridge University Press.

Miikkulainen, Risto, and Leow, Wee Kheng (1995). 'Visual Schemas in Object Recognition and Scene Analysis', in Arbib (1995).

Miller J. L., Kent, R. D., and Atal, B. S. (eds.) (1991). *Papers in Speech Communication: Speech Perception.* New York: Acoustical Society of America.

Miller, R. J. (1999). 'The Cumulative Influence of Depth and Flatness Information on the Perception of Size in Pictorial Representations', *Empirical Studies of the Arts* 17: 37–57.

Millikan, Ruth G. (1984). *Language, Thought, and Other Biological Categories.* Cambridge, Mass.: Bradford Books, MIT Press.

—— (1989). 'Biosemantics', *Journal of Philosophy* 86: 281–97.

—— (1995). 'Pushmi-Pullyu Representations', *Philosophical Perspectives* 9: 185–200.

Milner, A. David, and Goodale, Melvyn A. (1995). *The Visual Brain in Action*. Oxford: Oxford Psychology Series 27, Oxford University Press.

Mitchell, Melanie (1996). *An Introduction to Genetic Algorithms*. Cambridge, Mass.: Bradford Books, MIT Press.

Mollon, J. D. (1991). 'Uses and Evolutionary Origins of Primate Colour Vision', in Cronly-Dillon and Gregory: 306–19.

—— (2000). 'Cherries Among the Leaves: The Evolutionary Origins of Color Vision', in Davis: 10–30.

Mollon, J. D., and Jordan, Gabriele (1997). 'On the Nature of Unique Hues', in C. Dickinson, I. Murray, and D. Carden (eds.), *John Dalton's Colour Vision Legacy*. London: Taylor & Francis: 381–92.

Moore, G. E. (1903). 'The Refutation of Idealism', *Mind* 7: 1–30.

Nassau, Kurt (1997/1980). 'The Causes of Color', in Byrne and Hilbert (1997*b*): 3–29. Reprinted from *Scientific American* 243: 124–54.

Neander, Karen (1983). 'Abnormal Psychobiology', PhD dissertation, La Trobe University, Melbourne, Australia.

—— (2002). 'Types of Traits: The Importance of Functional Homologues', in Ariew et al.: 390–415.

Neumeyer, Christa (1991). 'Evolution of Colour Vision', in Cronly-Dillon and Gregory: 284–305.

—— (1998). 'Comparative Aspects of Colour Constancy', in Walsh and Kulikowski: 323–51.

Noë, Alva, and O'Regan, Kevin (2002). 'On the Brain-Basis of Visual Consciousness: A Sensorimotor Account', in Noë and Thompson: 567–98.

Noë, Alva, and Thompson, Evan (eds.) (2002). *Vision and Mind: Selected Readings in the Philosophy of Perception*. Cambridge, Mass.: Bradford Books, MIT Press.

Nozick, Robert (2001). *Invariances: The Structure of the Physical World*. Cambridge, Mass.: Harvard University Press.

Nuboer, J. F. (1986). 'A Comparative View of Colour Vision', *Netherlands Journal of Zoology* 36: 344–80.

Nundy, Surajit, and Purves, Dale (2002). 'A Probabilistic Explanation of Brightness Scaling', *Proceedings of the National Academy of Science Usa* 99: 14482–7.

Ogmen, Haluk, Breitmeyer, Bruno G., and Melvin, Reginald (2003). 'The What and Where in Visual Masking', *Vision Research* 43: 1337–50.

O'Hear, Anthony (1998) (ed.). *Contemporary Issues in Philosophy of Mind*. Cambridge: Cambridge University Press, *Philosophy*, supplementary volume 43.

Ölveczky, Bence P., Baccus, Steven A., and Meister, Markus (2003). 'Segregation of Object and Background Motion in the Retina', *Nature* 423: 401–8.

Passingham, R. E. (1998). 'Attention to Action', in A. C. Roberts, T. W. Robbins, and L. Weiskrantz (eds.). *The Prefrontal Cortex: Executive and Cognitive Functions*. Oxford: Oxford University Press.

Peacocke, Christopher (1984). 'Colour Concepts and Colour Experience', *Synthese* 58: 365–82.

—— (1989). 'Perceptual Content', in Almog et al.: 297–329.

Perry, John (1979). 'The Problem of the Essential Indexical', *Noûs* 13: 3–21.

—— (1999). 'Rip Van Winkle and Other Characters', *Cognitive Dynamics, European Review of Analytic Philosophy*, vol. 2: 13–39.

—— (2001). *Knowledge, Possibility, and Consciousness: The 1999 Jean Nicod Lectures.* Cambridge, Mass.: Bradford Books, MIT Press.

Pinker, Steven (1997). *How the Mind Works.* New York: W. W. Norton.

Preston, Beth (1998). 'Why is a Wing Like a Spoon? A Pluralist Theory of Functions', *Journal of Philosophy* 95.

Price, H. H. (1933). *Perception.* London: Routledge & Kegan Paul.

Prinz, Jesse (2000). 'The Ins and Outs of Consciousness', *Brain and Mind* 1: 245–56.

—— (2002). *Furnishing the Mind: Concepts and Their Perceptual Basis.* Cambridge, Mass.: MIT Press, Bradford Books.

Prinzmetal, W. (1995). 'Visual Feature Integration in a World of Objects', *Current Directions in Psychological Science* 4: 90–4.

Purves, Dale, and Lotto, R. Beau (2003). *Why We See What We Do: An Empirical Theory of Vision,* Sunderland, Mass.: Sinauer.

Pylyshyn, Zenon (1989). 'The Role of Location Indexes in Spatial Perception', *Cognition* 32: 65–97.

—— (2001). 'Visual Indexes, Preconceptual Objecthood, and Situated Vision', *Cognition* 80: 127–58.

Quine, W. V. O. (1960). *Word and Object.* Cambridge, Mass.: MIT Press.

—— (1969a). *Ontological Relativity and Other Essays.* New York: Columbia University Press.

—— (1969b). 'Natural Kinds', in Quine (1969a).

Regan, B. C., Julliot, C., Simmen, B., Viénot, F., Charles-Dominique, P., and Mollon, J. D. (2001). 'Fruits, Foliage and the Evolution of Colour Vision', *Philosophical Transactions of the Royal Society of London* B 356: 229–83.

Rensink, Ronald A. (2004). 'Visual Sensing Without Seeing', *Psychological Science* 15: 27–32.

Richardson, Alan W. (1998). *Carnap's Construction of the World.* Cambridge: Cambridge University Press.

Rizzolatti, G., Luppino, G., and Matelli, M (1995). 'Grasping Movements: Visuomotor Transformations', in Arbib.

Roberson, Debi, Davies, Ian, and Davidoff, Jules (2000). 'Colour Categories Are Not Universal: Replications and New Evidence From a Stone-Age Culture', *Journal of Experimental Psychology: General* 129: 369–98.

Rock, Irvin (1984). *Perception.* New York: W. H. Freeman, *Scientific American Books.*

Rosch Heider, Eleanor (1972). 'Universals in Color Naming and Memory', *Journal of Experimental Psychology* 93: 10–20.

Russell, Bertrand (1914). *Our Knowledge of the External World.* London: George Allen & Unwin.

Sacks, Oliver, (1998). *The Island of the Colorblind.* New York: Vintage Books, Random House.

Schacter, Daniel L. (1996). *Searching for Memory: The Brain, the Mind, and the Past.* New York: Basic Books, HarperCollins.

Schneider, G. E. (1969). 'Two Visual Systems', *Science.* 163: 895–902.

Scholl, Brian (2001). 'Objects and Attention: The State of the Art', *Cognition* 80: 1–46.

Searle, John (1983). *Intentionality.* Cambridge: Cambridge University Press.

—— (1992). *The Rediscovery of Mind.* Cambridge, Mass.: Bradford Books, MIT Press.

Sellars, Wilfrid (1963/1956). 'Empiricism and the Philosophy of Mind', in Sellars *Science, Perception and Reality*. London: Routledge & Kegan Paul: 127–96. Reprinted from Minnesota Studies in the Philosophy of Science I: 253–329.

Shapiro, Larry (2000). 'Multiple Realizations', *Journal of Philosophy*. 97: 635–54.

Shepard, Roger N. (1982). 'Geometrical Approximations to the Structure of Musical Pitch', *Psychological Review* 89: 305–33.

Shepard, Roger N. (1997/1992). 'The Perceptual Organization of Colors: An Adaptation to Regularities of the Terrestrial World?' in Byrne and Hilbert (1997b): 311–56. Reprinted from J. Barkow, L. Cosmides, and J. Tooby (eds.), *The Adapted Mind*. New York: Oxford University Press: 495–532.

Shimizu, Toru, and Karten, Harvey J. (1993). 'The Avian Visual System and the Evolution of the Neocortex', in Zeigler and Bischoff: 103–14.

Shoemaker, Sydney (1996/1990). 'Qualities and Qualia: What's in the Mind?' Ch. 5 of Shoemaker: 97–120. Reprinted from *Philosophy and Phenomenological Research* 50 (supplement): 109–31.

—— (1996/1991). 'Qualia and Consciousness', Ch. 6 of Shoemaker: 121–40. Reprinted from *Mind*. 100: 507–24.

—— (1997/1994). 'Phenomenal Character', in Byrne and Hilbert (1997a): 227–45. Reprinted from *Noûs* 28 (1994): 21–38.

—— (1996). *The First-Person Perspective and Other Essays*. Cambridge: Cambridge University Press.

Skyrms, Brian (1996). *Evolution of the Social Contract*. Cambridge: Cambridge University Press.

Smith, David Woodruff (1980). 'The Ins and Outs of Perception', *Philosophical Studies* 49: 187–217.

Squire, Larry R., and Kandel, Eric R. (1999) *Memory: From Mind to Molecules*. New York: Henry Holt, *Scientific American* Books.

Sterelny, Kim (2003). *Thought in a Hostile World: The Evolution of the Objective World*. Oxford: Blackwell.

Sternheim, C. D., and Boynton, R. M. (1966). 'Uniqueness of Perceived Hues Investigated with a Continuous Judgemental Technique', *Journal of Experimental Psychology* 72: 770–6.

Stevens, K. N., and Blumstein, S. E. (1978). 'Invariant Cues for Place of Articulation in Stop Consonants', *Journal of the Acoustical Society of America* 64: 1358–68. Reproduced in Miller et al. (1991): 281–91.

Stokes, Dustin (unpublished). 'Seeing and Desiring'.

Strawson, Galen (1989). 'Red and "Red" ', *Synthese* 78: 193–232.

Strawson, P. F. (1957). *Individuals: An Exercise in Descriptive Metaphysics*. London: Methuen.

—— (1974). *Subject and Predicate in Logic and Grammar*. London: Methuen.

—— (1979). 'Perception and its Objects', in Macdonald: 41–60.

Studdert-Kennedy M., and Shankweiler, D. (1970). 'Hemispheric Specialization for Speech Perception', *Journal of the Acousticalal Society of America*.: 579–94.

Sumby, W., and Pollack, I. (1954). 'Visual Contribution to Speech Intelligibility in Noise', *Journal of the Acoustical Society of America* 26: 212–15.

Surridge, Alison K., Osorio, Daniel, and Mundy, Nicholas I. (2003). 'Evolution and Selection of Trichromatic Vision in Primates', *Trends in Ecology and Evolution* 18: 198–205.

Sutton, John (2003). 'Memory'. *The Stanford Encyclopedia of Philosophy* (Summer 2003 edn.), URL = <http://plato.stanford.edu/archives/sum2003/entries/ memory/>.

Tarski, Alfred (1944). 'The Semantic Conception of Truth and the Foundations of Semantics', *Philosophy and Phenomenological Research* 4: 341–76.

Teller, Davida Y. (2002/1984). 'Linking Propositions', in A. Noë and E. Thompson: 289–317. Reprinted from *Vision Research* 24: 1233–46.

—— (2003). 'Color: A Vision Scientist's Perspective', *Behavioural and Brain Sciences* 26: 48–9.

Teller, D. Y., and Pugh, E. N. Jr (1983). 'Linking Propositions in Color Vision', in J. D. Mollon and L. T. Sharpe (eds.), *Colour Vision: Physiology and Psychophysics*. London: Academic Press.

Thompson, Evan (1992). 'Novel Colours', *Philosophical Studies* 68: 321–49.

—— (1993). *Colour Vision: A Study in Cognitive Science and the Philosophy of Perception*. London: Routledge.

—— (1995). 'Color Vision, Evolution, and Perceptual Content', *Synthese* 104: 1–32.

Thompson, Evan; Palacios, Adrian G; and Varela, Francisco J. (1992). 'Ways of Colouring: Comparative Colour Vision as a Case Study for Cognitive Science' (with Open Peer Commentary), *Behavioral and Brain Sciences* 15: 1–74

Travis, Charles (2004). 'The Silence of the Senses', *Mind* 113: 57–94.

Treisman, Anne (1993). 'The Perception of Features and Objects', in A. Baddely and L.Weiskrantz (eds.), *Attention: Selection, Awareness and Control*. Oxford: Clarendon Press.

—— (1996). 'The Binding Problem', *Current Opinion in Neurobiology* 6: 171–8.

Treisman, A., and Gelade, G. (1980). 'A Feature Integration Theory of Attention', *Cognitive Psychology*. 12: 97–136.

Trenholme, Russell (1994). 'Analog Simulation', *Philosophy of Science* 61: 115–31.

Tulving, Endel (2000). 'Concepts of Memory', in Tulving and Craik: 33–43.

Tulving, Endel, and Craik, Fergus I. M. (2000). *The Oxford Handbook of Memory*. New York: Oxford University Press.

Turner, R. Steven (1994). *In the Eye's Mind: Vision and the Helmholtz-Hering Controversy*. Princeton: Princeton University Press.

Tversky, Amos (1977). 'Features of Similarity', *Psychological Review* 84: 327–52.

Tye, Michael (1995). *Ten Problems of Consciousness*. Cambridge, Mass.: Bradford Books, MIT Press.

—— (2000). *Color, Consciousness, and Content*. Bradford Books: MIT Press.

Von Uexküll, Jakob (1957/1934). 'A Stroll Through the Worlds of Animals and Men: A Picture Book of Invisible Worlds' (illustrated by G. Kriszat), tr. C. Schiller', in Claire H. Schiller (ed.), *Instinctive Behavior: The Development of a Modern Concept*. NewYork: International Universities Press. Originally *Streifzüge durch die Umwelten von Tieren und Menschen*. Berlin: Springer.

Ungerleider, Leslie G., and Haxby, James V. (1994). ' "What" and "Where" in the Human Brain', *Current Opinion in Neurobiology* 4: 157–65.

Ungerleider, L. G., and Mishkin, M. (1982). 'Two Cortical Visual Systems', in D. J. Ingle, M. A. Goodale, and R. J. W. Mansfield (eds.), *Analysis of Visual Behaviour*. Cambridge, Mass: MIT Press 549–86.

Varela, Francisco J., Palacios, Adrian G., and Goldsmith, Timothy H. (1993). 'Colour Vision of Birds', in Ziegler and Bischoff: 77–99.

Walman, Josh, and Letelier, Juan-Carlos (1993). 'Eye Movements, Head Movements, and Gaze Stabilization in Birds', in Zeigler and Bischoff: 245–63.

Walsh, Vincent, and Kulikowski, Janusz (1998). *Perceptual Constancy: Why Things Look as They Do.* Cambridge: Cambridge University Press.

Walton, Kendall L.(1984). 'Transparent Pictures: On the Nature of Photographic Realism', *Critical Inquiry.* 11: 247–77. (Shorter version published in *Noûs* 18 (1984): 67–72.)

Webster, W. R. (2002). 'Wavelength Theory of Colour Strikes Back: The Return of the Physical', *Synthese* 132: 303–34.

Weiskrantz, Lawrence (1997). *Consciousness Lost and Found: A Neuropsychological Exploration.* Oxford: Oxford University Press.

Werker, Janet, and Tees, Richard (1984). 'Cross-language Speech Perception: Evidence for Perceptual Reorganization during the First Year of Life', *Infant Behaviour and Development* 7: 49–63. Reproduced in Miller et al. (1991): 733–47.

—— (1999). 'Influences on Infant Speech Processing: Toward a New Synthesis', *Annual Review of Psychology* 50: 509–35.

Werner, John S., and Wooten, B. R. (1979). 'Opponent Chromatic Mechanisms: Relation to Photopigments and Hue Naming', *Journal of the Optical Society of America* 69: 422–34.

Westphal, Jonathan (1986). 'White', *Mind* 95: 311–28.

Wheeler, M. A., Stuss, D. T., and Tulving, E. (1997). 'Toward a Theory of Episodic Memory: The Frontal Lobes and Autonoetic Consciousness', *Psychological Bulletin* 121: 331–54.

Wilson, Robert A. and Keil, Frank C. (1999). *The MIT Encyclopedia of the Cognitive Sciences.* Cambridge Mass: Bradford Books, MIT Press.

Wittgenstein, Ludwig (1922). *Tractatus Logico-Philosophicus,* tr. C. K. Ogden. London: Routledge and Kegan Paul.

—— (1977). *Remarks on Colour* (ed.) G. E. M. Anscombe, tr. L. L. McAliser and M. Schättle. Oxford: Basil Blackwell.

Wollheim, Richard (1973). 'The work of Art as Object', in Wollheim, *On Art and the Mind: Essays and Lectures.* London: Allen Lane 112–129.

Wong, J., Groenveld, Mark, F., and Hoyt, C., (1986). 'Travel Vision: A Collicular Visual System?', *Pediatric Neurology* 2: 239–62.

Woozley, A. D. (1967). 'Universals', in P. Edwards (ed.) *The Encyclopedia of Philosophy.* New York: Macmillan.

Wyszecki, Günter and Stiles, W. S. (1982). *Color Science: Concepts and Methods, Quantitative Data and Formulae.* 2nd edition. New York: John Wiley.

Yang, Zhiyong, and Purves, Dale (2003). 'A Statistical Explanation of Visual Space', *Nature Neuroscience* 6: 632–40.

Zatorre, R., Evans, Alan C., Meyer, Ernst, and Gjedde, Albert (1992). 'Lateralization of Phonetic and Pitch Discrimination in Speech Processing', *Science* NS 256: 846–9.

Zeki, Semir (1993). *A Vision of the Brain.* Oxford: Blackwell Scientific Publications.

Ziegler, H. P., and Bischof, H-J. (eds)., (1993). *Vision, Brain, and Behaviour in Birds.* Cambridge Mass: Bradford Books, MIT Press.

Zihl, J., von Cramon, D., and Mai, N. (1983). 'Selective Disturbance of Movement Vision after Bilateral Brain Damage', *Brain* 106: 313–40.

Index